T0133086

THE MEANINGS of *Menopause*

THE MEANINGS of *Menopause*

Historical medical and clinical perspectives

Edited by
Ruth Formanek

A△P THE ANALYTIC PRESS

1990   Hillsdale, NJ   Hove and London

Published by The Analytic Press, Inc., Hillsdale, NJ.

Distributed solely by

Lawrence Erlbaum Associates, Inc., Publishers
365 Broadway
Hillsdale, New Jersey   07642

Library of Congress Cataloging-in-Publication Data

The Meanings of Menopause: historical, medical, and clinical
perspectives / edited by Ruth Formanek.
          p.   cm.
    Includes bibliographic references.
    ISBN 0-88163-080-2
    1. Menopause. I. Formanek, Ruth
    [DNLM: 1. Menopause.   WP 580 M483]
612.6'65—dc20
DNLM/DLC
for Library of Congress   CIP

PRINTED IN THE UNITED STATES OF AMERICA
10 9 8 7 6 5 4 3 2 1

Contents

II. Psychosocial, Cross-Cultural, and Research Perspectives

III. Endocrinology, Clinical and Experiential Studies, and Literary Aspects

Acknowledgments

I am grateful to all those who shared their expertise by contributing to this book. I am also grateful to patients, students, friends, and relatives who shared their experiences and points of view with me. Eleanor Starke Kobrin of The Analytic Press has been a most astute and intuitive editor, who has improved the readability of all chapters. Miriam Formanek-Brunell, Claude Brunell, Jean Franco, Selma Greenberg, Anita Gurian, Helena Harris, Margot and Athan Karras, Susan Medyn, and Paul Stepansky were invaluable as critical readers of my chapter, and I thank them. Talks with colleagues and students helped me distill ideas, and I thank them for their questions.

Librarians and dealers of rare and out-of-print books on women's health were most helpful. I want to thank in particular Ben Gottlieb of the Long Island Book Center; the librarians of the New York Academy of Medicine Rare Book Room; Susan Alon of the Yale University Historical Library; Gordon E. Mestler of the Medical Library of the State University of New York Health Science Center at Brooklyn, Janet Wagner and Joyce Payne of the Hofstra University Library, and Margaret Jerrido, Associate Archivist of The Medical College of Pennsylvania. A Hofstra University Faculty Development Grant freed me from some of my duties and permitted me time to browse, think and write.

Contributors

Susan E. Bell, Ph.D., is Associate Professor of Sociology, Bowdoin College, Brunswick, Maine. She is also Research Associate in Sociology, Laboratory in Social Psychiatry, Harvard Medical School, Cambridge, Massachusetts.

Cheryl L. Bowles, R.N., Ed.D., is Associate Dean, Graduate College, and Professor of Nursing, University of Nevada, Las Vegas.

Nancy Datan, Ph.D., was Professor of Human Development at the University of Wisconsin-Green Bay and was a fellow in the American Psychological Association and the Gerontological Society of America.

Ruth Formanek, Ph.D. (editor), a psychologist, is Professor of Elementary Education, Hofstra University, Hempstead, New York. She is also in private practice in Hempstead.

Linda Gannon, Ph.D., is Professor of Psychology and Coordinator of Women's Studies, Southern Illinois University at Carbondale.

Madeleine J. Goodman, Ph.D., is Assistant Vice President for Academic Affairs and Professor of General Science and Women's Studies, University of Hawaii, Honolulu.

John G. Greene, Ph.D., a clinical psychologist, is Head of Department, Greater Glasgow Health Board, Mental Health Unit, Gartnavel Royal Hospital, Glasgow, Great Britain.

Helena Harris, Ph.D., is a psychoanalyst in private practice in New York City. She was formerly Associate Professor of Education, College of Staten Island, The City University of New York.

Marilyn Maxwell, M.A., is a doctoral candidate in American literature at New York University and teaches in the Hewlett-Woodmere (NY) schools.

Malkah T. Notman, M.D., is Clinical Professor of Psychiatry, Harvard Medical School, and is in private practice in Brookline, Massachusetts.

Suzanne B. Phillips, Psy.D., is a supervisor in the Postdoctoral Program in Psychoanalysis and Psychotherapy, Gordon Derner Institute of Advanced Psychological Studies, Adelphi University, Garden City, New York. She is a psychoanalyst in private practice in Northport, New York.

Dean Rodeheaver, Ph.D., a psychologist, is Associate Professor, Department of Human Development, University of Wisconsin-Green Bay.

Preface

Although menopause is an important stage of life, until recently it received only scant attention for several reasons. Through the centuries a host of negative meanings—about women and about aging—have accumulated, meanings that still cling to the term itself and evoke embarrassed laughter when menopausal symptoms are mentioned.

Middle and old age—in both women and men—have barely been studied, in contrast to the wealth of information available on infancy, childhood, and adolescence. Aging seems to evoke a fear of death, as well it might, and menopause, for many people, is a first marker of aging. It has been neglected in research and theory and has been practically absent in novels, dramas, and poetry.

The woman in middle or old age has been neglected in the media as well. If she is allowed to become visible, she is painted with a nasty brush: she is the vicious mother-in-law, the spinster, the old maid schoolmarm, the labile menopausal woman. Our language is rich in insulting descriptions of the older woman—for which there are no male equivalents—crone, hag, harridan. For adult women, regardless of age, there are additional terms: fishwife, shrew, virago, frump, hellcat. Nor do we lack denigrating expressions for the younger woman: she is irrational and suffering from PMS, a nymphomaniac, a strumpet, a slut. Insults abound not only in popular language: older and younger women alike have been chracterized, even by those in the helping professions, as hysterics, dependent and masochistic personalities, as double-binding mothers who smother their children, as "castrating bitches" and "involutional melancholics" responsible for the suffering of husbands. If you're female, especially when you get older, it's difficult to escape the name calling.

In view of the many negative perceptions of women in general, and of menopausal women in particular, it is not surprising that young people fear the advent of the menopause. Many women about to enter middle age become hyperalert to their emotional state, afraid of impending depression, instability, or irrational behavior, if not total breakdown. Research, however, has shown no association between menopause and either depression or insanity.

How many strange taboos and mysteries still surround menopause! As a stage of life and as a female experience, the topic has, until recently, remained in darkness, not to be discussed. And outdated ideas about the menopausal woman have managed to survive. In 1969, David Rubin's *Everything You Always Wanted to Know About Sex but Were Afraid to Ask* was serialized in newspapers and magazines and distributed by the Psychiatry and Social Science Book Club; it became a bestseller with more than a million copies in print. Rubin described the woman at the mercy of her decreasing hormone production:

> When a woman sees her womanly attributes disappearing before her eyes, she is bound to get a little depressed and irritable. . . . Having outlived their ovaries, they may have outlived their usefulness as human beings. The remaining years may be just marking time until they follow their glands into oblivion [p. 365].

What is the *reality* of menopause? It occurs at an average age of 51. Although in the past this was old age indeed, today's 51-year-old Western women can look forward to living another 30 years. In contrast to prophecies about impending mental and physical illness at menopause, the message from an ongoing, large-scale epidemiological study is that "the biological event, cessation of menses, has almost no impact on subsequent perceived physical or mental health. . . ." (McKinlay, 1989; McKinlay and Avis, 1989, p. 1). This is by no means the only view, as menopause is now being studied by social scientists, by physiologists, and, especially, by the medical establishment.

The current debate on menopause pits physicians and pharmaceutical manufacturers against nonmedical researchers, feminists, and consumers. For the medical establishment, the debate is narrower than it is for social scientists. For physicians, menopause is simply a question of hormone replacement therapy, which is currently advocated by most gynecologists for the prevention of cardiovascular disease and/or osteoporosis: "All postmenopausal women should be made aware of the consequences of untreated menopause and should be offered the opportunity to receive estrogens" (Gambrell, 1989). Gambrell also deals with the well-known association between estrogens and endometrial cancer. His own stand is evident in the title of his article: "Endometrial Cancer from ERT: An Unfounded Fear." It is no coincidence that articles advocating HRT and minimizing its dangers appear in the journal *Menopause Management*—which is published with an educational grant from Wyeth-Ayerst Laboratories, makers of hormones. Ayerst has been sponsoring the dissemination of information on its estrogens since the 1960s, when women were told that estrogens would keep them young and "Feminine Forever" (see Wilson, 1966; Fausto-Sterling, 1985). Educated consumers, on the other hand, have called attention to the lack of evidence of the safety of such potent medicines. It is possible, of course, that estrogens will indeed protect most women against the dangers of those diseases which show a rise in incidence after menopause—cardiovascular disease and osteoporosis. Only continued research will tell.

Medical and nonmedical views were expressed at the September 1989 meeting on menopause cosponsored by the New York Academy of Sciences and the North American Menopause Society. This interdisciplinary society was inaugurated at the meeting with a grant of $35,000 from several well-known manufacturers of hormones. The need for "menopause management," or the medicalization of menopause, was questioned by social scientists. That most women do *not* consult their physicians when they enter their natural menopause was a finding of the Massachusetts Women's Health Study, a five-year longitudinal study of the health of 2500 randomly sampled women. Women who entered natural menopause did not necessarily require medical care. Women who experienced surgical menopause appear to have been an atypical group who used the health care system, both before and after surgery (McKinlay and Avis, 1989).

Anthropologists at the meeting called attention to those studies whose results support the view that physiological symptoms of the menopause, as well as attitudes and beliefs associated with it, are influenced and defined by the culture in which they are found (Flint and Samil, 1989). Nonmedical and medical researchers, as well as feminists, emphasized the menopausal woman's need for information, either directly from counseling, newsletters, and books, or indirectly, from physicians and other clinicians.

Whereas physicians and pharmaceutical manufacturers adhere to a narrow view, nonmedical researchers have called attention to the variety of meanings of the menopause. Medical personnel refer to menopause as a "deficiency disease" or "endocrinopathy" in need of medical management. Nonmedical researchers have attempted to bridge the epistemological split in research between the medical concentration on an endocrine theory of menopause and behavioral scientists' commitment to an experiential factor theory (Ballinger, 1989). Each discipline has its own way of conceptualizing phenomena and its own approach to the creation of new knowledge. Thus, no one discipline can claim that only knowledge produced by its methods has validity. Menopause research has been limited by the lack of awareness by one discipline of the knowledge produced by another (Kaufert, 1989).

This book contains original work from many disciplines. It represents research and theory on menopause, its psychosocial, cross-cultural, and methodological perspectives; the endocrinology of menstruation and menopause, as well as clinical studies of both menopausal women and their spouses, and the treatment of menopausal women in English and American literature. We hope that our book will contribute to the dialogue on menopause across disciplines and thus advance knowledge.

Personal experience motivates and propels many books forward, and this one is no exception. I experienced menopause without any symptoms other than hot flushes, and I became aware of renewed energies—what Margaret Mead called "postmenopausal zest." One day, while browsing, I happened to see an out-of-print book published in 1729 and advertised as the first English book on menstruation

(translated from the Latin). I bought it because I couldn't resist its first
sentence:

> Wretched surely and unequal seems the condition of the Female
> Sex, that they who are by Nature destined to be the preservers of
> the human Race, should at the same time be made liable to so
> many Diseases. . . .

The author was a then-famous physician and mathematician, John
Freind, whose ideas on menopause are summarized in chapter 1 of this
book.

I continued my browsing and buying, and soon my collection on
women's health included out-of-print books by midwives, male and
female physicians, homeopaths, phrenologists, water curers, as well as
more recent works by women historians. Since the process of neither
menstruation nor menopause could be explained until the discovery
of sex hormones in the 1920s, speculations before then are totally
inaccurate yet titillating in their florid weirdness. Some of these ideas
live on and are discussed in chapter 1.

Speaking to friends, colleagues, and students, and hearing from
patients about their menopausal experiences, led me to see the
pressing need for more information about menopause. We hope that
this book will calm the apprehensions of premenopausal women and
their families and inform practitioners and students in the helping
professions, those involved in human development, and those whose
interest is in gender issues. *The Meaning of Menopause* represents the
thinking of specialists interested in menopause who offer the views of
their particular discipline, research, or clinical experience. The chapters need not be read in sequential order. The following brief summa-
ries of chapter contents will aid readers in establishing their own
priorities.

Chapter 1 traces the roots of older and newer perceptions of
menopause, beginning with the ancients. To explain menstruation,
Galen spoke of a "plethora," an abundance of blood, which required
periodic discharge; but in the aging woman, the blood vessels become
rigid and can no longer discharge the accumulated blood. It was feared
that the accumulated blood would now rise toward the brain and

cause the woman to go insane. This ancient view was most influential until the discovery of sex hormones in the 1920s.

In the 19th century, women were viewed as frail and ill. These views changed after the rise of feminism and women were permitted to enter medical schools. The medicalization and pathologization of menopause during the 19th century appears to have been based on ancient myths of women as insane, as well as on the idealization of motherhood, the view of the body as a closed-energy system, the decline in the status of midwives, and the concomitant rise of professional medicine. Physicians elaborated on illnesses that were said to befall women at both puberty and menopause; they perfected operations such as ovariotomy and hysterectomy, which were recommended as cures for all "female troubles," both mental and physical. Menopause was believed not only to render a woman vulnerable to depression, but to increase her chances of serious illness, especially cancer.

By the end of the 19th century, feminist reformers and women physicians began to formulate a more benign view of menopause: that it was a normal stage of life, that male physicians had overemphasized the pathology of their menopausal patients and overlooked the majority of women without serious symptoms, and that, most important of all, a postmenopausal woman could still lead a productive life.

In chapter 2, Susan Bell examines the intellectual roots of the medicalization of menopause in the 1930s and 1940s. An analysis of published papers written by prominent American medical specialists reveals three models for understanding menopause—biological, psychological, and environmental—and shows how each contributed to its medicalization. Bell examines the effects of the transformation that followed the discovery of sex hormones and the availability of a new drug (DES), first produced in 1938. Exploring the medicalization of menopause illuminates some of the special and complicated ways that women's experiences are vulnerable to medical control.

Helena Harris, in chapter 3, examines various psychoanalytical theories in regard to menopause: the traditional Freudian model, ego psychology, and object relations. Harris suggests that the traditional model, as exemplified by Helene Deutsch's account, has lost its validity with the lack of empirical confirmation of Freudian psychosexual stages on which it was based. Benedek's attempted integration of the newly emerging knowledge of hormones with a menopausal woman's emotional life now seems reductionistic. On the other hand, Benedek did consider the importance of feminine identity, self-esteem issues, and cultural values as all exerting an influence on the course of menopause. The object relations model underlies Lax's conceptualization of the menopause as evoking an "expectable" depression. A conflict between a wishful self-image and a deflated, failing self is the chief cause of this inevitable depression.

Harris suggests that more recent and nontraditional analytic theorists have used self-esteem in their formulations. She considers it essential to take into account how the individual woman responds to menopause, differences that may well depend on the relative stability of a woman's self esteem.

John G. Greene reviews in chapter 4 the now substantial body of empirical research on the effects of social and psychological factors on women during menopause. Studies reviewed are categorized as those relating to sociodemographic factors, those investigating the role of women's attitudes to the menopause, and those examining the effects of interpersonal factors within the woman's family and social situation. Studies using the methods of life event research are also examined.

A variety of influences are associated with an *increase* in nonspecific symptoms around the time of menopause, including low socioeconomic status, poor educational attainment, lack of employment, negative attitudes toward the menopause and its perceived consequences, quality of marital relations, limited social networks, stressful life events, and illness and death of family members. The effects of these factors appear to be more potent during the climacteric, a finding that suggests that as women enter the climacteric they become more vulnerable to such factors. Climacteric vulnerability thus is seen as mediating and exacerbating nonspecific symptoms at that time of life.

Chapter 5 was constructed after Nancy Datan's death in May, 1987, by her husband, Dean Rodeheaver, from her presentations, her publications, and his reminiscences. Datan and her associates had examined the relationship between culture and psychological well-being among women following menopause. The women in the study represented five Israeli subcultures—Moslem Arabs, North Africans, Persians, Turks, and Central Europeans—each reflecting different degrees of modernity. Despite variations in religious observance, family life, and work and childbearing history, the women universally welcomed the end of fertility. Furthermore, those women who had experienced the greatest amount of cultural transition – the Persians – also experienced the greatest stress in their experience of menopause. These results are discussed in terms of the "sense of coherence" provided by cultural stability and the ambivalence toward menstruation expressed in rituals of purity and uncleanness found in both traditional and modern cultures.

In chapter 6, Madeleine Goodman differentiates a gradual from an abrupt, surgical menopause. Menopause poses a problem to the researcher since it is neither uniformly described nor universally experienced, and positive evidence of its actual occurrence is not immediately available for study. Yet the study of menopause is of critical value in four areas: (1) menopause forms an important and neglected life-cycle milestone marking the closing of the reproductive years; (2) it is a key variable in the study of aging; (3) menopause and variations in its character have been epidemiologically associated, causally or as concomitants, with a wide variety of diseases and conditions; and (4) an understanding of menopause is critical for both men and women because it will enhance women's understanding of the workings of their bodies, aid the population at large in the overcoming of stereotypes about middle-aged women, and call attention to the dangers resulting from the treatment of menopause as a disease. Goodman pays special attention to recent large-scale population studies of middle-aged women.

Cheryl L. Bowles, in chapter 7, discusses the difference between *experience* and *symptom*, the meanings of menopause for women of different cultural backgrounds, and the similarity of attitudes toward both menarche and menopause. She reviews the few existing studies on the hot flash and the meanings individual women attach to this experience. She examines the medical community's view of menopause and includes discussion of the semantics and the impact of the Western medical model on societal views of menopause. Bowles reviews theoretical models of the menopause – biomedical, premorbid personality of the woman, coincidental stress, cultural relativist, and her own model. Bowles combines several of these models and emphasizes attitude formation. She hypothesizes that a woman with initially low self-esteem will be more vulnerable to a negative stereotype of menopause and will thus experience more symptoms during meno-pause.

Linda Gannon's chapter (8) discusses the endocrinological changes that occur during the menopausal transition. Menopausal symptoms are discussed in relation to endocrinological changes. Researchers and theorists have concluded that hot flashes, and perhaps atrophic vaginitis and osteoporosis, are caused by the changing hormonal environment of menopause, whereas other somatic and psychological symptoms are the result of aging as well as historical, cultural, and stress factors. The endocrinological and physiological aspects of those symptoms most clearly associated with menopause are discussed in detail. The chapter concludes with a discussion of the major treat-ments for menopausal symptoms, their side effects, and possible alternative treatments.

Malkah T. Notman, in chapter 9, suggests that we reconsider (1) those attributes thought to be characteristically feminine and (2) those experiences of mind and body that belong to women. Women's experiences must not continue to be thought of in terms of men's experiences, and women's particular ways of feeling, knowing, and judging must be acknowledged. Uniquely female experiences—men-struation, pregnancy, menopause—must be assessed rather than de-nied and minimized. Menopause has been subject to distortions and misconceptions, thought of as a loss and evoking mourning. Any difficulty suffered by middle-aged women has been blamed on the menopause. Hormonal changes and their mysterious consequences are blamed for conditions that are actually the result of lack of exercise, poor nutrition, and other changes accompanying aging.

Notman includes several case histories of women referred to for therapy for menopausal "problems." On exploration, it becomes clear that these problems were not caused by menopause, but rather illustrate the great variety of issues that women patients bring to therapy.

In chapter 10, Marilyn Maxwell offers a literary perspective. Owing to almost universal taboos, menopause was seldom treated explicitly as a central theme in Western fiction prior to the 20th century. However, depictions of middle-aged women in literature have often reinforced the female stereotype of madness, depression, nymphomania/frigidity. A variety of characterizations of middle-aged, presumably menopausal, fictional women are analyzed, beginning with Chaucer, Shakespeare and Pope, and continuing to Wharton, Woolf, and Lessing.

Suzanne Phillips, in chapter 11, considers men's views in the light of their parallel positions to women in midlife. From her perspective as a therapist, Phillips also discusses gender differences in intimate relationships, preexisting personality traits, and the conscious and unconscious interactive patterns between men and women in such close relationships. Building on clinical data and a review of theoretical formulations, Phillips presents the results of a questionnaire on men's views of menopausal women. In her examination of close relationships in midlife, she finds in both partners evidence of confusion, crisis, and collusion, along with more positive factors—concern, empathy, and complementarity.

REFERENCES

Ballinger, S. E. (1989), Stress as a factor in lowered estrogen levels in the early post-menopause. Paper presented at joint meeting of New York Academy of Sciences and North American Menopause Society, New York City.

Fausto-Sterling, A. (1985), *Myths of Gender*. New York: Basic Books.

Flint, M., & Samil, R. S. (1989), Cultural and subcultural meanings to the menopause. Paper presented at joint meeting of New York Academy of Sciences and North American Menopause Society, New York City.

Freind, J. (1729). *Emmenologia* (trans. T. Dale). London: Cox.

Gambrell, R. D., Jr. (1989), Endometrial cancer from ERT: An unfounded fear. *Menopause Mgmnt.*, 2:13–15.

Kaufert, P. A. (1989), Methodological issues in menopause research. Paper presented at joint meeting of New York Academy of Sciences and North American Menopause Society, New York City.

McKinlay, S. M. (1989), The Massachusetts women's health study: A longitudinal study of the health of mid-aged women and the epidemiology of the menopause. *Psychol. of Women*, 16:1–4.

——— Avis, N. E. (1989), Midlife women and the health care system. Paper presented at joint meeting of New York Academy of Sciences and North American Menopause Society, New York City.

Rubin, D. (1969), *Everything You Always Wanted to Know About Sex But Were Afraid to Ask*. New York: McKay.

Wilson, R. A. (1966), *Feminine Forever*. New York: Mayflower-Dell.

Prologue

The Space Crone

BY URSULA K. LE GUIN

The menopause is probably the least glamorous topic imaginable; and this is interesting, because it is one of the very few topics to which cling some shreds and remnants of taboo. A serious mention of menopause is usually met with uneasy silence; a sneering reference to it is usually met with relieved sniggers. Both the silence and the sniggering are pretty sure indications of taboo.

Most people would consider the old phrase "change of life" a euphemism for the medical term "menopause," but I, who am now going through the change, begin to wonder if it isn't the other way round. "Change of life" is too blunt a phrase, too factual. "Menopause," with its chime-suggestion of a mere pause after which things go on as before, is reassuringly trivial.

But the change is not trivial, and I wonder how many women are brave enough to carry it out wholeheartedly. They give up their reproductive capacity with more or less of a struggle, and when it's gone they think that's all there is to it. Well, at least I don't get the Curse any more, they say, and the only reason I felt so depressed sometimes was hormones. Now I'm myself again. But this is to evade the real challenge, and to lose, not only the capacity to ovulate, but the opportunity to become a Crone.

In the old days women who survived long enough to attain the menopause more often accepted the challenge. They had, after all, had practice. They had already changed their life radically once before, when they ceased to be virgins and became mature women/wives/matrons/mothers/mistresses/whores/etc. This change involved not only the physiological alterations of puberty—the shift from barren childhood to fruitful maturity—but a socially recognized alteration of being: a change of condition from the sacred to the profane.

With the secularization of virginity now complete, so that the once awesome term "virgin" is now a sneer or at best a slightly dated word for a person who hasn't copulated yet, the opportunity of gaining or regaining the dangerous/sacred condition of being at the Second Change has ceased to be apparent.

Virginity is now a mere preamble or waiting room to be got out of as soon as possible; it is without significance. Old age is similarly a waiting room, whre you go after life's over and wait for cancer or a stroke. The years before and after the menstrual years are vestigial: the only meaningful condition left to women is that of fruitfulness. Curiously, this restriction of significance coincided with the development of chemicals and instruments that make fertility itself a meaningless or at least secondary characteristic of female maturity. The significance of maturity now is not the capacity to conceive but the mere ability to have sex. As this ability is shared by pubescents and by postclimacterics, the blurring of distinctions and elimination of opportunities is almost complete. There are no rites of passage because there is no significant change. The Triple Goddess has only one face: Marilyn Monroe's, maybe. The entire life of a woman from ten or twelve through seventy or eighty has become secular, uniform, changeless. As there is no longer any virtue in virginity, so there is no longer any meaning in menopause. It requires fanatical determination now to become a Crone.

Women have thus, by imitating the life condition of men, surrendered a very strong position of their own. Men are afraid of virgins, but they have a cure for their own fear and the virgin's virginity: fucking. Men are afraid of crones, so afraid of them that their cure for virginity fails them; they know it won't work. Faced with the fulfilled Crone, all but the bravest men wilt and retreat, crestfallen and cockadroop.

Menopause Manor is not merely a defensive stronghold, however. It is a house or household, fully furnished with the necessities of life. In abandoning it, women have narrowed their domain and impoverished their souls. There are things the Old Woman can do, say, and think that the Woman cannot do, say, or think. The Woman has to give up more than her menstrual periods before she can do, say, or think them. She has got to change her life.

The nature of that change is now clearer than it used to be. Old age is not virginity but a third and new condition; the virgin must be celibate, but the crone need not. There was a confusion there, which the separation of female sexuality from reproductive capacity, via modern contraceptives, has cleared up. Loss of fertility does not mean loss of desire and fulfillment. But it does entail a change, a change involving matters even more important—if I may venture a heresy— than sex.

The woman who is willing to make that change must become pregnant with herself, at last. She must bear herself, her third self, her old age, with travail and alone. Not many will help her with that birth. Certainly no male obstetrician will time her contractions, inject her with sedatives, stand ready with forceps, and neatly stitch up the torn membranes. It's hard even to find an old-fashioned midwife, these days. That pregnancy is long, that labor is hard. Only one is harder, and that's the final one, the one that men also must suffer and perform.

It may well be easier to die if you have already given birth to others or yourself, at least once before. This would be an argument for going through all the discomfort and embarrassment of becoming a Crone. Anyhow it seems a pity to have a built-in rite of passage and to dodge it, evade it, and pretend nothing has changed. That is to dodge and evade one's womanhood, to pretend one's like a man. Men, once initiated, never get the second chance. They never change again. That's their loss, not ours. Why borrow poverty?

Certainly the effort to remain unchanged, young, when the body gives so impressive a signal of change as the menopause, is gallant; but it is a stupid, self-sacrificial gallantry, better befitting a boy of twenty than a woman of forty-five or fifty. Let the athletes die young and laurel-crowned. Let the soldiers earn the Purple Hearts. Let women die old, white-crowned, with human hearts.

If a space ship came by from the friendly natives of the fourth planet of Altair, and the polite captain of the space ship said, "We have room for one passenger; will you spare us a single human being, so that we may converse at leisure during the long trip back to Altair and learn from an exemplary person the nature of the race?"—I suppose what most people would want to do is provide them with a fine, bright, brave young man, highly educated and in peak physical condition. A Russian cosmonaut would be ideal (American astronauts are mostly too old). There would surely be hundreds, thousands of volunteers, just such young men, all worthy. But I would not pick any of them. Nor would I pick any of the young women who would volunteer, some out of magnanimity and intellectual courage, others out of a profound conviction that Altair couldn't possible be any worse for a woman than Earth is.

What I would do is go down to the local Woolworth's, or the local village marketplace, and pick an old woman, over sixty, from behind the costume jewelry counter or the betel-nut booth. Her hair would not be red or blonde or lustrous dark, her skin would not be dewy fresh, she would not have the secret of eternal youth. She might, however, show you a small snapshot of her grandson, who is working in Nairobi. She is a bit vague about where Nairobi is, but extremely proud of the grandson. She has worked hard at small, unimportant jobs all her life, jobs like cooking, cleaning, bringing up kids, selling little objects of adornment or pleasure to other people. She was a virgin once, a long time ago, and then a sexually potent fertile female, and then went through menopause. She has given birth several times and faced death several times—the same times. She is facing the final birth/death a little more nearly and clearly every day now. Sometimes her feet hurt something terrible. She never was educated to anything like her capacity, and that is a shameful waste and a crime against humanity, but so common a crime should not and cannot be hidden from Altair. And anyhow she's not dumb. She has a stock of sense, wit, patience, and experiential shrewdness, which the Altaireans might, or might not, perceive as wisdom. If they are wiser than we, then of course we don't know how they'd perceive it. But if they are wiser than we, they may know how to perceive that inmost mind and heart which we, working on mere guess and hope, proclaim to be humane. In any case, since they are curious and kindly, let's give them the best we have to give.

The trouble is, she will be very reluctant to volunteer. "What would an old woman like me do on Altair?" she'll say. "You ought to send one of those scientist men, they can talk to those funny-looking green people. Maybe Dr. Kissinger should go. What about sending the Shaman?" It will be very hard to explain to her that we want her to go because only a person who has experienced, accepted, and acted the entire human condition—the essential quality of which is Change—can fairly represent humanity. "Me?" she'll say, just a trifle slyly. "But I never did anything."

But it won't wash. She knows, though she won't admit it, that Dr. Kissinger has not gone and will never go where she has gone, that the scientists and the shamans have not done what she has done. Into the space ship, Granny.

THE MEANINGS of *Menopause*

I
History
and
Theory

Continuity and Change and "The Change of Life"

Premodern Views of the Menopause

RUTH FORMANEK

Until recently, neither menstruation nor menopause was spoken of in polite society. Although these are by no means the only taboo subjects in our culture—incest is an example of another—no jokes, amusing anecdotes, or proverbs touch on menstruation or menopause. Only women among themselves talked about these events, remarking about unexpected or unusual aspects—menopause came either too early or too late, childbirth occurred after menopause, when it should not have happened any more. Or the expected symptoms were discussed: insanity, depression, hypochondriasis, cancer.

Birth was the one event of the female reproductive cycle that could be talked about in mixed company. Birth, of course, was not solely a female happening; it depended on the contribution of the man, whose procreative role carried many meanings and was the basis, at least in part, of his prestige. But evidence of the beginning of the woman's procreative capacity—menstruation—was kept hidden, as was its ending. Menopause, moreover, was perceived negatively since it also represented aging. Thus, attitudes toward menopause became doubly pejorative, demeaned women, and lowered their self-esteem and sense of worth.

Remnants of ancient myths, taboos, and superstitions still influence contemporary medical and nonmedical attitudes toward the menopause, although our view of menstruation is no longer that of years gone by. The ancients feared that a menstruating woman could turn beer sour, spoil wine and milk, make mares miscarry, dim mirrors, blunt razors, and kill bees (Chadwick, 1932). Present-day attitudes toward menopause, however, still suggest the influence of old fears of the suppression of menstruation (amenorrhea), especially that the blood not discharged might wreak havoc in the brain. In the 19th century, obsolete views of amenorrhea were elaborated and ultimately merged with newer ideas. One of these newer, socially constructed ideas asserted the existence of a link between being female and being in physical and mental ill health. Women's health began to be obsessively debated by the whole society, with allegations of their frailty and illnesses, and the 19th century was called by some the "age of the womb" (Stage, 1979).

The idea of female weakness was extremely influential in determining women's self-perceptions, expectations, and self-experience and thus created a new reality. Although we no longer view women as frail and ill, the idea that menopause is linked to emotional and mental problems still lives on, leading many women to expect depression to strike when they enter menopause. Even though sex hormones were discovered more than half a century ago, and both menstruation and menopause can now be adequately understood, old ideas continue to prevail, especially when societal power relationships demand their survival.

Information on menopause is sparse, one reason being that in the past most women died early—before they reached middle age. In 1789, for example, the life expectancy of a girl child at birth was 36.5 years; it had increased to 40.5 years in 1850, to 44.5 years in 1890. Nevertheless, most deaths occurring in infancy or childhood, women born in 1789 who were able to survive until they were 20 years old could expect to live to 56 years (Shryock, 1960) and, presumably, experience menopause. Although life expectancy rose during the course of the 19th century, menopause was barely mentioned in the texts of the time. Whatever knowledge we do have of the perceptions of menopause through the centuries comes to us almost exclusively from male sources and must therefore be assumed to include major gender biases. With the exception of the writings of women physicians and the Mosher (1980) survey conducted between 1892 and 1920, no extant documents from women – letters, diaries, journals – offer us first-hand knowledge. In addition to gender bias, class bias can be inferred – physicians were describing primarily their middle-class patients. Moreover, 19th-century attitudes were strongly influenced by the views of religious "purity" tracts. Thus it is in the context of middle-class aspirations that perceptions of women and sexuality during this period must be understood (see Haller and Haller, 1974).

An exploration of attitudes toward menopause through the centuries poses other difficulties: (1) systematic references to the subject are virtually absent; (2) books and papers that might be relevant are out of print; (3) the terms denoting menopausal changes are often unclear and euphemistic; (4) one cannot reliably assess the significance of extant sources, nor be certain about the origins of repeated themes. As a result, our understanding of how menopause was perceived during some time periods remains hidden in darkness.

The word menopause is of recent origin and first appeared in the 1870s. It is derived from the Greek words for *month* and *cessation.* Before the term was coined, menopause was referred to as "cessation," "the changes," "Indian summer," a "physical Rubicon," or some other euphemism. Today menopause is still referred to by some medical writers as an "endocrinopathy" or "deficiency disease" (Utian, 1987). In this book, the term *climacteric* will refer to "that phase in the aging process of a woman marking the transition from the reproductive stage of life to the non-reproductive phase" (Utian and Serr, 1976). *Menopause* refers to the final cessation of menses within the climacteric phase. Within the climacteric, women can be classified as to pre-, post-, or perimenopausal, depending on their menstrual status.

PRE -19TH CENTURY VIEWS: GALEN TO THE 18TH CENTURY

Probably the earliest reference to menopause is found in the Old Testament. When Abraham's wife, Sarah, overheard a messenger inform her husband that she would have a child, she laughed and said that she was past the time during which women can bear children.

In Galen's time, and until sex hormones were discovered in the

1920s, descriptions and explanations of menstruation and menopause were all influenced by the theory of "humors," especially the concept of "plethora." Although not all ancient physicians agreed on their number, Galen named four humors: yellow bile, black bile, phlegm, and blood. Physiological and clinical observations could be explained by the presence or absence of the four humors. What interests us most is Galen's view of blood. The ancients thought that each humor could be present in abundance or in diminished quantity. Excess of one humor was called "plethora," or fullness. Signs of a blood plethora were a heavy and reddish urine, especially during a fever. The opposite was an exaggerated evacuation of blood, which caused pallor and was thought to be due to protracted uterine bleeding. Anemia was not mentioned as a disease, but the term *chloros*, which means pale yellow, was used to indicate skin color and became "chlorosis," the "green sickness" (see Napheys, 1871), said to occur during menarche and menopause.

Until the end of the 17th century, amenorrhea, or "suppressed menstruation," was considered the chief cause of women's illnesses. According to Rowland's (1981) translation, it was believed to be caused by "the heat or the cold of the uterus or the heat or cold of the humors . . . inside the uterus, or excessive dryness of their complexion, or being awake too much, thinking too much, being too angry or too sad, or eating too little" (p. 61). In this medieval account, menopause is not mentioned and may not have been differentiated from amenorrhea. Amenorrhea's symptoms included

> a feeling of weight from the navel down to the privy member. And the ache of their kidneys, backbone, forehead, neck, eyes, and infection of the waters, that is to say, their changing into the wrong color . . . And such women have, at times, an unreasonable appetite for food not suited to them, such as coal or rinds or shells, and their complexion is a bad color or grows pale. And sometimes it terrifies the heart so much that it causes women to fall down in a faint as though they had the falling sickness. And they lie in that sickness for a day or two as though dead. And sometimes they have dizziness with great confusion in the brain and think that everything is turned upside down . . . [p. 63].

Treatment for amenorrhea included blood-letting at the veins of the big toe and cuts on the legs below the calf, cupping under the nipples or under the kidneys at the back, bathing in herbs, drinking wine, walking, working, eating well, the insertion of suppositories with medication.

Ancient themes stressed that: (1) the moon exerts an influence on menstruation; (2) blood that stops flowing during menstruation represents a danger to health; (3) sexual desire is affected by amenorrhea and will influence the health of an infant; (4) a healthy lifestyle is beneficial; (5) symptoms are pervasive and include neurological ones, and (6) bleeding is the most effective treatment.

In contrast to these older themes, 18th-century perceptions of menstruation and menopause were influenced by a commitment to logic and direct observation of nature, although the views of Galen persisted. The first book on menstruation in English was written by John Freind, a famous English scholar, historian, mathematician, and physician. First published in Latin in 1703, the book was translated in 1729. Freind's model of the body was rooted in 18th-century geometry and classical mechanics: he referred to such concepts as velocity, the sine of the angle of incidence, momentum, pressure of liquids, inertia, conservation, and the like.

According to Freind (1729), menstruation either rendered women ready for conception, or it afforded nutriment to the fetus. It was not caused by the moon but by a "plethora." Women, "inasmuch as they heap up a great quantity of Humours, by living continually at home, and not being used to hard Labour, or exposed to the Sun, should receive a discharge of this Fulness, as a Remedy given by Nature" (p. 13). The uterus was the most suitable of all the vessels in a woman's body for the discharge of the blood. However, in cases of suppression, when the vessels of the uterus had become tenacious and blocked passage of the blood, "the plethorick Blood is very often discharged by the Nostrils or the Lungs . . ." (p. 40), or a "looseness" substituted for the discharge of menstrual blood.

As an "iatromathematician," Freind explained changes in the menses and their eventual cessation. To him, nature ran along mathematical lines: since the menses usually begin at the "second Septenary . . . they cease at the seventh, or the square of the number seven" (p. 1). Change in the menses came about "as old Age creeps on, the Humours become rigid and hard; so that a Plethora can neither be accumulated at that Age, nor if it be, can it be discharged, because of the tenacity of the Vessels" (p. 59). After the seventh septenary, the vessels of the uterus would be too strong for the momentum of the blood to break through them. Thus, nature has wisely ordered that the menses should decrease with increasing age.

These views of the menopause clearly predate its later medicalization: Since it is as nature ordered, "no very bad symptoms happen in elderly Women, although the Menses should be wanting . . . the sensible Evacuations are encreased in old Age. . . . many Women, as soon as they are destitute of their Menses, contract a fuller habit, and grow fat" (p. 62).

What is most important in Freind's account is his differentiation of menopause from the suppression of menstruation (amenorrhea) and his assertion that menopause preserves the health of the older woman—it was not an illness.

THE 19TH CENTURY

Transition from Midwives to Physicians

In early America, before the professionalization of medicine, women assumed responsibility for illness in the family. Advice and assistance were available from kin and community, and newspapers and almanacs offered medical advice. Yet medical practice was still grounded in oral tradition. By the late 18th century, physicians had begun to publish guides to domestic practice. The best known and most widely read of these manuals, written in lucid, everyday language, was by William Buchan. Published originally in 1769 in Edinburgh and two years later in Philadelphia, it remained popular through the mid-1800s, going through at least 30 editions (Starr, 1982).

Buchan (1771) emphasized healthful living. Women at all ages, he wrote, are greatly injured from the want of exercise and free air. . . . the confinement of females, besides hurting their figure and complexion, relaxes their solids, weakens their minds, and disorders all the functions of the body. Hence proceed obstructions, indigestion, flatulence, abortions, and the whole train of nervous disorders. These not only unfit women for being mothers and nurses, but often render them whimsical and ridiculous. Proper food and drink for women are particularly important "at the time they are out of order" [p. 332].

More cautious than some earlier physicians, Buchan advised against therapy with nauseous drugs to bring on menstruation in cases of amenorrhea or menopause. Rather than ingest powerful drugs to deal with their "last great crisis," women were to eat healthy foods, exercise in fresh air, and live in a protected setting. Buchan feared that the "stoppage of any customary evacuation, however small, is sufficient to disorder the whole frame, and often to destroy life itself. . . . many women either fall into chronic disorders, or die about this time." Yet other women survived cessation and "often become more healthy and hardy than they were before, and enjoy strength and vigour to a very great age" (p. 335).

Buchan's natural approach resembles that of most midwives who, beginning at this time, were slowly forced out of their work with women by male physicians. Manuals on midwifery had urged care in regard to menopausal problems. The suppression of menses is due to two causes, they wrote: "violent passions of the mind, and the application of cold to the surface of the body" (Burns, 1820, p. 124). Some women believed they were "with child," rather than suppose they were feeling the consequences of cessation and thus of old age. No medicines were necessary and the use of "emmenagogues," which aimed to prolong the menstrual discharge was considered foolish and hurtful.

According to another midwifery manual (by an "American Practitioner," 1826), however, menopause was one of the most dangerous periods of a woman's life. Dropsy might occur and dormant complaints come forward: A litte lump in the breast, hardly felt for years, might now be converted into a cancer, which would destroy life if not removed. In some women, the breasts would collapse, emaciation take place, the skin shrivel and lose its softness, color, and suppleness. Treatment consisted of frequent small bleedings, cooling laxatives, and the avoidance of excitement.

Later in the 19th century, midwives, in contrast to physicians-,viewed the menopause as nonpathological (Cazeaux, 1863), even salutary. So-called hysterical women, for years martyrs to uterine functions, were described as taking a new lease on life when menopause began (Playfair, 1880).

The Social Construction of the Female Invalid

To understand such complex and irrational phenomena as the 19th-century American and Western European perception of women as frail and ill, and of the menopausal woman as vulnerable to mental and physical illness, we must first understand the historical and social contexts in which they occurred. Although it is beyond the scope of this chapter to answer them, let us pose the following questions: Why and how did these perceptions arise when and where they did? What was the nature of the social environment that influenced their development? What was the effect of the professionalization of medicine and the rise of gynecology, gynecological surgery, and psychiatry on perceptions of women?

Three different approaches are possible: (1) that a patriarchal society determined the perception of women and thus of menopause; (2) that the professionalization of medicine largely determined those perceptions; or (3) that men's irrational fear of women provided the underlying impulse to viewing women in general as ill and menopausal women in particular as insane. Most likely, all these views combine to provide an explanation.

By the middle of the 19th century, social instability, urbanization, and the new industrial economy had erased traditional patterns of life and created anxieties and confusions that were expressed in concern with women's health. In American cities, the sphere of the middle-class woman became constricted when machines could do what heretofore women had done—spinning, weaving, sewing. Women's traditional domestic role was being assumed by immigrant servants.

Middle-class families began to limit their size; industrial work was taboo for middle-class women; working-class women tended to be either agricultural workers or domestics. In 1850, only 13% of the paid labor force was female (Stage, 1979).

Women were needed primarily in their role as mothers. While men's freedom to move became part of their self-identification, women's expected passivity led them to doubt their own adequacy. The more men succeeded in the world, the less middle-class women were needed economically. Thus, as American men became increasingly obsessed with work during the 19th century, and as earning money was equated with possessions, the danger for women was that they themselves might become merely possessions. This dilemma was compounded by the ideology of 'Mother,' which made women accountable for the advancement of civilization, that is, for the rearing of sons (Meyer, 1965).

The cult of motherhood overvalued women's reproductive capacities. Menopause, representing sterility, was feared, and the woman who could no longer give birth was devalued. As women aged, their problems increased. As families limited their size and medicine began to add years to life, the job of mother constituted a smaller and smaller fraction of the lifespan. Old age had had a respected place in the old days but now had lost it. How was a woman to fill the void created when her children left her home? She was only 50.

Perhaps one escape for a woman was to be ill. It permitted her to withdraw from the world and gave her something to do: to try to regain her health (see Meyer, 1965). But illness was not only characteristic of the woman who had married and become a mother. Unmarried women also took to their beds and became invalids. The woman who had been a mother had lost her place, but the "spinster" had never had one.

In America and Western Europe, attitudes toward the menopause were part of a larger issue: attitudes toward women and their physical and mental illnesses. Showalter (1985) has argued that the image of the insane woman in the 19th century was part of the cultural framework in which ideas both of femininity and of insanity were constructed. She has pointed to the preponderance of women in English public lunatic asylums between the 17th and the middle of the 19th century. And present-day feminists have shown the existence of an expected

alliance between being a woman and being insane. Women are still
viewed as "situated on the side of irrationality, silence, nature, and
body, while men are situated on the side of reason, discourse, culture,
and mind" (Showalter, 1985, p. 4).

Illness and social class factors intertwined: the way middle- and
upper-class women lived predisposed them to illness. Illness, in turn,
predisposed them to feeling in delicate health and to living and
behaving as they were expected to. In particular, women were expected to experience menstrual and menopausal problems, dislocated
or fallen wombs, hysteria, and the like. Illness became fashionable
(Wood, 1974). Illness was also exploited both by its victims and by
physicians "as an advertisement of genteel sensibility and an escape
from the too pressing demands of bedroom and kitchen" (Ehrenreich
and English, 1978, p. 2).

Medicine's Role in the Popular Perception of Menopause

An influential idea underlying 19th-century medical conceptualizations was derived from classical mechanics. It viewed the body as a
closed-energy system in which all organs competed for the limited
amount of available blood.

> The general stock of nutriment circulating through an organism
> has to support the whole. Each organ appropriates a portion of
> this general stock for repair and growth. Whatever each takes
> diminishes by so much the amount available for the rest. All
> other organs therefore, jointly and individually, compete for
> blood with each organ. So that the welfare of each is indirectly
> bound up with that of the rest . . . [Spencer, 1986, p. 75].

Medicine was strongly influenced by this view of the closed-energy
system, with its emphasis on conserving body fluids. Physicians vastly
exaggerated the role of the uterus and, later, that of the ovaries, and
viewed women's internal organs as engaged in competition for the
limited quantity of blood available. Although a man's sexual activity
could deplete his body of fluids, and thus of energy, sexual expression
was partly under the control of his will; whereas menstruation and

menopause were uncontrolled, unpredictable, mysterious, simultaneously fascinating, frightening, and repulsive to men. No doubt, ancient fears of women, expressed in myths of the harpy and witch, fueled men's perceptions of women's reproductive functioning.

Kuhn (1962) has suggested that we view premodern science in relation to its internal development rather than from our present-day vantage point. Physicians, like other scientists, must be viewed as prisoners of their own theories. In the 1850s, medical science had left physicians few alternatives to the measures then in use (most of which we now consider cruel—blood letting, using powerful emetics and cathartics) except to admit to themselves and their patients that they were helpless (see Morantz, 1974).

Treatment was equally harsh for men and women alike. Concern with disorders of male reproductive functions was similarly vastly exaggerated and medical treatments for men's reproductive problems equally cruel. Major societal, religious, moral and medical concerns pertained to masturbation. One of its more serious consequences was believed to be "spermatorrhea," or the frequent and involuntary loss of semen. This condition was believed to cause loss of memory, epilepsy, and insanity, if not an early death. Men with this condition were described as "profoundly melancholy . . . often [with] an aversion to either sex—and impotent . . ." (Napheys, 1883, p. 85). Among the treatments for spermatorrhea were cauterization, cold baths, spermatorrheal rings with sharp points on their inner surface. These were worn at night; the pain caused by the points was to wake the man as soon as an erection began. Other treatments were adhesive plasters applied to the back of the penis, or tying hands and feet to the bed posts, or surgical treatment that interrupted the circulation of blood to the genitals and prevented erection.

The treatment of men's "illnesses" thus paralleled the treatment of women's. Yet, despite treatment similarities, physicians had different attitudes toward their male and female patients. It was believed essential for men to conserve their fluids to ensure that their bodies, especially their brains, retained sufficient moisture. Men needed only to produce sperm and discharge it at specified times, a process that could be brought under control through the prevention of masturbation.

Women, on the other hand, needed to be sure that their wombs retained an adequate supply of blood; their brains' need for fluids was secondary. The regularity of menstruation was considered important, and irregularity of discharge was believed to harm women's ability to procreate. To aid the establishment of the "catamenial function," which was said to last between the menarche and age 18 and was essential to future motherhood, young women were discouraged from pursuing higher education (Clarke, 1873). It was also feared that blood not discharged during the menstrual years, and, later, during menopause, could enter the brain and cause insanity.

Thus one can conclude that, in addition to cultural constructions of women as ill and the needs of new medical specialties—gynecology, gynecological surgery, and psychiatry—the harsh treatments of both female and male reproductive problems were a result of limited knowledge of the body's functioning. These limitations in knowledge were not confined to reproduction alone. Overall national health improved only slightly over the 19th century, and it even deteriorated in the large cities. Tuberculosis, pneumonia, typhoid, and children's diseases were the chief killers. Only smallpox became less common as a result of vaccination, and the use of quinine against malaria was the only medical intervention that had a specific impact on morbidity (Shryock, 1960). Although sanitation improved in the cities, medicine was unable to effect cures for infectious diseases until the 1930s, when sulfa drugs were discovered (Thomas, 1983). By this time, sex hormones had been discovered and thus permitted an understanding of reproductive processes.

The Rise of Gynecology

As the century progressed, menopause was perceived more and more negatively. Although clearly differentiated from amenorrhea, menopause seemed to have inherited the endless list of illnesses earlier believed to follow from amenorrhea. Moreover, a link was now solidly constructed between menopause and insanity, which continues in our own times as the link between menopause and depression (Formanek, 1987a,b). Ancient ideas of blood raging in the body without finding an escape, as well as equally ancient and negative views of older women in general, unquestionably aided the construction of this link. By the middle of the 19th century, ovulation had become associated with menstruation, although the function of the ovaries was not understood until the 20th century, and older explanatory concepts such as the plethora persisted.

In the course of the 19th century medicine became a profession and developed specialties. The view of women as objects, inferior to men, suffering in silence from undiagnosable illnesses, and unable to bear children underlies the conceptualizations that led to the specialties of obstetrics and gynecology. The development of this specialization owes much to Charles Meigs, a professor of midwifery and the diseases of women and children in the Jefferson Medical College at Philadelphia. He was a member of the American Medical Association and the American Philosophical Society; vice president of the College of Physicians of Philadelphia, and widely read and plagiarized in popular marriage manuals. Although menopause was not considered an indication for medical attention, either by midwives or by Buchan (1771) and his generation of physicians, for the 19th century gynecologist, menopause and other "diseases" of women became a source of fascination. Their innovative treatment held the promise of a career leading to both prestige and increasing income.

Meigs's (1854) views on women were that "women are clearly different from men; if we view the statue of Venus and compare it to that of Apollo, we note that she has a head almost too small for intellect, but just big enough for love" (p. 63). In line with the *Zeitgeist*, Meigs admired women for their pure and pious nature and their civilizing influence over men. The woman's uterus, an organ of great power, he believed, influences her whole constitution. He wondered "whether *she* was not made in order that *it* [i.e., the uterus] should be made, and whether it may not on occasion become a disturbing radiator in her economy . . ." (p. 4). Thus there is a direct connection between reproductive functioning and the mind, the latter affected by changes in the former. Not only was gynecology given an impetus by such views of women, but psychiatry similarly focused on the womb in its conceptualization of hysteria (Drinka, 1984).

According to Meigs (1854) a menopausal woman's emotional state derives from changes in her reproductive system: change in the "caliber of the vagina is associated with . . . melancholy, which led to suicidal propensities and attempts . . ." (p. 466). In addition to melancholy, cancer might result from the cessation of menstruation. Thus, Meigs's view was consistent with that of other physicians, who now emphasized woman's special predisposition both to physical illness and to insanity.

Men's fear of women's insanity, which was believed to be due to the malfunctioning of women's reproductive organs, seemed to motivate physicians to attempt more radical treatment—to become gynecological surgeons (Barker-Benfield, 1976). American doctors pioneered ovariotomy, hysterectomy, and the repair of the vesicovaginal fistula, the latter accomplished by J. Marion Sims. Sims's (1884) autobiography details his experiments on the slave women he had bought and operated on—as often as 30 times on the same woman—for the repair of the fistula. It is unclear whether the women submitted to repeated operations because they were slaves, or because they suffered, or for the laudanum (opium) given to them postoperatively. The pattern that emerges, however, seems to be the same for all such operations: they were perfected on slaves or on poor women, and then performed on middle-class women who could pay their surgeons (see Buxton, 1968).

Case Histories of Menopausal Women

Aside from a page or two in medical texts, menopausal women were not mentioned in detail. Tilt's books (1851, 1882) are the exception. An influential British gynecologist, Edward John Tilt was president of the Obstetrical Society of London. Tilt's (1882) *The Change of Life in Health and Disease*, widely read on both sides of the Atlantic, was based on case records from 500 "upper class" menopausal women. The following case histories appear in an earlier version (Tilt, 1851).

A 48-year-old needlewoman, with auburn hair and blue eyes, tall and stout, has always lived in the country. As her menstrual flow began to be irregular and was attended by heat and perspiration, she felt "a great darting pain in the forehead, and a dizzy stupid feeling in the head, with a great tendency to sleep" (p. 142).

Another woman's menstruation ceased with "terminal flooding," and she became troubled with symptoms of "faintness, flushes, perspirations and . . . bleeding piles. She looks exhausted, stupid, and bewildered . . . her head feels as heavy as lead, with noises and great giddiness. . . ." Tilt treated her with henbane and ordered a plaster of opium and camphor to be placed over the pit of the stomach and the lower part of the chest. She improved, grew stouter. Sedatives, not alcohol, will arrest "in its bud that tendency to mental derangement which . . . occurs more frequently in women than in men" (p. 147).

I was lately consulted by a lady aged 53, of middle stature, sanguine complexion, brown hair, and hazel eyes. She menstruated abundantly for the first time in her thirteenth year, and the function has since been pretty regularly performed, the discharge being usually abundant. While the function was ceasing she was twice seized with flooding, and felt better in health afterwards. Menstruation ceased at 51, and was soon followed by diarrhoea, which came on at irregular intervals, but did not interfere with the appetite and strength of the patient. When that supplementary discharge subsided, heaviness of the head, with giddiness, came on, together with flushes of heat and drenching perspirations. For these distressing symptoms she had consulted several medical men, and had taken large doses of quinine, acetate of lead, and gallic acid, but without benefit. I ordered her to be bled twelve ounces. The vertigo, flushes, and perspirations abated considerably. I next recommended that the bowels should be kept open by Seidlitz powders; several glasses of effervescing lemonade to be taken in the course of the day, and a tepid bath for an hour every week. Meat once a day, no beer nor porter, one glass of sherry at dinner, and more exercise to be taken in the open air. In a month all the painful symptoms had completely disappeared, and the patient remained well for several subsequent months, when, without any apparent cause, the same symptoms broke out again, as with a sudden burst. I ordered eight ounces of blood to be withdrawn, and prescribed the former treatment, with similar good effect; and I should do so again—diminishing as much as possible the quantity of blood to be withdrawn—if a neglect of the prescribed diet, or some unforeseen nervous excitement, should bring on a relapse [p. 131].

These cases appear to be typical of the medical treatment accorded menopausal women during the second half of the 19th and early 20th centuries. They may be typical of the attitudes of physicians as well— one is struck by Tilt's misogynist descriptions of women as dizzy, stupid, and bewildered, especially those women who were not members of the upper classes.

The descriptions of Tilt's cases and their treatment point to Tilt's beliefs:

1. Puberty and menopause are both periods of crisis that last several years.

2. The course of menarche presages the course of menopause.

3. "Flooding" is a type of terminal menstrual period that, according to the plethoric theory, improves the woman's subsequent state of health. That is, an accumulation of blood must be discharged or she will be ill.

4. Blood is only one type of discharge. When menstruation ceases, diarrhea (or nosebleeds or perspiration) may substitute for it.

5. Mental symptoms and hot flushes and perspiration are due to the undischarged blood now entering the brain.

6. Nervous excitement must be avoided at menopause since it may attract blood to the brain. ("Nervous" most likely means "sexual.")

7. Treatment consists of: (a) bleeding, by cupping, leeching or other methods; (b) by paying attention to a woman's general health: a bland diet, limited alcohol intake, keeping her bowels open and bathing once a week; (c) prescriptions were not specific ones but those used for most illnesses and ranged from the ineffective to the harmful.

By 1882, Tilt, among others, began criticizing contemporary gynecological surgery. Many female complaints, such as dysmenorrhea or sterility, were cured by means of J. Marion Sims's new operation— slitting of the womb. Maliciously, Tilt adds that "Dr. Sims' most promising pupil was busy sewing up the wombs he had helped his teacher to divide . . ." (p. 4). In America, Tilt stated, "the womb is to have no peace." He was also critical of the less dangerous pessary, a mechanical device that was to support and rectify the position of the womb and prevent prolapse.

Tilt had now revised his earlier speculations and was presenting a new view of menopause. He found the origin of menopausal illness to lie in the ovaries, which disturb the viscera, the center of nerve power and the cerebrospinal system. He retained the notion of the similarity between menarche and menopause and suggested that menopausal disturbances resemble the assumption of power by the ovaries at puberty.

His book presents statistics on a very long list of diseases attending menopause—over 100! They include epigastric faintness and sinking, fainting, prolonged and intense debility, chlorosis, palpitations. Diseases of the brain include nervous irritability, headache, pseudo-narcotism, and hystericism. A pseudo-narcotic woman "feels silly, as if her head were one dead lump" (p. 142), is forgetful, loses her way in the streets, falls asleep during the day, feels stunned, and so on. To document the menopausal woman's vulnerability to insanity, Tilt used hospital admission statistics to show the relative frequency of insanity at different ages: 437 out of 1320 women admitted to a hospital became insane between the ages of 40 to 45; pregnancy and lactation explained the presence of insanity before the age of 40. Menopausal insanity was of several types: delirium, mania, melancholia, suicidal tendencies, uncontrollable impulses and perversion of moral instincts, uncontrollable peevishness, dipsomania, impulse to deceive, demonomania, erotomania, apoplexy, hemiplegia, and so forth.

In contrast to his earlier speculations of a direct connection between the uterus and the brain, Tilt's theory presumed not one but two channels of communication between the reproductive apparatus and the brain: the blood vessels and the nerves. Many mental diseases were *not* the result of a plethora. On the contrary, the brain was imperfectly stimulated by too little blood. Not content with viewing women as "silly" and "stupid," he also saw the similarity between their reproductive organs and that of frogs: just before frogs copulate, their nervous system is most irritable. "When women are under the influence of increased ovarian action they are also more irritable, more easily impressed by cold, noise, other physical agents, and emotional stimuli" (p. 173).

Popular Sex and Marriage Manuals

Nineteenth-century sex and marriage manuals seemed to justify, even promote, the prevailing social and moral fabric of Victorian America.

They compensated for the lack of tradition in urban life and helped the middle cass to understand its sexual relationships (see Haller and Haller, 1974). By popularizing medical opinion on menopause, these manuals added both to its medicalization and to the confusion about its meanings.

Usually written by physicians, the manuals frequently went into hundreds of editions. Although menopause was mentioned in them, albeit briefly, writers were generally more fascinated with the young woman at menarche: "Every one must have noticed what an astonishing change occurs in a young female at that time. The bust becomes full, the pelvis enlarges . . ." (Hollick, 1853, p. 109). And most repeated the old idea that menstruation purifies the body of harmful substances. Hollick even found a new use in industry for this evacuative ability: ". . . females can work, without injury, at certain employments in the metals, where poisonous fumes are evolved, and which would kill men, the deleterious matter being carried off in this way" (p. 115). Menopause presumably put an end to such bodily purification and rendered the woman vulnerable to disease.

When the manuals mentioned menopause, women were apprised of its dangers. Physicians stated that the extent of discomfort and disease during menopause was due to the abuse a woman had earlier inflicted on her constitution, thus blaming women for their own illnesses. "Abuse" included sexual passion, immodest dress, the use of stimulating foods, prurient reading, contraception, or masturbation. All of these were said to increase the sufferings of the menopausal woman because nature compelled "the payment of her violated laws" (Dråke, 1902), by means of malignant disease or years of invalidism.

In line with medical advice to the menopausal woman current at mid-19th century, it was suggested that women

> avoid all intense mental application, or strong emotions, and not think of the change that is taking place. Some persons make themselves very unhappy in this way, and greatly increase the danger of their situation. They cannot help thinking of their past condition, and dreading the future. Their thoughts, especially when associated with others peculiar to certain temperaments, keep up the excitement in the womb, and protract the struggle . . . [Hollick, 1853, p. 235].

Cessation of menses was not necessarily a dangerous time, but evils might arise from sexual excess and women should avoid amorous thoughts that might be evoked by viewing "lascivious pictures," reading love stories, and anything that might "cause regret for charms that are fled, and enjoyments that are ended forever" (Hayes, 1869, p. 221).

American "purity" literature influenced the content of the manuals. This literature stressed both piety and purity as vital components of the female character and encouraged passionlessness. According to the doctrine of separate spheres, the sexes were differentiated on the basis of their opposite personality traits: lust and carnality were male; spirituality and moral superiority, female. This new view differed from those of earlier times, when women were permitted, if not encouraged, to be more lustful, licentious, and insatiable than men (Woloch, 1984; see also Maxwell, this volume). Women not only were passionless, but derived their knowledge of sexual physiology from prescribed sources: "Learned everything I know from good sources and in a pure and sacred way. Had access to Cowan's *Science of a New Life*, Napheys' *Physical Life of Woman* and from the best pages of [phrenologist] Fowler" (Mosher, 1980).

Until the end of the 19th century, popular manuals helped disseminate negative stereotypes of the menopausal woman. After that time, more positive perceptions of women, initiated by reformers and feminists were published. The earlier manuals depicted menopausal women as cognitively and emotionally damaged, paranoid, depressed, hypochondriacal, and impossible to live with:

> . . . she grows more confused, and imagines that she is watched with suspicious and unkind eyes, and often she worries herself by such unfounded fancies into a most harassing state of mental distress. Society loses its attractions, and solitude does but allow her opportunity to indulge to a still more injurious extent such brooding phantasms. Every ache and pain is magnified. Does her heart palpitate, as it is very apt to do? Straightway she is certain that she has some terrible disease of that organ, and that she will drop down dead some day in the street. Is one of her breasts somewhat sore, which, too, is not unusual, she knows at once it is a cancer, and suffers an agony of terror from a cause wholly

imaginary. . . . she becomes fretful, and yet full of remorse for
yielding to her peevishness . . . she annoys those around her by
groundless fears, and is angered when they show their annoy-
ance. . . . She is utterly wretched, without any obvious cause of
wretchedness [Napheys, 1871, p. 296].

Her symptoms included:

a sense of choking, a feeling of faintness, shooting pains in the
back and limbs, creepings and chilliness, a feeling as if a hand
were applied to the back or the cheek, a fidgety restlessness,
inability to fix the mind on reading or in following a discourse,
and a loss of control over the emotions . . . nature is employing
all her powers to bring about the mysterious transformation in
the economy by which she deprives the one sex forever of
partaking in the creative act after a certain age, while she only
diminishes the power of the other [p. 297].

Antimedical Alternatives

The medical view of the pervasive frailty and illness of women was not
shared by such critics as homeopathic physicians, phrenologists, and
water curers, some of whose ideas on women's health resembled those
found in the earlier manuals of midwifery. Although urban, Eastern,
middle-class women had substituted the physician for the midwife,
many did not trust the bleeding, strong medicines, and pessaries
advocated as treatment by physicians and sought less dangerous
treatment alternatives for their illnesses. Many women consulted
quacks who advocated such fads as eating cereals (Grahamism),
animal magnetism, Galvanism, water cures, or homeopathy. Middle-
class women also joined ladies' physiological societies where health
and medicine were discussed, and attended spas (see Woloch, 1984).
   The success of patent medicines, such as Lydia Pinkham's Vegetable Compound, first marketed in 1875, is evidence of the distrust
women felt toward physicians' harsh medicines and dangerous gynecological operations. The misconceptions of menopause were still

embedded in mistaken ideas of women's functioning. This was true for the alternatives to medicine as well.

The Compound's formula consisted of a variety of roots and seeds, all suspended in 19% alcohol. The label on the bottle stated its uses for "all female weaknesses, including Leucorrhea, Painful Menstruation, Inflammation, and Ulceration of the Womb, Irregularities, Floodings." Ads for the compound suggest that Lydia Pinkham agreed with prevailing medical opinion about the close bond between "female complaints" and insanity. The ads promised that, with the use of the Compound, women would no longer be ill. Not only operations, but murders too could now be avoided: ". . . a Stratford, Conn., clergyman, killed by his own wife . . . [owing to] insanity brought on by 16 years of suffering with female complaints." Regardless of condition—dysmenorrhea, prolapsed uterus, nonspecific pain, or menopausal troubles associated with insanity—Lydia Pinkham's Vegetable Compound promised to provide health and happiness (see Stage, 1979).

Not only reformers and the general public, but many physicians believed in the curative properties of water and became critical of mainstream medicine:

> The Best Joke of the Season [was] perpetrated the other night in the Pathological Society. One of its members had been treating a female in a pauper hospital for Ulceration of the Os Uteri with all the paraphernalia of speculum, topical cauterization, astringent and anodyne washes, etc., after the most approved fashion, until, as usual, she died. . . . Whereupon the organ and its appendages were removed from the body, and taken to the Society for . . . inspection. . . . after diligent search, the uterus was declared to be a perfect . . . organ, the only deviation from health being the local injury of the textures, resulting from the mistaken remedies which had been applied for a disease which had no existence. The blunder can only be accounted for by the theory that the disease had been cured, of which the patient is nevertheless reported to have died . . . [from the *Water Cure Journal*, 1853].

Physicians' increasing wealth was criticized as well. Trall (1862) reported that, at a festival held by a New York medical society, women were toasted as "the last best gift of God to man, and the chief support of the doctors." Forty-thousand physicians with an aggregate income of 100 millions of dollars, "three fourths of this sum. . . . our physicians must thank frail women for . . ." (p. 67).

Water Cure advocates differed from mainstream medical practitioners in that they discarded harsh medical treatments and relied on the use of baths, a regimen of drinking water, eating grains, fruits and vegetables, two rather than three meals per day, avoiding gross, heavy, stimulating foods, and wearing loose clothing rather than corsets. Application of water to the surface of the body had, they believed, a particularly cathartic effect. It was said to result in the purification of the blood and tissues. By means of fiery rashes, boils, sweatings, and purulent defecations, the system relieved itself. Menopausal patients were advised to walk barefoot and take air baths for such troubles as impaired digestion, headache, tendency of blood to run to the head, nervous affections ranging from simple nervous irritability to serious mental disorder, and the like. These symptoms were said to subside when menstruation definitely ceases; often, however, a woman's health might be permanently affected. Treatment was a harmless series of "full ablutions" twice a week, with water temperature and duration exactly specified (Bilz, 1898).

Phrenologists were indirectly motivated to take a stand on the treatment of women's reproductive health. They had branched out from their original interest in the contours of the skull and the inheritance of both mental and emotional traits to suggest that the health of the mother was vitally important to the welfare of her offspring. As part of this effort, they tended to demedicalize menstruation, pregnancy, and menopause and to emphasize leading a natural life, taking exercise, being in the open air and avoiding the often abused luxuries of refined society.

In contrast to water curers and phrenologists, homeopaths generally accepted the prevailing views of menopause and its symptoms, and described

a febrile state of system . . . headache, of a hammering, beating character, with roarings or whistlings in the ears . . . sensitive to sound and light . . . she desires to sit away from her family for quiet . . . nervous apprehensions and anxieties . . . frequently weeping without a cause . . . fretful or peevish and irritable, or pre-occupied with despondent ideas about herself . . . vacillation of feelings . . . dyspeptic symptoms, constipation, hysterical symptoms . . . [Leadam, 1851, p. 55].

Medicines, such as aconite, belladonna, ignatia, pulsatilla, sepia, and coffea, were administered in minute dilutions (see Leadam, 1851). Hahnemann, the inventor of homeopathy, advocated taking one part of a drug, adding to it 99 parts milk sugar or alcohol, and grinding or shaking the mixture. The result was "the first potence." Homeopaths then further diluted drugs to the 6th, 12th, and 30th power. It seems unlikely that their effects were more than those of a placebo, in contrast to Lydia Pinkham's Vegetable Compound which, owing to its high alcohol content, could at least improve the user's mood.

One can conclude that advocates of alternative approaches, despite their critique of mainstream medical treatments, brought with them neither new views of the menopause nor relief for whatever symptoms women consulted them for.

Late 19th-Century Views

Toward the end of the 19th century, physicians increasingly stressed menopausal women's vulnerability to nervous and mental, as well as physical, illness. This emphasis was reflected in the Surgeon-General's *Index Catalogue* (1888), which directs those searching for information on the cessation of menstruation to "See also: insanity in women, and uterus (cancer of)" (p. 154).

Physicians also began to search for explanations for variations in the manifestations of menstruation and menopause and examined demographic variables. These included climate, urban-rural, and social class factors. Like fruits, women were said to reach puberty earlier in hot than in cold climates, in densely populated manufacturing towns than on farms. Girls brought up in luxury or sensual indulgence were said to menstruate earlier than those reared in poverty (Carpenter, 1851).

Physicians also continued to expect menopausal women to become ill with latent diseases: rheumatism, syphilis, hemorrhoids, diarrhea, constipation, insomnia, and tachycardia. Some physicians, however, correctly asserted that these conditions could be due to increasing age and not to the menopause (Reed, 1901). According to Reed, about one woman in 10 would be annoyed by hot flashes, which are a "subjective sensation and . . . not real" (p. 739). Sometimes a curious mental exaltation would occur early in menopause, and a woman would meddle with business affairs that did not concern her. Reed held that, in general, mental changes during menopause resulted from the woman's compressing into two years a man's 20 years of gentle change. During this limited span, she must change her attitude toward life and love, the big world, and the great future.

> It is evolution for him; it is revolution for her. She is suddenly brought to perceive that her charms, her youth, her sex itself, are passing from her. She is invited, with cruel abruptness, to be to her husband merely an intellectual companion or a sexless helpmeet, when she has been of late the object of his embraces and the mother of his babes. One third of her adult life is still before her, full of promise of placid enjoyment and great usefulness, but to her, remembering the glory of conquest and surrender, the future stretches a dreary waste of empty years [p. 742].

Thus procreative functioning was associated with sexual functioning (for similar views by Freud, see Harris, this volume).

Beard (1888) proposed a new nosological entity "neurasthenia," or nervous exhaustion, which he viewed as due to the negative effects of modern civilization. By invoking such effects, Beard abandoned medical tradition, which had viewed women's reproductive organs as vulnerable to illness from no particular cause or one that had called attention to the deleterious effects of restrictive clothing, higher education, or rich foods. The shift from viewing disease as inherited, or as caused by nature, to finding its cause in deleterious social conditions was consistent with the progressive ideology of the time. It enabled people to change the conditions under which they lived and thus to eradicate the causes of illness. Manifestations of stress and other conditions were included in neurasthenia: sick headache; changes in the expression of the eye; noises in the ears; mental irritability; hopelessness; morbid fears, for example, mysophobia (fear of contamination); siderodromophobia, due to the "perpetual jarring, shaking and noise that completely break up the nervous equilibrium," which was found especially among railway-engine mechanics; anthropophobia (fear of society); gynephobia (fear of women); pantaphobia (fear of everything); also blushing, insomnia, tenderness of the teeth and gums, desire for narcotics, heaviness of the loins and limbs, pain in the feet, convulsive movements, and so on.

Although most of these symptoms could affect both men and women, Beard believed that women's illnesses could be either the causes or effects of neurasthenia, especially for women between the ages of 15 and 16, and again between 45 and 50. Women's nervous symptoms were not to be regarded as the result of uterine disease; rather they were actually the result of exhaustion. Irritability of the ovaries and the uterus was analogous to cerebral or spinal irritation, which does not yield to local treatment. Therefore "general" treatment was recommended.

Beard's rival in the advocacy of "general" rather than local treatment was S. Weir Mitchell, a Philadelphia society physician, who also focused on the plight of women who had developed "neurasthenic" lifestyles. He suggested that women suffered from exhausted nerves caused by unhappy love affairs and loss of social position. Mitchell's rest cure for "hysterical" women—many, no doubt, diagnosed as suffering from menopausal symptoms—required six weeks of isolation, with the patients lying on their backs in dimly lit rooms. Reading or visitors were prohibited; foods, though bland, were offered to induce weight gain. Massages lasted an hour each day. The secret of the rest cure lay not in the bland foods, the massages, or the intellectual and social deprivation, but in the doctor himself. Mitchell was authoritarian, his manner gentle and sympathetic one moment and commanding the next (Ehrenreich and English, 1978). Patients were isolated from their families and other social contacts, and most likely they developed idealizing transferences. Those women who were strong or who had feminist leanings left Mitchell, and his rest cure failed (see Gilman, 1973).

Insanity in menopausal women was associated with social class and its treatment was "general": "In some few cases with great nervous fretting and poor nutrition, a period of rest and seclusion away from home may avert absolute insanity. This treatment, with high feeding, is indicated especially for women who have long been overworked . . ." (p. 741). On the other hand, it was thought that patients who had nothing to do might become psychotic but could be cured by means of useful work, which would renew a woman's zest for life and bring peace to her mind.

Certainly the most influential of all physicians in associating menopause with insanity, or "involutional melancholia," was the German psychiatrist Kraepelin (1909). "Involutional melancholia," like neurasthenia, also combined symptoms and became an "illness." Women at menopause were said to be vulnerable to this first-onset depressive episode. Involutional melancholia constituted one-third of all functional psychoses, the other two being dementia praecox and manic-depressive psychosis. Its onset was gradual during the climacterium; it was marked by hypochondriasis, pessimism, and irritability and led to a full-blown depressive syndrome. Prominent symptoms included agitation, restlessness, anxiety and apprehension, occasionally bizarre delusions or paranoid ideation, insomnia, anorexia, and feelings of guilt and worthlessness. This concept, based on the prevailing notion of a connection between brain and uterus and aided by misogynist attitudes toward older women, was extremely influential and continued well into the 20th century, with entries in both DSM I and II. Since no empirical studies could find a basis for its existence, involutional melancholia was ultimately deleted from DSM III and is no longer used as a diagnostic entity.

WOMEN DOCTORS AND THE NEW PERCEPTION

Toward the end of the 19th century, many female physicians treated women's illnesses as male physicians had done. They used the same textbooks with the same explanations, the same medicines and operations. However, some women physicians were also influenced by alternative approaches and advocated healthful living, with simple food and less constricting clothing. What women physicians added in particular was a new attitude toward women's functioning: they advocated normal conduct during both menstrual periods and menopause. A new, more positive perception of menopause was strongly urged by Eliza W. Farnham, a social reformer who argued for the natural superiority of women. In regard to menopause, Farnham radically disagreed with prevailing medical opinion. Most women, Farnham (1864) stated, experience a secret joy in their advancing age but have been "so overruled by the universal masculine judgment as to see in it only a loss of Power . . . That day is forever past, thank God. . . . We shall soon cease the wailing and lamentation over the first gray hair and the first wrinkle at the eyes" (p. 57). According to her, a woman's life is divided into three periods, each of which is an advance over the last: the first period is the youthful one; the second, the maternal; and the third, "the regenerative, or spiritual, in which the others culminate, and where the ultimate brightest glory of earthly Womanhood alone is seen or enjoyed. Who can dread to reach this?" (p. 57). The third period, which begins with menopause, is characterized by "the opening of wider channels for the overflow of the affectional and spiritual nature . . ." (p. 57) and "the transfer of the finer powers, capacities, and sensibilities . . . from the corporeal to the psychical level" (p. 63). But woman must pay for her new, exalted state with "perturbations of the heart, nerve, and brain, appalling at times, in the darkness wherein she has to grope her lonely way" (p. 63). Farnham seems to have subscribed to the limited-energy model of the body: Once energies are no longer needed for reproductive functioning, they may be converted to the spiritual.

Female physicians, unlike their male colleagues, also held a more reasonable attitude toward the patient and her complaints. The woman physician seemed to be more attuned, empathic, and soothing to her female patient than was the male physician. They did not ascribe a woman's menopausal complaints to her high living and sexual licentiousness, but stated that men had caused many of women's illnesses: "alcoholism of the fathers; gonorrhea contracted by wives from husbands; sterility due to licentiousness in which the innocent woman may have no share; enforced celibacy due to bad social arrangements . . . childbirths too close together" (Jacobi, 1895, p. 482).

Nor did female physicians concentrate only on women's allegedly diseased reproductive system. Rather—and this is the major change from earlier perceptions—women physicians saw women in roles beyond that of reproduction alone. Thus, by the end of the century, another view of menopause had established itself. Several women physicians and one novelist wrote about menopause.

A.M. Longshore-Potts

Longshore-Potts lectured throughout the English-speaking world on medical subjects. Her new ideas about menopause must have been welcomed by her female audience despite her retaining some old myths: ". . . like the fruit-trees in the orchard, she ceases to bear. But her existence is maintained for other purposes; for woman has a variable mission—her sphere of usefulness is not limited to one work, however important that one may be" (1895, p. 97).

This statement carried important social and political implications. Longshore-Potts went even further, asserting that no medical assistance was necessary unless the woman hemorrhaged and that annoying hot flashes could be corrected by attention to the woman's general health. Longshore-Potts viewed women as human beings rather than merely as a housing for the uterus. She sympathetically described the course of a woman's life

> . . . until ten, twelve, or even fifteen children have been born, with an accumulation of troubles to correspond, and at times they have been discouraged, and almost, or quite, insane, and they have felt that there was no justice in God's dispensation if woman was assigned a life of pain, sorrow, and ceaseless toil, and if that was to be the whole of woman's pleasure here on earth. But after these years have passed, and the climax of her womanhood has been reached, when there are no more children to be born, no more teeth to come, no more measles or whooping-cough, and no more babies' deaths to break her heart. Now the numerous sons are grown up to fill useful and important posts, daughters are married, and "Mother" is left alone again to the renewed loved of her husband . . . [p. 101].

No 19th-century male physicians had referred either to a woman's roles other than that of childbearing and childrearing or to the relationship of a middle-aged woman to a loving husband. Longshore-Potts went on:

> Now his love for her may occupy his heart and mind, though at one time business cares had quite suppressed it, and the twenty years to come may be like the harvest-home of their existence, the most quiet and contented time; and now it is they such enjoy themselves. Now they have leisure to read, think, and talk on subjects congenial to their age and development; now is the time for them to lay aside the more worldly cares, and to let the intellect have opportunity to grasp what may be learned in social life, or from public lectures . . . [p. 102].

Thus the time of middle age—of menopause—became one for husband and wife to enjoy each other.

Mary Melendy

A graduate of Hahnemann Medical College in Chicago and a lecturer on diseases of women and children at the American Health University, Melendy reassured women about the change of life. She told them that not all women suffer during their 40s and 50s, and there is no need for apprehension. She reminded them that there is lower mortality among women at this period than among men of the same age and also lower mortality among women during this decade than during any other after the age of puberty; that women who safely pass this period have a better chance of living to a ripe old age than have men. She emphasized the importance of living unimpaired by fashionable dress, by dissipation, or by excesses, and of eating nutritious food. For relief of hot flashes, heartburn, and sleeplessness, she prescribed fasting. Melendy (1903) recommended pure air and moderate exercise to restore the system, and cautioned that "the mind should not continually dwell upon self, but should be diverted with pleasant company, reading, riding, etc. The atmosphere of music also is very beneficial. Elevate the spirit, and the body will grow strong" (p. 177).

A woman could be as healthy at 50 as at 15. Despite her good health, however, indulgence in sexual relations is not recommended. In any case, she believed, most women lose interest in sexual passion.

> The reproductive organs have finished their work . . . Sometimes, however, the opposite is the case, and the passions increase in intensity, and become more violent than at any other time of their lives. . . . This condition . . . should always be looked upon with serious apprehensions, for it is against nature, and may be the indication of some grave disease" [p. 179].

Melendy could, apparently, go so far but no farther.

Clelia Duel Mosher

Most of our knowledge about women physicians' views of the menopause comes to us through their writings and is based on their informal observations and clinical experience. One empirical study, however, has been unearthed, *Study of the Physiology and Hygiene of Marriage with some Consideration of the Birth Rate*, begun in 1892. The survey, found in 1973 in the Stanford University Archives, was published in 1980. Mosher, its author, was a physician and researcher who questioned 45 American women, 70% of whom were born before 1870. Most of the women were in their late 30s, married, and well educated, who responded to questions about their experiences of, and attitudes toward menstruation, sexuality, health, birth control, and the like.

To the question, How was your mother's health affected by the climacteric (change of life)? 16 women responded: Three mothers were described as symptom free; one mother's health had improved, and 12 mothers had suffered from physical and mental symptoms ranging from minor to major. None apparently complained of the well-known hot flashes and perspiration. Reported symptoms were unrelated to the hormonal process of menopause: deafness, rheumatism, bilious colic, the "morbid emotional excitement" that required morphine. One woman reported that her mother's health had been ruined at menopause, it "seemed as if she would lose her mind. Wandered back to her old home nearby in the night bcause she was sleepless" (No. 13). Because most respondents were relatively young, only five could report on their own menopause. Of the five, two were symptom-free, two had physical symptoms, and one wrote a lengthy statement:

> About 1909 . . . my menses began to decline and in the course of a year ceased altogether, without *any nervous disturbance whatever*. During this time I was doing heavy intellectual labor — published a statistical and sociological book in 1906, another in 1908 and another in 1912; gained some weight (from average of 110 to 120) and did my own housework beside lecturing frequently in public. My health has steadily improved during the last seven years and I am [at 53] much stronger and capable of doing both more physical and mental work every day than any woman of my acquaintance and more than most women of forty. I can walk 15 miles without feeling it and lift my own weight. Although my *passionate* feeling has declined somewhat and the orgasm does not always occur, intercourse is still agreeable to me [p. 26].

Since the dates roughly correspond to Mosher's (1980) life and career milestones, this anonymous statement may be her own. Another woman alluded to prevailing attitudes that menopause represents the end of sexuality and her decreasing "passionate feeling." Case No. 21, when asked, What, to you, would be an ideal habit? answered, "Once a month until after the change [menopause], then not at all."

The Mosher Survey describes a variety of reactions to the menopause, ranging from improvement in health, to the absence of symptoms, to mild or severe problems. The responses of these women furnish a contrast to the uniformly severe symptoms described by male physicians.

Marion Harland

Some women writers continued to express the old myths about menopause, albeit in softer versions. Harland, a prolific American novelist and wife of a physician, however, also took cognizance of the difference among women in regard to their experience of menopause. For some women, she wrote, it is a time resembling "Indian Summer,"

while for others it is "the Valley of the Shadow of Death." Harland
(1882) also accurately and vividly described its vasomotor symptoms:
"The blood surges to the head at the slightest provocation, making the
eyes dim, and the ears to ring and roar. . . . swift waves of heat flash
and throb from feet to crown, and one lives for a gasping minute in a
furnace heated seven times hotter than an August noon" (p. 316).

Emma F. Angell Drake

Drake, a physician, addressed middle-aged women to help them
acquire the "correct view concerning the climacteric" (1902, p. xiii).
Menopause, she wrote, is not "a terrible physical Rubicon" (p. 28), as
many physicians would have women believe. She spoke against the
medicalization of menopause: "The well are not noticed, but they
outnumber the former class [the sick] fifty to one" (p. 30). Like
Farnham, Drake suggested that there are three stages of a woman's life
and divided the third period into two parts, the meridian and the
decline. For most women at menopause, some of their very best work
is yet to be done; Drake referred to Queen Victoria, feminists Frances
Willard and Julia Ward Howe, and other productive middle-aged
women. She also listed variables influencing the course of menopause,
such as age, childbirth, heredity, ethnic group, occupation, and
temperament. Menopausal symptoms might occur in some women,
she said, but surely not in all, and, in addition to the usual ones, she
included "a marked exaltation of the faculties and an exuberance of
the imagination" (p. 65).

Thus, by the end of the 19th century, two views of the menopause
seemed to exist. One, held by male physicians and their followers,
stated that menopause was a disease in need of medical treatment; the
other, newer view elaborated by women physicians and feminists,
stated that menopause was not synonymous with disease and that
women could continue to live productively after their reproductive
years were over.

EARLY 20TH CENTURY

Although Gregorio Maranon's book on the climacteric was published
in 1919 in Spain, his sentiments barely differed from those of male

American or English gynecologists at the end of the 19th century. By the time the book was translated into English in 1929, sex hormones had been discovered, and Maranon's speculations, although they were about hormones, were out of date. He considered menopause to be an "endocrine crisis," and he advanced, in his "pluriglandular interpretation," that the ovaries, the thyroid, and the suprarenal are the fundamental glandular elements causing this crisis. The ovary's internal secretions at the beginning of the climacteric cause changes: "The woman grows corpulent . . . the character changes . . . sweet feminine ways are lost. She becomes aggressive. The voice may become rough. A light or heavy tracing of a moustache may appear, with more or less down on the chin and perhaps on the limbs and trunk" (p. 57).

According to Maranon, the climacteric was multiply determined: by the energy of the ovary; by the structure of the genital apparatus; by the manner of sexual activity; by social condition; by weight, color of hair, and temperament; by climate and race; and by state of health, especially lesions of the genital apparatus. Menopause would, he believed, be accelerated by celibacy, frequent pregnancies close together, miscarriage, and exhausting lactations. He saw a correspondence between early menopause and "premature senility," the latter evidenced by tooth decay.

According to Maranon, obese women with genital or thyroid insufficiency entered menopause early. Very dark women, he wrote, are usually hyperthyroid, hyperpituitary and hyperovarian, and passionate. Bizet's Carmen, for example, exerts a "primitive and blind sexual attraction. . . . Bizet added a contralto voice, also with true biologic precision, as it belongs to the hyperpituitary temperament" (p. 109).

Influenced by Freud, Maranon was most interested in the psychology of menopausal women and considered sexuality to have a benevolent influence on their whole being. Thus, the climacteric, which represents the end of a woman's sexual functioning, carried with it, for him, psychic complications (e.g., mania, melancholia, neurasthenia, hysteria, epilepsy, sexual sadness, increase or decrease of sexual feeling, and emotional instability).

Maranon contributed the view that menopausal symptoms, which are due to glandular malfunctioning, also interact with marital difficulties. Using examples from literature, Maranon saw menopause as often preceded by an "impatience over trifles." Symptomatic portraits are painted in drama as well. In Feuillet's comedy, "La Crise", for example, Julia, the heroine, "in the fullness of her sexual life and therefore within the shadow of its close," reflects on her discontent with her husband, "doubtless the best of men. But nothing that he says or does pleases me. His watch charms irritate me above every-thing else. . . . My husband has the insufferable habit of jingling them while he is talking—making an unbearable clinking . . ." (Maranon, 1929, p. 200).

Julia's husband, a dignified magistrate, reports to Julia's physician the changes he has observed in his wife:

> For ten years I have said I possessed a treasure in my wife. Then suddenly sweet Julia takes on the air of a martyr—obedient but irritated. This woman of the world, this refined woman now speaks a language full of sharp, bitter words, harsh and peevish maxims. I find in her conversation . . . a banal melancholy, a sharp poetic flavor, with a socialistic tendency which fills me with uneasiness [p. 201].

The physician interrupts: "The wife of a magistrate! Horrors!" and suggests that the cause of Julia's changed behavior and socialist leanings is her age. Another menopausal woman is equally irritated by her husband: "With what absolute perfection he managed his knife and fork! I could have stood it if he would ever . . . put his elbows on the table, or bite into an apple before peeling it, or make a noise when drinking!" (p. 202).

According to Maranon, late menopause was caused by the abnor-mally conserved internal secretion of the ovary. Such women keep their youthful feeling, their beauty, and premenopausal freshness, together with an "amorous restlessness" (p. 214). That younger men arouse such women suggests that they instinctively seek in another's youth the warmth that their own waning powers require. Some of Maranon's ideas resonate with Helene Deutsch's writings on the menopause (see Harris, this volume).

The Discovery of Sex Hormones

Sex hormones were discovered primarily because men, especially aging men, hoped to find ways of maintaining sexual interest and energy. Although research interest dates back as far as 1849, it was in the 1920s that the active ovarian hormone was identified and bioassay techniques for estrogenic hormones invented. Estrogen was found in the urine of pregnant women, and, in 1930, estrone was isolated. The isolation of estriol and progesterone followed (see Carter, 1983).

The discovery of sex hormones ushered in a new era in which many of the observed phenomena of mammalian reproduction could now be explained. Yet, despite this new knowledge, old ideas continued to thrive. One of the most persistent of these ideas, the link between menopause and depression, remained in the medical literature until recently, and physicians continued to ascribe any complaints of a middle-aged woman to her "change of life."

CONCLUSIONS

Knowledge—along with biased and inaccurate information—about menopause accumulated over the centuries, although the topic of menopause continued to be taboo. The absence of discussion about menopause kept it shrouded in obscurity, while hearsay, speculation, and reasoning by analogy kept misconceptions based on ancient ideas alive.

The cyclicity of women's functioning remained mysterious until the discovery of hormones in the 1920s. Before that time, creative but false analogies led to the wrong conclusions and, sometimes, to problems. One such analogy most likely resulted in unwanted pregnancies: it was thought that estrus, the animal's fertile period, was the equivalent of menstruation. Thus, if animals were fertile only during estrus, then women were believed to be fertile only during menstruation. Sexual intercourse during the middle of a woman's menstrual month was therefore recommended to those couples wishing to *limit* their families.

A new era seemed to dawn when women became physicians and

feminism began to demand societal changes. The idea that a woman's life was not totally determined by the activity of her uterus, that she was not solely the victim of her "diseased" uterus, but that she could have a productive life before *and* after menopause, surely had a major impact on her self-esteem. Fortunately, we have by now abandoned such ideas as the humoral account of menopause, the "plethora;" the competition between brain and womb for blood; the need for strong "emmenogogues" to bring on menstruation in cases of amenorrhea, as well as its confusion with menopause; the conversion of menstrual blood into another body fluid, and, most important of all, that menopause represents a major interference with the health and life of the women, signaling the end of her usefulness.

Some ideas, however, were prematurely abandoned and are now believed to contain some truth, in particular that with menopause a woman loses her protection against some previously latent diseases. Studies have found that the incidence of heart disease or gout, for example, increases post-menopausally. (On the connection between menopause and osteoporosis, see Gannon, this volume.)

A few old and inaccurate ideas about menopause are retained today although only by a minority: for instance, that menopause is a deficiency disease and that all middle-aged women, regardless of symptoms, need hormone replacement therapy; that menopause represents the end of a woman's sexual life; that menopause is a critical period lasting about two or three years, after which no symptoms (for example, hot flushes) will occur; and that emotional instability and depression are associated with menopause.

The 20th century has seen the discovery of hormones, which solved the riddle of both menstruation and menopause. It also saw the synthesis of hormones and their advocacy as hormone replacement therapy (HRT) for the menopausal woman, as well as HRT's falling into disrepute after a link with endometrial cancer was discovered. Today we more cautiously reaccept HRT for some menopausal women despite a continuing lack of knowledge about its long-term effects.

The 20th century also has seen the beginnings of systematic studies of the menopause, a distinction between clinical and epidemiological data and between natural and surgical menopause, and the relationship of menopause to social class and cultural factors, etc. (see Bowles, and Goodman, and Greene, this volume).

The connection between menopause and aging is still confounded, and symptoms are ascribed to the former when they may be due to the latter. Much research on this issue and on others needs to be done. Despite new epidemiologic studies, too little attention is, even now, given to the variety of women's experiences of the menopause (see Notman, this volume). Moreover, very little is known about men's attitudes toward their menopausal spouses (but see Phillips, this volume). Now that taboos have lifted, and both international and national menopause societies have been formed, our knowledge will be more firmly based. Thus, ancient pejorative perceptions of both menopause and of the older woman will be replaced by more rational ones.

REFERENCES

American Practitioner (1826), *The London Practice of Midwifery, including the Treatment during the Puerperal State and the Principal Infantile Diseases*. Concord, NH: Isaac Hill.

Barker-Benfield, G. J. (1976), *The Horrors of the Half-known Life. Male Attitudes Toward Women and Sexuality in Nineteenth-Century America*. New York: Harper & Row.

Beard, G. M. (1888), *A Practical Treatise on Nervous Exhaustion (Neurasthenia)*. New York: E. B. Treat, 1971.

Bilz, F. E. (1898), *The Natural Method of Healing*, Vol. 2. Leipzig: F. E. Bilz.

Buchan, W. (1771), *Domestic Medicine*. Exeter: J. & B. Williams, 1836.

Burns, J. (1820), *Principles of Midwifery, Including the Diseases of Women and Children*. Vol. 1. Philadelphia, PA: Parker, Warner, Carey & Son.

Buxton, C. L. (1968), Preface to *The Story of My Life* by J. Marion Sims. New York: DaCapo Press.

Carpenter, W. B. (1851), *Principles of Human Physiology*, ed. F. G. Smith. Philadelphia, PA: Blanchard & Lea.

Carter, C. S. (1983), *Hormones and Sexual Behavior*. Stroudsburg, PA: Dowden.

Cazeaux, P. (1863), *A Theoretical and Practical Treatise on Midwifery Including the Diseases of Pregnancy and Parturition* (trans. W. R. Bullock). Philadelphia, PA: Lindsay & Blakiston.

Chadwick, M. (1932), The psychological effects of menstruation. *Nervous & Mental Disease Monogr*. No. 56. New York: Nervous & Mental Dis. Pub.

Clarke, E. (1873), *Sex in Education*. Boston: Osgood & Co.

Drake, E. (1902), *What a Woman of Forty-Five Ought to Know*. Philadelphia, PA: Vir.

Drinka, G. F. (1984), *The Birth of Neurosis*. New York: Simon & Schuster.

Ehrenreich, B. & English, D. (1978), *For Her Own Good*. Garden City, NY: Anchor Press/Doubleday.

Farnham, E. (1864), *Woman and Her Era*. New York: Davis.

Formanek, R. (1987a), Learning the lines. In: *Psychoanalysis and Women*, ed. J. Alpert. Hillsdale, NJ: The Analytic Press, pp. 139–157.

———— (1987b), Depression and menopause: A socially constructed link. In: *Women and Depression*, ed. R. Formanek & A. Gurian. New York: Springer.

Freind, J. (1729), *Emmenologia* (trans. T. Dale). London: Cox.

Gilman, C. P. (1973), *The Yellow Wallpaper*. Old Westbury, NY: Feminist Press, 1975.

Haller, J. S., Jr., & Haller, R. M. (1974), *The Physician and Sexuality in Victorian America*. Urbana: University of Illinois Press.

Harland, M. (1882), *Eve's Daughter, or Common Sense for Maid, Wife and Mother*. New York: Anderson & Allen.

Hayes, A. M. (1869), *Sexual Physiology of Woman and Her Diseases*. Boston, MA: Peabody Medical Institute.

Hollick, F. (1853), *The Marriage Guide or Natural History of Generation*. New York: Strong.

Index-Catalogue of the Library of the Surgeon General's Office (1888), U.S. Army, Vol. 9.

Jackson, J. C. (1860, June), Female diseases. *The Laws of Life*, 3(6):81.

———— (1866, March), The constitutional degeneracy of American women. *The Laws of Life*, 9:33.

Jacobi, M. P. (1895), *A Pathfinder in Medicine*, ed. Women's Medical Assn. of New York City. New York: Putnam's Sons, 1925.

Kraepelin, E. (1909), *Psychiatrie*. 8th ed. Leipzig: Barth.

Kuhn, T. S. (1962), *The Structure of Scientific Revolutions*. Chicago: University of Chicago Press.

Leadam, T. R. (1851), *Homoeopathy as Applied to the Diseases of Females and the Most Important Diseases of Early Childhood*. London: Leath.

Longshore-Potts, A. M. (1895), *Discourses to Women on Medical Subjects*. National City, San Diego, CA.

Maranon, G. (1929), *The Climacteric: The Critical Age* (trans. K.S. Stevens). St. Louis, MO: Mosby.

Meigs, C. D. (1854), *Woman: Her Diseases and Remedies*, 3rd ed. Philadelphia, PA: Blanchard & Lea.

Melendy, M. M. (1903), *Perfect Womanhood for Maidens-Wives-Mothers*. K.T. Boland.

Meyer, D. (1965), The positive thinkers. In: *Women and Womanhood in America*, ed. R. W. Hogeland (1973). Boston, MA: D. C. Heath.

Morantz, R. (1974), The lady and her physician. In: *Clio's Consciousness Raised*, ed. M. Hartman & L. W. Banner. New York: Harper & Row.

Mosher, C. D. (1980), *The Mosher Survey, Sexual Attitudes of 45 Victorian Women*, ed. J. MaHood & K. Wenburg. New York: Arno Press.

Napheys, G. H. (1871), *The Physical Life of a Woman: Advice to the Maiden, Wife and Mother*. Philadelphia, PA: Maclean.

_____ (1883), *The Transmission of Life, Counsels on the Nature and Hygiene of the Masculine Function*. Philadelphia, PA: Watts.

Playfair, W. S. (1880), *A Treatise of the Science and Practice of Midwifery*. Philadelphia, PA: Lea.

Reed, C. A. L. (1901), *A Text-book of Gynecology*. New York: Appleton.

Rowland, B. (1981), *Medieval Woman's Guide to Health: The First English Gynecological Handbook*. Kent, OH: Kent State University Press.

Showalter, E. (1985), *The Female Malady*. New York: Pantheon.

Shryock, R. H. (1960), *Medicine and Society in America: 1660-1860*. Ithaca, NY: Cornell University Press.

Siegel, R. (1968), *Galen's System of Physiology and Medicine*. Basel, Switzerland: Karger.

Sims, J. M. (1884), *The Story of My Life*. New York: Da Capo Press, 1968.

Smith-Rosenberg, C. (1974), *Disorderly Conduct*. New York: Oxford University Press, 1985.

Spencer, H. (1896), *System of Synthetic Philosophy*. London: Williams & Norgate.

Stage, S. (1979), *Female Complaints: Lydia Pinkham and the Business of Women's Medicine*. New York: Norton.

Starr, P. (1982), *The Social Transformation of American Medicine*. New York: Basic.

Thomas, L. (1983), *The Youngest Science*. New York: Viking Press.

Tilt, E. J. (1851), *On the Preservation of the Health of Women at the Critical Periods of Life*. New York: Wiley.

_____ (1882), *The Change of Life in Health and Disease*. New York: Bermingham.

Trall, R. T. (1862, Nov.), Women and the medical profession. *The Hygienic Teacher and Water-Cure Journal devoted to Physiology, Hydropathy, and the Laws of Life*, 34:103.

Utian, W. (1987), The fate of the untreated menopause. *Obs. Gyn. Clin. N. Amer.* 14:1-11.

_____ Serr, D. (1976), Report on workshop: The climacteric syndrome. In: *Consensus on Menopause Research*, ed. P. A. van Keep et al. Lancaster, PA: MTP Press.

Woloch, N. (1984), *Women and the American Experience*. New York: Knopf.

Wood, A. D. (1974), The fashionable diseases: Women's complaints and their treatment in nineteenth-century America. In: *Clio's Consciousness Raised*, ed. M. Hartman & L. W. Banner. New York: Harper & Row.

2

Changing Ideas

The Medicalization of Menopause

SUSAN E. BELL

The complicated roots and paradoxical consequences of defining human experiences as medical problems and giving medical personnel the task of treating them have been explored by numerous sociologists (Freidson, 1970; Zola, 1972; Conrad and Schneider, 1980a). Schneider and Conrad argue that the process of medicalization has both a "cultural resonance" and an "organizational form" (p. 3) compatible with the values and structures of modern American society. Thus, to understand particular cases of the expansion of medical jurisdiction, this broader context must be taken into account. At the same time, "concrete detail" is important. In their view, the "proper study" of medicalization "requires careful attention to specific historical events and their participants" (Schneider and Conrad, 1980, p. 8).

According to Conrad and Schneider (1980b), medicalization occurs on three levels: conceptual, institutional, and interactional. On

An earlier version of this paper appeared in *Social Science and Medicine* (1987), 24:535–542. Reprinted by permission of Pergamon Journals Ltd.

Suggestions from Roberta Apfel, Peter Conrad, Sue Fisher, Liliane Floge, Diana Long, Sol Levine, Constance Nathanson, Catherine Kohler Riessman, and Rosemary Taylor helped to strengthen the argument of this paper. Research assistance from Scott Lauzé is gratefully acknowledged. Funded by a grant from the Faculty Research Fund, Bowdoin College.

the conceptual level, medicalization occurs when a medical vocabulary or model is used to define a problem. Often, medical "discoveries" are published in professional journals by a small segment of "elite" members of the profession.[1] On the institutional level, medicalization comes about when professionals legitimate an organization's work, serving as "gatekeepers" or "formal supervisors." On the level of doctor-patient interaction, medicalization occurs when individual physicians define or treat patients' complaints as medical problems.

In Schneider and Conrad's (1980) view, particular cases of medicalization are more likely to come about when they are championed by elite members of the profession. After a "discovery" has been published, its fate depends on, among other things, "who the authors are, their professional status and identities, the prestige of the journal in which the 'discovery' is published, and the scientific 'value' of the evidence and research strategies used, as well as the practical utility of the discovery . . ." (p. 12). From this viewpoint, if work is published in prestigious journals, it has a greater likelihood of being read. If champions of a "discovery" are on the faculty of prestigious medical schools, they can be influential through education; and if they are staff members at research institutes or participants in medical and scientific societies, their views are more likely to be solicited by government policy makers. These people usually are not organized, even though they may appear so to others; more often than not, "their common view is . . . a product of similar scientific perspectives and research procedures" (p. 14). In sum, the views of elite members of the profession are important and influential in the process of medicalization.

The values and organizational structure of American society make the experiences of women especially compatible with medicalization. Riessman (1983) has examined the special vulnerability of women. In a review of five domains (childbirth, reproductive control, menstruation, weight, and mental health), she describes reasons that women's experiences have been medicalized, including the correspondence

---

[1]The term elite is used here as defined in *A Modern Dictionary of Sociology* (Theodorson and Achilles, 1969). It refers to those persons who constitute the highest stratum within a socially identifiable hierarchy, who are recognized as outstanding and considered the leaders in this hierarchy. An elite influences values, attitudes, and behaviors held within the hierarchy and in society generally.

between women's biology and the theoretical model guiding modern medical practice.

This chapter explores the medicalization of menopause on the conceptual level. It traces how and why a medical vocabulary was constructed and used to define menopause as a "deficiency disease" by a small, elite segment of American medical professionals in the 1930s and 1940s. It shows that this conceptual transformation was made possible by a number of interrelated processes that occurred during this period. First, it explores the role of intellectual developments in laboratory science and research medicine. It then looks at how the process of medicalization was influenced by the fit between women's biology and the theoretical model guiding medicine, on one hand, and the persistence of values and structures of sexist society on the other.

The medical approach fashioned in the 1930s and 40s has been remarkably consistent. The view of menopause as a disease has continued virtually unchanged in the medical literature (Kaufert, 1982; Voda, Dinnerstein, and O'Donnell, 1982; Kaufert and McKinlay, 1985). Exploring the genesis of the disease orientation to menopause is requisite to understanding the persistence of this approach today, despite attempts within and outside medicine to challenge it (McCrea, 1983).

Smith-Rosenberg (1973) argues convincingly that in the nineteenth century physicians viewed menopause as a "physiological crisis" that could lead either to tranquility or to disease, depending on a woman's prior behavior and her "predisposition to malignancy." In the twentieth century, menopause itself became defined and treated as a disease.[2] North American social scientists disagree about whether this transformation occurred in the 1930s (Lock, 1982) or the 1960s (Goodman, 1980; McCrea, 1983). A close reading of the medical literature supports the argument that conceptually at least the medicalization of menopause took place in the 1930s and 40s.

The medicalization of menopause is examined here through an

---

[2]To date, studies of menopause in the nineteenth and early twentieth centuries, with the exception of Smith-Rosenberg (1973), examine women as they were depicted in "traditional male historical sources," such as advice books and writings of prominent male physicians, theologians, and educators (Smith-Rosenberg, 1985, p. 25). Women's experiences of menopause—expressed in their unpublished letters and diaries—have yet to be explored.

analysis of papers about menopause published by 37 physicians in medical journals between 1938 and 1941. All of them investigated, in addition, the possibility of using DES, a synthetic estrogen, to treat menopause, which subsequently became the first widely used estrogen replacement therapy. Between 1938, when DES was first synthesized, and 1941, when it was approved for marketing, 178 physicians submitted material to the Food and Drug Administration for its review of the safety of DES. Of these, 141 physicians either were not interested in menopause or did not publish papers about menopause during this period of time. The remaining 37 comprise the physicians whose work is analyzed here. They were neither all the physicians who experimented with DES nor all the physicians who published papers about menopause. The 37 physicians were all those who both experimented with DES and published papers about menopause between 1938 and 1941.[3]

Judging from their professional status and identities, it is clear that the 37 physicians were members of the medical elite and that therefore their perspectives about menopause were more likely to gain acceptance. In her study of specialization in medicine, Stevens (1971) has shown that there was stratification within the medical profession at this time. According to data in the 16th edition of the *American Medical Directory* (1940), thirty of the physicians whose work is examined here (81.1%) were full-time specialists, compared with less than a quarter (23.5%) of all physicians in the U.S. in 1940.[4] Twenty-

---

[3]Of the 178 physicians, 39 completed questionnaires in the capacity of "experts" about the safety of DES in humans; 124 contributed clinical reports as "supplemental" material; 15 supplied both types of data to the FDA. A list of the 37 physicians analyzed here is available from the author. See Bell (1986).

[4]See Stevens, 1971, p. 181. A variety of specialists were involved in this process. Of the 37 whose writings are included in this essay, 24 (64.9%) were gynecologists and 8 (21.6%) were specialists in internal medicine (2 of the 32 were not full-time specialists). Five of the physicians (13.5%) did not list specialties in this edition of the *American Medical Directory*. Of these five physicians, two were enrolled in residency programs and one had, in addition to an M.D., a Ph. D. in physiology.

From their published writings, it is not clear whether and to what extent there were varying political and theoretical interests along subdisciplinary lines regarding DES among the 37. Of the four specialists who were opposed to the release of DES for sale, three (Samuel H. Geist, Raphael Kurzrok, and Udall J. Salmon) were obstetrician/gynecologists, and the fourth (Ephraim Shorr) was a specialist in internal medicine.

five of the full-time specialists (83.3%) were board certified, compared with 40% of all full-time specialists in the U.S. at that time (estimated by Stevens, 1971, p. 218). In comparison with others, the physicians in this group fell within the highest stratum in medicine.

Additionally, these physicians were influential in education and policymaking; all of them published papers about menopause in medical journals. Seventeen (45.9%) had teaching appointments at medical schools. Moreover, officials at the Food and Drug Administration had designated thirty of them as "experts" and requested that they complete questionnaires giving clinical evidence of the safety of DES. Their answers (along with the answers of some other physicians exploring the use of DES beyond menopause) formed the basis of the government's decision about the safety of DES (Bell, 1986).

MEDICAL PERSPECTIVES AND AMBIVALENCE ABOUT SCIENCE

Medical specialists interested in menopause had ambivalent views about science, which are revealed in their professional publications and which were influential in the transformation in their thinking about menopause. They believed that with the help of science, they could understand the hormonal causes of aging and thereby make their treatment of aging women more systematic and successful. Yet, at the same time, they questioned whether science could adequately explain the problems of individual patients (Pratt, 1939). Research scientists were able to provide medicine with theories, tools, and methods; medicine was able to accept them in a somewhat limited way. As it had earlier in the century, "[t]he superimposing of science onto medicine added not brute force, but new complexities, new strains and new possibilities" (Maulitz, 1979, p. 104).

The medicalization of menopause on the level of conceptualization depended on the "discovery" of a theory of etiology. This was made possible by the paradigm of sex endocrinology. In the 1930s, biochemically trained researchers were able to lay "the foundations of an analytical base for a reliable science of endocrinology" (Hall and Glick, 1976, p. 230). Research scientists in the field of sex endocrinology were able to explain and reproduce the mechanisms of "almost all of the female sexual functions" in animals, on the basis of "experimental evidence" that included "quantitative aspects of hormone balance" (Allen, Danforth, and Doisy, 1939, pp. 452–53). They developed theories about the role of hormones in sex differentiation, reproduction, and sexuality, as well as tools for research consisting of pure hormone extracts and synthetic substitutes (including DES) (Pratt, 1939). They discovered and explained the "form, function and behavior of the sexes" in a "dispassionately empirical way," releasing women from responsibility for behavior by attributing its cause to biological processes (Hall, 1977, p. 18). They also introduced standard methods for research, including the use of controls, correlation of data obtained by different observers, and collection and quantification of large numbers of observations (Pratt, 1939). Their work raised the possibility of treating hormonal deficiencies in women with hormone replacement therapy, basing treatment on a standardized measurement of hormones.

Treatment with estrogen replacement therapy depended on more than a scientific theory. A prerequisite was the availability of substances that could be used in clinical research and clinical practice. Prior to the synthesis of DES in 1938, medical research was hampered by the scarcity of pure estrogenic substances. DES heralded an advance because unlike natural estrogens and previously synthesized hormone substitutes, it could be easily purified. The specialists imagined that DES would enable them to standardize and systematize their estrogen research on women (Shorr, 1940; Sevringhaus, 1941). Further, until DES was synthesized, estrogen therapy was extremely expensive, since the natural estrogens were difficult to extract, purify, and stabilize and were most potent when injected (Dodds, 1941). DES was easy to produce and to purify, and it was effective orally; so it was readily prescribed. If the initial laboratory findings were corroborated, clinical research would no longer be impeded by the scarcity of pure compounds, and estrogen therapy would no longer be limited to a few financially advantaged patients.[5] Medical specialists incorporated science into their research and practice because, despite their ambivalence, they believed that the theories and tools provided by sex endocrinologists could help to improve medical practice. First, if theory preceded the "application of endocrines to medical practice,"

---

[5]For a discussion of the development of DES, see Bell (1986).

they believed gynecology would become more scientific and physicians would make fewer mistakes (Douglas, 1940). Second, the specialists thought that pure extracts such as DES would allow them to standardize therapeutics, making their work more systematic and less subject to individual variation and inadvertent overdosage. The use of worthless "cures" could be replaced by effective endocrine extracts and synthetic substitutes (Hall, 1975). Finally, use of the scientific method would enable physicians to judge therapeutic success on the basis of "objective" tests instead of on the ambiguous "subjective" impressions of individual doctors and patients (Pratt, 1939). For example, laboratory tests, such as the vaginal smear, aided diagnosis and treatment by allowing a physician to determine if a woman's symptoms were caused by estrogen deficiency and to determine the effectiveness of estrogen therapy (Shorr, 1940). In sum, medical specialists believed that science would help gynecology become safer (Shorr, 1940; Sevringhaus, 1941).

The impact of the introduction of the tools and methods of science on the power of medicine was uncertain, but it could potentially increase medicine's "cultural authority" (Starr, 1982). The use of "detached technologies," such as microscopes and chemical and bacteriological tests, produced data "seemingly independent of the physician's as well as the patient's subjective judgment." Use of these technologies also made it possible to "remove part of the diagnostic process from the presence of the patient into 'backstage' areas where several physicians might have simultaneous access to the evidence" (Starr, 1982, p. 137). These sorts of technologies strengthened gynecology's claim to "objective judgment."

Medical specialists, however, were ambivalent about how thoroughly to incorporate sex endocrinology into their work. One reason for their ambivalence was their concern for safety. Although medical specialists could use the work of sex endocrinologists in their clinical research and clinical practice, they raised questions about how and under what circumstances to do so. They warned of the dangers of too much "clinical aloofness" (Novak, 1939, p. 428) and the questionable value of "mass statistics" (Pratt, 1938, p. 566) in the practice of medicine. Medical specialists questioned whether the theories and methods of science could adequately explain the signs and symptoms of individual patients. An eminent gynecologist at Johns Hopkins, Emil Novak (1939), displayed the ambivalence of medical specialists toward science when he wrote:

> It has seemed to me that clinicians are developing a sort of
> inferiority complex in the study of endocrine problems, so awed
> are they by the brilliant contributions which have been coming
> from the laboratory, and so dependent have they become upon
> the laboratory workers for the ammunition which they so sorely
> need in their own clinical world. . . . And yet there are certain
> advantages which the clinician enjoys over the laboratory
> worker [p. 423].

Although objectivity was important, they thought it should be tempered by the ability to see patients as individuals and to watch their individual responses closely. Good medicine depended on clinical judgment in conjunction with science.

Specialists' ambivalent views of science surfaced in their review of the safety of DES. Within two years after its synthesis, there was "practically unanimous agreement" about the efficacy of DES (Novak, 1940, p. 594). However, there was serious disagreement about its toxicity. Reports of the incidence of toxic reactions (including nausea, vomiting, and skin rashes) ranged widely from 5% to 80% (Council on Pharmacy and Chemistry, 1939). The debate about safety focused on a number of problems, including the use of the vaginal smear as a method for evaluating DES.[6] This controversy reflected specialists' differences of opinion about objective versus subjective measures in clinical medicine (Shorr, Robinson, and Papanicolaou, 1939; MacBryde, Freeman, and Loeffel, 1941). By 1941 the majority of specialists investigating DES deemed it safe on the basis of clinical observations; a minority determined that it was unsafe, on the basis of evidence from the vaginal smear (Bell, 1984). The safety of DES, according to the majority, could be ensured only if it was used for a limited number of conditions and by prescription only.[7]

A second reason for specialists' ambivalence about science was political. Paradoxically, the introduction of science could lead to the

---

[6] These problems included two serious side effects: long-term liver damage and cancer (Bell, 1986).

[7] Warnings by a minority of specialists proved prescient. In 1971, an association between the use of DES during pregnancy and cancer in young women exposed prenatally was reported (Herbst, Ulfelder, and Poskanzer, 1971). For more on this effect see Apfel and Fisher (1984).

diminishment of medicine's cultural authority, by diverting research funds from the clinic to the laboratory (Maulitz, 1979), increasing dependence on "capital equipment and formal organizations" (Starr, 1982, p. 30), and creating dependence on the laboratory for clinical diagnosis and treatment.[8] Medicine's insistence on clinical judgment served to protect its authority.

Medical specialists' attempts, then, to superimpose science onto medicine were cautious and complex. The advances in sex endocrinology offered them the possibility of systematizing, standardizing, and improving their work, which they welcomed. In this respect, science enhanced their cultural authority. Yet they resisted science, worrying that incorporating it into medicine would lead to too much distance between doctor and patient, perhaps even to the point where diagnosis would be made in the laboratory instead of the clinic (Maulitz, 1979). Reliance on the laboratory for diagnosis could lead to unsafe medical practice. It could also reduce medicine's power. They believed that clinical judgment was an essential and valuable tradition in medicine. Their adherence to clinical judgment also protected their cultural authority (Starr, 1982).

MEDICAL PERSPECTIVES ON MENOPAUSE

Specialists' ambivalence about science — their adoption of the scientific paradigm alongside their uncertainty about its role in medicine — had major consequences. It influenced their discussions about the types of changes occurring during menopause, recommendations for treatment, and the new definition of menopause as a disease. Specialists' views about women also shaped these discussions.

The paradigm of sex endocrinology allowed specialists to see the biological causes of menopause more exactly than before: to see that it was a normal phase of the female life cycle. For most women (85% was

---

[8]At different historical periods, organized medicine has both welcomed and felt threatened by the introduction of science. For example, the infusion of bacteriology in the early twentieth century, which historian Russell Maulitz (1979, p. 93) deems "pivotal in the history of scientific medicine," was greeted by clinicians with "creative ambivalence."

the figure most often cited) menopause was "physiologic," not "pathologic" (Pratt, 1939, pp. 1286–1287). However, clinical studies of menopause consisted almost exclusively of patients: women seeking medical
help for their menopausal symptoms (Pratt, 1939). Thus, specialists'
conclusions about menopause were drawn from a biased sample
(McKinlay and McKinlay, 1973; Goodman, 1980). Even though the
specialists argued that most women negotiated menopause successfully, these women were not included in their studies.

The paradigm of sex endocrinology also enabled them to distinguish
biological changes from psychological and environmental ones. Paradoxically, however, the paradigm contained the possibility for reducing
their medical work to measuring hormones and treating hormonal
deficiencies to the exclusion of social, psychological, and environmental factors in individual women's experiences. The new science tended
to narrow their vision at the same time that it focused it more clearly.

Sex endocrinology also provided them with a cheap estrogen
replacement therapy, DES. Medical specialists debated which scientific methods to use in their evaluation of DES, as well as the relative
merits of clinical judgment and science in determining the safety and
efficacy of the new hormone substitute. They worried about how to
prevent such problems as overdosage or inappropriate use. Although
they wrote that most menopausal women were normal, DES offered
them the possibility of treating all menopausal women. While they
were beginning to define menopause as a deficiency disease they were
introducing a new cure for it. Their ambivalent and complicated views
of science and menopause surfaced in their discussions and their use of
DES (Bell, 1984, 1986).

BIOLOGICAL MODEL OF MENOPAUSE

Medical specialists developed three models for understanding the
causes (and cures) of menopausal complaints: biological, psychological, and environmental.[9] Most commonly, they studied biological

---

[9]Typologies described by Koeske (1982) and Perlmutter and Bart (1982) in their
analyses of attitudes toward menopause today helped me to see these three themes in
medical specialists' work in the 1930s and 1940s.

changes and described menopause as a physiological process caused by the cessation of ovarian function. Although many physiological changes take place at this time in a woman's life (involving the endocrine, reproductive, nervous, circulatory, metabolic, digestive, and cutaneous systems), they believed that loss of ovarian function was "the most important single event" during this period (Shorr, 1940, p. 453).

Discoveries by sex endocrinologists in the laboratory helped specialists to identify the role of lowered estrogen levels in menopause, yet the only group of symptoms they agreed were caused by this decrease were vasomotor—hot flushes and sweats (Novak, 1940, p. 590). Individual experiences varied widely, and, apart from these two signs, the myriad signs and symptoms associated with menopause presented a confusing and variable puzzle that even the new objective tests could not solve. So many other conditions were associated with menopause (but not necessarily to loss of ovarian function) that J.P. Pratt (1938), Chief of Gynecology and Obstetrics at the prestigious Henry Ford Hospital in Detroit, commented that the list of symptoms commonly attributed to menopause "would not be complete unless nearly all the index in a textbook of medicine were included" (p. 564).

The loss of estrogen could lead to many other effects, according to these physicians. Estrogen deficiency could cause hot flushes and sweats that awakened "the patient at night and [caused] her to catch cold." Other symptoms could "produce a feeling of insecurity, in extreme cases inducing the patient to stay at home and lead a hermit existence" (Frank, 1941, p. 856).

If a specialist believed that menopausal symptoms were caused by a lack of estrogen, estrogen replacement therapy was the logical solution; it would supply "the patient with the hormone she [lacked]" (Salmon, Geist, and Walter, 1941, p. 1843). Therapy would let "her down more gently and gradually" and remove "temporarily the immediate cause of the symptoms" (Novak, 1940, p. 591.) Estrogen therapy, according to this view, replaced a biological deficiency (Geist and Salmon, 1939; Salmon, Geist, and Walter, 1941; Frank, 1941). In a lecture to the New York Academy of Medicine, Robert T. Frank, Clinical Professor of Gynecology at the College of Physicians and Surgeons (Columbia), compared the treatment of menopause to the treatment of two deficiency diseases. In his view, "the estrogenic relief of the menopause" was "a major triumph, second only to the treatment of hypothyroidism by thyroid medication and of diabetes by insulin" (Frank, 1941, p. 863). In other words, menopause, like hypothyroidism and diabetes, was a deficiency disease and therefore it, too, could be treated with a replacement therapy.

The focus on biological changes acknowledged and explained the presence of menopausal symptoms in all women and the particularly uncomfortable experiences of some. It then provided a simple solution for relieving a woman's symptoms. Estrogen replacement therapy smoothed the "stormy period" (Shorr, 1940, p. 455) of menopause directly (by reducing symptoms) and indirectly (by reducing symptoms that interfered with a woman's lifestyle). Yet, when used as the sole explanatory model of menopausal symptoms, it risked reducing the problems faced by aging women to biologically determined ones and reinforcing the traditional view of women as biologically different and inferior.[10] Further, the biological model located the problem and the solution in the individual. Simultaneously, the biological model showed that individual women could not control their symptoms and located the problem and solution within their individual bodies. Treating them hormonally would give women relief from symptoms and restore them to their customary social lives. Simply put, the biological model individualized women's experiences.[11]

---

[10]Belief that women's reproductive systems direct their behavior can be traced to ancient times, where it can be seen in the writings of Plato (Fausto-Sterling, 1986). The Victorians, according to Smith-Rosenberg (1985) "asserted gender complimentarity and male dominance as 'eternal verities' rooted in human biology" (p. 186), using religious metaphors and the language of romanticism. Regarding menopause, opinions "have always had a moralizing quality, whereby women have been seen as inferior due to their hormonal changes" (Perlmutter and Bart, 1982, p. 188). Far from obviating the situation of menopausal women, the biological model lent scientific credibility to earlier philosophical or religious theories of female inferiority.

[11]Whether or not experiences are considered individual and private beforehand, the process of medicalization precludes their identification as anything else. As Zola (1972, p. 500) points out, by "locating the source and the treatment of problems in an individual, other levels of intervention are effectively closed." Medicalization puts problems where only medical personnel can discuss them; "the language of medical experts increases mystification and decreases the accessibility of public debate" (Conrad and Schneider, 1980a, p. 249).

PSYCHOLOGICAL MODEL OF MENOPAUSE

Specialists also recognized that psychic and emotional disturbances formed an "important part of the menopausal syndrome" (Pratt, 1938, p. 57). According to Frank (1941), the symptoms of menopause would be "most stormy in nervous, neurotic and unbalanced women and less marked in the well-poised and stable individual" (p. 856). In other words, instead of estrogen withdrawal, a woman's personality pattern could be the underlying cause of symptoms. If this was the case, the specialists argued, psychotherapy, not estrogen therapy, was warranted. As a specialist at Boston's prestigious Lahey Clinic wrote, physicians could not "expect to change the personality of a nervous, complaining individual whose complaints preceded the menopause" (Allan, 1938, p. 834).

The focus on psychological symptoms continued a tradition of attributing the cause of women's experiences during menopause to their previous behavior (Smith-Rosenberg, 1973) but used new psychiatric concepts and terminology to do so. When used as the only explanation for women's menopausal symptoms, this model blamed women and placed responsibility for alleviating symptoms on them: if women got rid of their neuroses, their menopausal symptoms would disappear. This model could lead physicians to overlook the biological nature of menopausal symptoms and to treat women improperly with psychotherapy alone. However, this model potentially offered a corrective to the narrow biological one by suggesting that gynecologists should look beyond ovarian function in understanding menopause. Like the biological model, however, it located the problem and solution within the individual.

ENVIRONMENTAL MODEL OF MENOPAUSE

Infrequently, specialists identified the etiological role of environmental factors in producing menopausal symptoms. Novak (1940) warned against "the easy assumption of menopausal etiology of symptoms in women of the fifth decade." He argued that often these symptoms were "explainable more rationally as the result of the stress and strain resulting from the rearing of large families of children, or because of domestic, economic, or marital problems. . . ." For these women, he recommended "reassurance . . . as well as of correcting so far as possible any detrimental environmental factors which may exist" (p. 589). Greenhill (1940), pointed out that menopause was a time of transition out of the childbearing and childrearing roles into another, which many women dreaded. He wrote that "a large proportion of women are of the opinion that at the change of life their libido will be at an end, that they will be unattractive and perhaps repulsive to their husbands, that they will grow fat and flabby. . . ." (p. 535). He recommended that physicians should disabuse women of these fears, and advise them that the period lying ahead would allow them to pursue new interests, and remind them of the "importance of a proper mode of living, including sufficient rest, sleep, some exercise, fresh air, reading of good books and other activities to occupy [their] time" (p. 535).

The environmental model widened the vision of medicine to include more than a woman's personality and physiology in diagnosing and treating menopausal symptoms. It acknowledged the social and cultural aspects of the passage into menopause for women in American society and the attendant stresses and strains of their new status. Women's complaints, according to this model, were the manifestations of changing circumstances in their social lives, not the result of estrogen deficiency. Women were responding to real events, not imagined ones. Even here, however, specialists recommended changing individual habits (reading, sleeping, and exercising) instead of the environment of women's lives more generally. While the etiology might be identified as external, in contrast to the biological and psychological models that targeted internal sources of the symptoms, the solution was nevertheless identified as internal.

To summarize, the medicalization of menopause at the conceptual level depended on a number of interrelated processes. A theoretical framework and methodology for understanding the role of estrogen in menopause became available in the 1930s. In addition, a new technology—DES—was produced in 1938 and could be used to test the theories of menopausal etiology. Together, these developments enabled medical specialists to discern the role of biology, psychology, and environment in women's experience, to construct three models of menopausal changes, and to control treatment.

With the help of science, and despite their ambivalence toward it, medical specialists transformed the definition of menopause and simultaneously preserved and enhanced their cultural authority. They transformed the meaning of menopause and defined it as a medical problem with a medical solution; they labeled it a "deficiency disease." The implications of this transformation of menopause did not go unnoticed or unchallenged in the medical community. An obstetrician/gynecologist at Duke registered a warning in his textbook of endocrine gynecology: "There seems to be an increasing tendency to consider this physiological period of sexual regression as a disease. If this be so, then we must accept, perhaps, the statement . . . that 'not senescence, but life has become a disease' " (Hamblen, 1939, p. 177).[12] To label menopause as a deficiency disease had even graver consequences for women, as Kaufert and McKinlay (1985) observed: "once menopause was defined as a deficiency condition, its treatment with estrogen was not only legitimate, but became an obligation" (p. 129). Although it is beyond the scope of this chapter, it is important to note that menopause became medicalized on all three levels – conceptual, institutional and interactional – in the 1960s, and by 1975 estrogens were the fifth most frequently prescribed drugs in the United States (MacPherson, 1981; McCrea, 1983). There were physical as well as social effects for women of medicalizing menopause. In the 1970s, ERT was linked to an increased incidence of endometrial cancer in postmenopausal women. Kaufert and McKinlay (1985) have superbly explored the medical controversy over the link between estrogen replacement therapy and cancer since that time.

The medicalization of menopause also strengthened the cultural authority of medicine. The specialists' underlying message was that all menopausal women should seek medical help. Physicians could then distinguish the "cause" of their symptoms and prescribe estrogen replacement therapy, psychotherapy, or talking and reassurance. Diagnosis and treatment would be based on the theories, methods, and tools of sex endocrinology, substantiating the claim of the specialists as scientists. Simultaneously, they would use clinical judgment in each case, strengthening the role of the physician in this process instead of weakening it by becoming entirely dependent on laborato-

---

[12]Hamblen was not one of those investigating DES.

ries and objective tests. Furthermore, women could obtain DES only if a physician prescribed it. DES was not sold over the counter. The decision to market DES under restricted conditions had emerged in the course of the specialists' negotiations with the Food and Drug Administration over the safety of DES. The specialists hoped to make estrogen therapy safer by restricting the use of DES and by limiting its distribution. This decision also had the effect of protecting the interests of medicine by giving it control over the distribution of DES (Bell, 1986).

MEDICAL PERSPECTIVES ON WOMEN

Ironically, the disease orientation to menopause was introduced by medical specialists who intended to reassure women that most often menopause was a normal physiological event. Their success in demonstrating the biological basis of this event had social, and especially sexist, implications. Unwittingly, the specialists had promoted a new view of menopause as pathological and abnormal, and consequently reinforced the stereotypical picture of women already in existence.

The medicalization of menopause reflected and reinforced traditional views about the role of hormones in women's behavior.[13] For example, two gynecologists at the Lying-In Hospital at the University of Chicago shared the view that for the "majority" of women menopause was normal, but they wrote that ". . . the cessation of ovarian function brings in its wake a bizarre train of symptoms which may completely upset the normal equilibrium of even the well-balanced individual" (Davis and Boynton, 1941, p. 341). These symptoms included many associated with menopause, but not necessarily with loss of ovarian function: languor, headaches, vertigo, weight changes, impairment of memory, emotional instability, depression, extreme irritability, apprehension, delirium, suicidal tendency, insomnia, digestive disturbances, neuralgia, trend toward masculinity, melancholia, agitation, and others (Pratt, 1939; Frank, 1941).

Cultural norms about the "proper" role of aging women were also reflected in and reinforced by the medicalization of menopause (Smith-

---

[13]See Kaufert (1982) on this point.

Rosenberg, 1973; Bart and Grossman, 1978). Specialists' prescriptions for their menopausal patients, such as reading good books, getting sufficient rest, and engaging in social and helpful activities, encouraged menopausal women to behave in socially appropriate ways (Pratt, 1938; Greenhill, 1940). Specialists' image of women was also narrow and class specific (Kaufert, 1982). Although they acknowledged poverty in their repeated references to the economic barriers posed by the high cost of estrogen therapy, their prescriptions for women were based on the belief that menopausal women had economic resources and leisure time. Their descriptions of women also assumed that all women lived in traditional nuclear families. Menopausal women, according to them, were married and had stayed at home raising children who had since left home (Novak, 1940; Greenhill, 1940). These were the women who could follow their advice to rest, relax, and do good works.

The medicalization of menopause at the conceptual level, like the medicalization of other women's experiences, had mixed effects for women (Riessman, 1983). On one hand, women's complaints of hot flushes, sweats, and other symptoms were legitimated, explained, and in some cases relieved, by medicine on the basis of scientific evidence, instead of dismissed as figments of their imagination.[14] On the other hand, medicalization reinforced traditional stereotypes of aging women and categorized their symptoms as evidence of individual deficiencies. Medicalizing menopause had the effect of extending medicine's control over women's experiences, individualizing and privatizing their experiences and strengthening cultural norms about the "proper" behavior of aging women.[15]

Menopausal women's experiences were particularly vulnerable to medicalization in a number of ways. First, women's biology fit with the theoretical model (the paradigm of sex endocrinology) of specialist medicine. Compatibility between medical theory and women's biology is one of the reasons Riessman (1983) gives for women's special vulnerability. The cessation of ovarian function could be identified

---

[14]This term is borrowed from Posner (1979), who shows how the contemporary medical orientations to menopause *also* dismiss women's experiences as largely figments of their imagination.

[15]See Kaufert (1982) and the readings in Voda et al. (1982) on this point.

and controlled in the bodies of women using the techniques and tools favored by medical specialists in the 1930s. DES pills could be taken daily. They had an effect that both women and their doctors could "see." Women felt better, and physicians could discern changes not only clinically but also using laboratory tests.

Second, the paradigm of sex endocrinology enabled specialists to distinguish biological problems from psychological and environmental ones. This gave increased scientific respectability to the role of physician as counselor and advisor to women. Women's fears about their changing status received acknowledgment from their doctors. At the same time, women were told what kinds of behavior would be appropriate for them.

In this role, male physicians reflected and reinforced their dominant social status at the same time as they reflected and reinforced the subordination of women—giving expert advice about how to grow old gracefully. Women's structural subordination to men, and its replication in interactions between male physicians and female patients, is another reason for women's special vulnerability to medicalization (Riessman, 1983).

DISCUSSION

A small segment of elite specialists transformed the meaning of menopause, defining it as a medical problem and labeling it as a deficiency disease. The specialists' implicit message was that all menopausal women should see physicians, who could prescribe the appropriate therapy. In recommending that even talking to a physician could be therapeutic and that all women should seek medical advice, specialists were defining menopause as a medical problem—not just for some women, but for all women. With the help of science, medical specialists discovered and came to appreciate the complex social, psychological, and biological roots of menopausal symptoms. Still, they argued that clinical judgment was a critical tool for untangling these roots in individual patients. Science could distinguish physiological causes from others, but only medicine could monitor the effects of hormone therapy in individuals and counsel fearful patients.

The specialists' emphasis on both "objective" science and "subjective" clinical judgment served a number of purposes. It enabled them to increase standards of medical care by incorporating new theories, methods, and tools. Simultaneously, it preserved the role of medicine in diagnosis and treatment instead of relying solely on the laboratory. This increased the cultural authority of medicine in the definition of menopause and the meaning of women's experiences.

On the conceptual level, then, menopause was medicalized in the 1930s and 1940s. This was made possible and shaped by developments in laboratory science and research medicine, as well as by the persistence of sexist values about menopausal women. By attending to concrete historical details, this chapter has demonstrated how one aspect of women's experience became the focus of the medical gaze and why a new orientation could be forged, as well as why it took the direction it did.

REFERENCES

Allan F. N. (1938), The treatment of artificial menopause. *Surg. No. Am.*, 18:831–840.

Allen E., Danforth C.H. & Doisy E., eds., (1939), *Sex and Internal Secretions*, 2nd ed. Baltimore, MD: Williams & Wilkins.

American Medical Association (1940), *American Medical Directory*. Chicago, IL: American Medical Association.

Apfel, R. J. & Fisher, S. M. (1984), *To Do No Harm*. New Haven, CT: Yale University Press.

Bart P. B. & Grossman M. (1978), Menopause. In: *The Woman Patient*, ed. M. T. Notman & C. C. Nadelson. New York: Plenum Press, pp. 337–354.

Bell S. E. (1984), Medical perspectives on gender and science: The case of DES. Presented at the Sixth Berkshire Conference, Smith College, Northampton, MA, June 2.

_____ (1986), A new model of medical technology development: A case study of DES. In: *Research in the Sociology of Health Care*, ed. J. Roth & S. Ruzek. Greenwich, CT: JAI, pp. 1–32.

Conrad P. & Schneider J. W. (1980a), *Deviance and Medicalization*. St. Louis, MO: Mosby.

_____ (1980b) Looking at levels of medicalization: A comment on Strong's critique of the thesis of medical imperalism. *Soc. Sci. Med.*, 14A:75–79.

Council on Pharmacy and Chemistry (1939), Stilbestrol: Preliminary report of the Council. *J. Amer. Med. Assn.*, 113:2312.

Davis M. E. & Boynton M. W. (1941), Indications, clinical use and toxicity of 4'4' Dihydroxy-diethyl Stilbene. *J. Clin. Endocrinol.*, 1:339–345.

Dodds, E. C. (1941), The new oestrogens. *Edinburgh Med. J.*, 48:1–13.

Douglas G. F. (1940) Endocrine considerations of a few gynecological conditions. *J. Internat. Coll. Surg.*, 3:543–547.

Fausto-Sterling, A. (1986), *Myths of Gender*. New York: Basic Books.

Frank R. T. (1941), Treatment of disorders of the menopause. *Bull. NY. Acad. Med*, 17:854–863.

Freidson E. (1970), *Profession of Medicine*. New York: Dodd, Mead.

Geist S. H. & Salmon V. J. (1939), Indications for estrogen therapy. *NY State J. Med.*, 39:1759–1767.

Goodman M. (1980), Toward a biology of menopause. *Signs*, 5:739–753.

Greenhill, J. P. (1940), Gynecology. In: *Year Book of Obstetrics and Gynecology*, ed. J. DeLee & J. P. Greenhill. Chicago, IL: Year Book Publishers.

Hall D. L. (1975), Sex and the good endocrinologist. Presented at the Boston Colloquium in the Philosophy of Science, Boston, MA.

_____ (1977), The social implications of the scientific study of sex. Presented at the symposium on Scholar and the Feminist IV: Connecting Theory, Practice, and Values. New York, Barnard College, April 23, pp. 11–20.

_____ & Glick T. F. (1976), Endocrinology: A brief introduction, *J. Hist. Biol.*, 9:229–233.

Hamblen E. C. (1939), *Endocrine Gynecology*. Springfield, IL: Charles C. Thomas.

Herbst, A. L., Ulfelder, H. & Poskanzer, D. C. (1971), Association of maternal stilbestrol therapy with tumor appearance in young women. *New Eng. J. Med.*, 284:871–881.

Kaufert P. A. (1982), Myth and the menopause. *Soc. Hlth. Illness*, 4:141–166.

_____ McKinlay S. M. (1985), Estrogen replacement therapy: The production of medical knowledge and the emergence of policy. In: *Women, Health, and Healing*, ed. E. Lewin & V. Olesen. New York: Tavistock, pp. 113–138.

Koeske R. (1982), Toward a biosocial paradigm for menopausal research: Lessons and contributions from the behavioral sciences. In: *Changing Perspectives on Menopause*, ed. A. M. Voda, M. Dinnerstein & S. R. O'Donnell. Austin: University of Texas Press, pp. 3–23.

Lock M. (1982), Models and practice in medicine: Menopause as syndrome or life transition? *Cult. Med. Psychiat.*, 6:261–280.

MacBryde C. M., Freeman H. & Loeffel E. (1941), The synthetic estrogen diethyl-stilbestrol: Clinical and experimental studies (II). *J. Amer. Med. Assn.*, 117:1240–1242.

MacPherson K. I. (1981), Menopause as disease: The social construction of a meta-phor. *Adv. Nurs. Sci.*, 3:95–113.

Maulitz R. C. (1979), "Physician versus bacteriologist": The ideology of science in clinical medicine. In: *The Therapeutic Revolution*, ed. M. J. Vogel & C. E. Rosenberg. Philadelphia: University of Pennsylvania Press, pp. 91–107.

McCrea F. B. (1983), The politics of menopause: The "discovery" of a deficiency disease. *Soc. Problems*, 31:111–123.

McKinlay S. M. & McKinlay J. B. (1973), Selected studies of the menopause. *J. Biolsoc. Sci.*, 5:533–555.

Novak E. (1939), Clinical employment of the female sex hormones. *Endocrinol.*, 25:423–428.

——— (1940), The management of the menopause. *Amer. J. Obstet. Gynecol.*, 40:589–595.

Perlmutter E. & Bart P. B. (1982), Changing views of the change: A critical review and suggestions for an attributional approach. In: *Changing Perspectives on Menopause*, ed. A. M. Voda, M. Dinnerstein & S. R. O'Donnell. Austin: University of Texas Press, pp. 189–199.

Posner, J. (1979), It's all in your head: Feminist and medical models of menopause (strange bedfellows). *Sex Roles*, 5:179–189.

Pratt J. P. (1938), Treatment of the menopause. *South. Med. J.*, 31:562–567.

——— (1939), Sex functions in man. In: *Sex and Internal Secretions*, ed. E. Allen, C. H. Danforth & E. A. Doisy. Baltimore, MD: Williams & Wilkins, pp. 1263–1334.

Riessman C. K. (1983), Women and medicalization: A new perspective. *Soc. Policy*, 14:3–18.

Salmon V. J., Geist S. H. & Walter R. I. (1941), Treatment of the menopause: Evaluation of estrogen implantation. *J. Amer. Med. Assn.*, 117:1843–1849.

Schneider J. W. & Conrad P. (1980), The medical control of deviance: Contests and consequences. In: *Research in the Sociology of Health Care*, Vol. I, ed. J Roth. Greenwich, CT: JAI, pp. 1–53.

Sevringhaus E. L. (1941), Treatment of the menopause. *J. Amer. Med. Assn.*, 116:1197–1199.

Shorr E. (1940), The menopause. *Bull. NY Acad. Med.*, 16:453–474.

——— Robinson F. H. & Papanicolaou G. N. (1939), A clinical study of the synthetic estrogen stilbestrol. *J. Amer. Med. Assn.*, 113:2313–2318.

Smith-Rosenberg C. (1973), Puberty to menopause: The cycle of femininity in nineteenth-century America. *Feminist Studies*, 1:58–72.

——— (1985), *Disorderly Conduct*. New York: Knopf.

Starr P. (1982), *The Social Transformation of American Medicine*. New York: Basic Books.

Stevens R. (1971), *American Medicine and the Public Interest*. New Haven, CT: Yale University Press.

Theodorson, G. A. & Achilles, G. (1969), *A Modern Dictionary of Sociology*. New York: Harper & Row.

Voda A., Dinnerstein M. & O'Donnell S., ed. (1982), *Changing Perspectives on Menopause*. Austin: University of Texas Press.

Zola, I. K. (1972), Medicine as an institution of social control. *Soc. Rev.*, 20:487–504.

3

A Critical View
of Three Psychoanalytical
Positions on Menopause

HELENA HARRIS

Psychoanalytic views on menopause span some 85 years and several important theoretical positions. The traditional psychoanalytic (Freudian) model was dominant from the beginning of the century until mid-century, when it became modified by ego psychology and subsequently by object relations theory. These theoretical shifts produced shifts in clinical concepts concerning the psychological difficulties related to menopause. The following discussion compares various theoretical positions.

TRADITIONAL FREUDIAN MODEL

Helene Deutsch (1924) the first psychoanalyst to write on the menopause, reveals her classical orientation with her opening words on the subject: "Woman's last traumatic experience as a sexual being, the menopause, is under the aegis of an incurable narcissistic wound" (p. 56).

She seems to suggest that trauma is the pervasive condition of women because they are sexual beings. However, in all fairness to Deutsch, it should be remembered that her views on the subject appeared in the first book by an analyst on female psychology – a book published in the atmosphere of a Vienna where the echos of Victorianism were still audible. Although Deutsch revised some of her views in 1945, her interpretation of the meaning of the menopause continued to be influenced by her original position. Psychoanalytically, her thinking about the menopause was based entirely on the stages of psychosexual development described by Freud (1905). The course of menopause was wholly determined by the vicissitudes of libidinal development.

Menopause, she writes, represents a "retrogressive phase in the history of the libido" (p. 56), marking as it does a regression to infantile libidinal positions. Throughout her discussion, Deutsch draws similarities between puberty and menopause—similarities entirely lacking in empirical foundation. In contrast to puberty, according to Deutsch, the libido at menopause goes "into reverse" because of the impossibility of genital "cathexis." However, an extended struggle ensues "before this withdrawal of libido from the genitals has been completed . . ." (p. 57). This struggle occurs because of the forward thrust of the libido during puberty as compared with its backward movement at menopause, with the menopausal woman attempting to retain all the values of puberty just at a time when the ultimate "devaluation of the genitals as an organ of reproduction" is imminent. The inevitable loss of this struggle inflicts a "severe narcissistic blow."

The courses of puberty and of menopause are further paralleled in physical development insofar as both are set off by biological signals. As a result, similar changes in behavior occur. The woman experiencing menopause

> believes herself able to make a fresh start in life. . . . feels ready for any passion. . . . starts keeping a diary as she did when she was a girl. . . . changes her behavior to her family as she did before, leaves home for the same psychical reasons as girls do at puberty, etc. . . . many women who are frigid during the reproductive period now become sexually sensitive, and others become frigid for the first time. . . . Others who have hitherto put up well with frigidity now begin to demonstrate all its typical concomitant phenomena; changes of mood, unbalanced behavior and irritability set in and make life a torment for the woman herself and those about her [p. 58].

Fantasy productions in puberty and in menopause are also said to be similar, with fantasies of rape and prostitution occurring at both periods of life. On the deepest fantasy level, a breaking through of the incest ban occurs at both times, a situation induced at menopause by libidinal regression.

Symptoms of depression in menopause, expressed by anxiety, giddiness, palpitations, high pulse rates, and the like resemble difficulties that appear at puberty. At menopause, depression is the result of the "irrevocable blow to female narcissism" induced by the "remobilized castration complex." Various physical symptoms are also said to resemble each other, including disturbances of the gastrointestinal tract, vasomotor disturbances, eczemas, and anomalies of growth. In making this latter claim, Deutsch cites a Vienna specialist in internal medicine.

Deutsch's citation of medical authority raises the question of the credibility of her account of the menopause. In the absence at that time of any precise research information, medical myths exerted an unwarranted influence on her as well as on others. Deutsch, it has been pointed out (Formanek, 1987), while retaining 19th-century pejorative medical myths about the menopause, explained its significance by the use of Freud's account of psychosexual development. Among the myths she retained were: (1) the similarity between the course of puberty and menopause; (2) the correlation between the ending of menstruation and the ending of women's sexuality, together with inappropriate sexual desires; (3) the presence of multiple symptoms, especially depression, ascribed to menopause; (4) the woman's presumed yearning for a continuation of her ability to reproduce.

Although Freud never wrote specifically on the subject of menopause, a number of passing references to the topic probably influenced Deutsch in her work. Over a period of about 45 years, from 1894 to 1937, Freud revealed a fairly consistent attitude about the menopause as a source of psychological difficulty to women. Anxiety neurosis was the condition to which he felt women to be especially vulnerable at this time.

In Freud's view, anxiety neurosis was induced by an increase in libido, an increase that he felt to be the expectable consequence of menopause. Through the years, this position is articulated over and over again. He writes of "the horror which, at the time of menopause, an aging woman feels at her suddenly increased libido . . ." (Freud, 1894, p. 111). Later on he (Freud, 1912) states that "the damming up of this increase in libido accounts for the onset of neurosis" at the time of menopause (p. 236), and in 1917 he again attributes the onset of anxiety disorders at menopause to "a considerable increase in the production of libido" (p. 403).

In discussing ego enfeeblement as a consequence of physical illness, Freud views illness of any kind as tending to increase the force of instincts beyond the ego's capacity. However, menopause is cited as an outstanding example of this condition: "The normal model of such processes is perhaps the alteration in women caused by the disturbances of menstruation and the menopause . . ." (Freud, 1926, p. 242). Finally, in 1937, he again refers to the increased libido at certain times of life, of which menopause is one, when previously non-neurotic people may become neurotic because of their difficulty in "taming" instincts that are "considerably reinforced" (p. 226).

It is evident from Freud's writings that menopause is regarded as a source of psychological disturbance. Although anxiety neurosis was supposed to be the probable outcome, Freud also revealed a belief in menopause as an actual physical illness. In summary, the accumulated weight of Freud's passing allusions to the subject of menopause is consistent with medical misconceptions of the times — misconceptions that were also expressed in Deutsch's work.

EGO PSYCHOLOGY MODEL

Benedek (1973), writing from an ego psychology orientation, takes a more optimistic view of the menopause, regarding it as a developmental phase — as a "progressive psychologic adaptation" (p. 322). However, she does consider aging an "involutional process" biologically. Hormonal imbalance, she states, results in certain physiological disturbances, including insomnia, vasomotor instability, palpitations, hot flushes, and other common symptoms of menopause. Nevertheless, internal physiological changes are seen as stimulating a psychological process that "enables the individual to master further, and anew, environmental stimulations" (p. 325).

In contrast to Deutsch, Benedek includes in her discussion empirical data beyond the treatment room. She cites surveys of "large groups of women" in which 85% "pass through climacterium without interrupting their daily routine" (p. 325). In the remaining 15% menopause could not be established as the cause of the symptoms observed. When pathology does occur during the menopause, Benedek concludes on the basis of her own clinical experience, it usually existed previously. The climacterium, she writes, "adds only one factor: it diminishes that part of the integrative strength of the personality which is dependent upon stimulation by gonadal hormones" (p. 336). However, depression, if it appears at menopause, may be related not to physiology but to the woman's psychosexual history.

The decline of hormonal production accounts for menopause's being seen by Benedek as a developmental phase—a phase in which pathology is not necessarily present. Hormonal decline, she suggests, desexualizes emotional needs, thus freeing subliminatory energies that further the integration of personality.

Cultural patterns also play a part in the extent to which developmental advantages at menopause may be achieved. Citing anthropological studies of societies in which women gain status and greater freedom after menopause, Benedek speculates about the possibility of emotional gains that might occur under these circumstances. "Much of the exaggerated fear of menopause appears to be culturally determined," she observes (p. 327). In Western culture, she suggests, women's emancipation in recent years has changed our expectations in a positive direction about the declining sexual functions associated with aging.

Like Deutsch, however, Benedek draws certain dubious psychological parallels between puberty and menopause. Furthermore, old prejudices are somewhat disguised beneath the new knowledge about hormones that Benedek adds to her discussion: "The rebellion of puberty appears to be repeated when the internal frustration of the declining hormonal function activates aggressive, hostile and regressive behavior" (p. 333). Many psychological aspects of the climacterium are said to be a repetition of puberty, the result of emotional tensions that originated in conflicts about feminine identity.

Although Benedek's point about the psychological effects of conflicts being related to feminine identity seems well taken, her use of the new knowledge about hormones is ambiguous. She seems to use

hormones to explain both positive and negative outcomes at menopause. Hormonal processes seem to become an all-purpose causal
factor in her psychological explanations of menopausal changes.
Although Freudian psychosexual developmental formulations provide the foundation of her discussion, hormonal production and
processes are interwoven with psychoanalytic theory in her account of
the menopause.

OBJECT RELATIONS MODEL

Object relations theory influences the discussion on the menopause
presented by Lax (1982). Psychological dimensions such as self-image
and ego interests are viewed in the light of "phase-specific physiological
changes" that are expressed in such symptoms as vasomotor dis-
charges, hot flashes, palpitations and other cardiac discomforts, insomnia, and so on. During the climacteric, a number of interrelated
factors will determine a woman's response to this phase of life. Lax
writes:

> The manner and extent to which a woman responds to the
> climacteric will depend on the severity of her physiological
> symptoms, the nature of past experiences, her internalized object
> relations, her psychic structure, the strength of her libidinal
> investments, the width of her conflict-free ego sphere, the nature
> and strength of her ego interest, the extent of her healthy
> narcissism, the nature of her current object relations, and the
> nature of her famililial and social setting [p. 157].

Because of the number and complexity of factors involved, a
negative outcome seems to be inevitable. Menopause is a period of
psychic crisis during which "disequilibria occur in all . . . areas of
psychic functioning" (p. 156). Lax states explicitly that depression is
the "expectable" climacteric reaction, a theme that is basic to her
position.

Where cultural influences are concerned, however, there is greater
variability in outcome. Socioeconomic factors may have differing
effects and lead either to a new and healthy integration or to a

pathological development. Lax cites research in which working women of lower socioeconomic status were found to exhibit more physiological distress than women of the higher socioeconomic group. In addition, the latter group were able to maintain a more positive self-image during menopause than did women belonging to lower socioeconomic groups.

Lax emphasizes the effect of cultural influences on self-image in general. In our youth-oriented culture, she writes, women experience both the physical symptoms of menopause as well as the visible effects of the aging process as a narcissistic assault. Most women, she claims, react to these changes with shame and with a "painful sense of mortification." Self-image inevitably suffers as a result of the "special narcissistic investment in their appearance" that women in our culture have practiced in the years preceding menopause.

The "highly narcissistically cathected ego goals" of a young woman's strivings are contrasted with those of the menopausal woman. Because of the menopausal woman's inability to achieve goals that she formerly took for granted, a temporary state of disequilibrium may result. A conflict between a wishful self-image and a deflated, failing self is the chief cause of the depression that Lax views as inevitable. Anger becomes directed toward the deflated, failing self with an accompanying loss of self-esteem and shame. A sense of loss is expressed in mourning for the youthful self of one's past.

The end of the childbearing years are said to be experienced by many women as a profound loss even though realistically there may no longer be a wish for a child. The awareness that one is no longer able to bear a child frequently induces either a conscious or an unconscious depression, according to Lax. Women who have never had a child especially feel a sense of loss and are more prone to depression. It is a time of maximum threat by the "biological clock."

In spite of the negative tone suggested by Lax's labeling depression as an expectable climacteric reaction, she manages to conclude her discussion on an optimistic note. If a woman successfully engages in a mourning process for the wishful self-image of her youth, she will renounce these no longer attainable goals. A woman in relatively good mental and physical health will be able to work through difficulties and reconstitute a meaningful life for herself. She may then develop an identification with an idealized matriarchal model "whose character-

istics of generativity, generosity, and compassion become her own
goals . . ." (p. 165). Object relations are thus enriched when such a
working through occurs.

DISCUSSION

In comparing the three analytic positions reviewed, it is useful to
consider those psychoanalytic concepts employed in each case to
explain the significance of the menopause.

Deutsch used Freud's account of psychosexual development to
explain its significance. The validity of her conclusions, therefore,
rests on the current status of that developmental position. How
adequate is that position today? On the whole, contemporary infant
research fails to confirm Freudian psychosexual development. In fact,
current infant research does not even frame its questions in a stage-
theory context. Stern (1985), for example, rejects stage theories in
general, and Beebe's (1986) work, revealing the exquisite subtlety of
mutual regulation in the mother-infant dyad, also calls into question
a stage-theory orientation.

Development, contemporary infant research suggests, is far more
complex than the simplistic movement of "cathexis" along a single
track (oral, anal, phallic, genital) traveling to, or getting stuck at,
certain way stations (fixations) and later going into "reverse" at
menopause, as Deutsch claims. Deutsch's entire account of the menopause consists, it seems, of grafting a body of mythology—19th-
century pejorative medical myths—onto an aspect of Freudian theory
now under considerable scrutiny and question.

Although Benedek also uses the developmental framework of
psychosexual development, her ego psychology orientation allows her
to take a somewhat broader view insofar as she regards menopause as
offering the opportunity for a progressive psychological adaptation.
Such pathology as does occur at menopause she attributes to preexisting psychosexual development.

Benedek's account of the menopause was strongly influenced by the
relatively new knowledge about hormonal influences. Hormones seem
to provide her with an all-purpose causal factor, explaining both

negative and positive outcomes. Yet Benedek's position is internally consistent despite its apparent ambiguity. She writes:

> It is our conclusion that, normally, the woman reaches the highest level of her psychosexual integration at the height of her hormonal cycle. This integration, in emotion and behavior, changes as the women responds to the inner perception of the hormonal decline [Benedek, 1973, p. 329].

In other words, hormone production affects the capacity for emotional integration.

In spite of Benedek's strong emphasis on physiological factors, her ego psychology orientation leads to a consideration of the subject of feminine identity and the conflicts surrounding it at the menopause. Consequently, there is a perceptible shift in her work in the direction of self-esteem issues throughout a woman's life and how they are expressed at the menopause. Her recognition of cultural factors that affect expectations about menopause also results in consideration of self-esteem issues because women's sense of their own value as they age is so strongly influenced by the culture's concepts about aging.

Lax, influenced by object relations theory, moves the discussion even further in the direction of self-esteem issues. While it is true that she places great emphasis on "phase-specific physiological changes," which tend to make depression an "expectable" climacteric reaction, her consideration of sociocultural factors results in the emergence of self-image as an important variable in women's reactions. She focuses especially on the effects of our youth-oriented culture on a woman's self-image over the life span.

Her object relations orientation shapes the nature of the psychoanalytic concepts used to explain menopausal reactions. In contrast to both Deutsch and Benedek, who make use of developmental explanatory concepts, Lax emphasizes the nature of object relations. For example, she envisions a positive outcome for women in relatively good mental and physical health. A successful working through of the difficult issues depends on object relations that have been enriched through identification with an idealized matriarchal model. A woman's self-esteem is thus enhanced through this identification process.

The focus on self-esteem in the work of both Benedek and Lax strongly suggests the conceptual framework of self psychology. It raises the question of whether a self-psychological orientation might not offer some insight on the subject of menopause. Self psychology has not as yet addressed the issue of the climacterium, and there has been little discussion about the differences in male and female self development, generally. Lang (1984), writing about gender issues states: "In the psychology of the self no specific elaboration has yet been made of the significance of gender identity in the nuclear self, nor of the specific processes by which this aspect of the self is consolidated within the matrix of selfobject relationships . . ." (p. 51).

In Lang's discussion of the consolidation of the feminine self, the selfobject function emerges as central. Her emphasis on this concept, a fundamental one in self psychology, allows us to speculate and extrapolate as to the implications for menopause. Defined as a function, the selfobject relationship is a cognitive-affective representation that permits the woman to consolidate certain features of real relationships with people into her own personality. As Lang expresses it, "The selfobject relationship is the crucial mediatior between external and psychic reality" (p. 55).

As far as menopause is concerned, the selfobject function could provide an explanatory basis for differing adaptations to this phase of life. According to self psychology theory, the selfobject relationship is fundamental and crucial in early life. The nurturance and support by primary caretakers result, optimally, in a self-soothing capability that is retained throughout life. It is a capacity that enables us to take the ups and downs of life in stride. A woman's self-soothing capacity at menopause would be central and critical.

There are many other ways in which the selfobject function would provide an explanatory foundation for the viewing of menopausal reactions. Alternative explanations to those offered by the previous writers are possible. All of the previous writers mention a woman's psychosexual history as one of the determining factors in either positive or negative reactions. But selfobject relationships constitute an important aspect of every psychosexual history. The extent to which a woman was valued and admired throughout her growing up will determine her level of self-esteem as an adult. How did her parents react to her oedipal strivings? Their reactions of either pride or threat

to her budding, assertive sexuality become integrated into her personality by way of the selfobject function and become a factor in her
self-esteem. And the issue of self-esteem, as we have seen, gained
increased explanatory importance in the work of both Benedek and
Lax.

Self-esteem regulation, another central concept in self psychology,
is intimately related to the selfobject function. Self-image is affected to
some degree throughout life by the self-reflections we are able to read
in the eyes of others. Granted that the aging process has its difficulties
and that menopause is merely one of the early landmarks along that
path, the woman with a strong sense of self-esteem will be more
adequately prepared. No matter what the physiological difficulties or
the negative cultural pressures, she will be able to cope more adequately than a woman with a vulnerable sense of self-esteem.

Examples from the work of Benedek and Lax illustrate several of
these points. Benedek has written of how conflicts about feminine
identity result in emotional tensions in puberty, tensions that are
repeated in menopause. The study and investigation of selfobject
functions throughout the female life cycle would enable us to understand better what aspects of selfobject development might account for
such tensions. Also, feminine identification is a matter of either
positive or negative feelings about being a woman—one aspect of
self-esteem. Lax writes about the enrichment of object relations for
postmenopausal women who have successfully worked through certain self-image difficulties. She cites the identification with an idealized
matriarchal model as one way of achieving this goal. The ability to
idealize in this case would depend on the developmental history of
idealization as an aspect of the selfobject function.

These suggestions of how self psychology might view the menopause are intended only as indications of a direction that study and
investigation might take. Such investigation might provide us with a
more detailed account of the development of self-esteem and its
specific effect on adaptation to menopause.

In this review of the work of Deutsch, Benedek, and Lax, self-
esteem clearly has emerged as the central issue. This is not to dismiss
the fact that profound physiological changes also occur. Nevertheless,
women respond very individually to menopause. The difference in

response seems to depend on the relative stability of their self-esteem. It is likely that the application of self psychology concepts to the study of menopause will further enhance our understanding of the subject.

REFERENCES

Beebe, B. (1986), Mother-infant mutual influence and the precursors of self and object representations. In: *Empirical Studies of Psychoanalytic Theories, Vol.* 2, ed. J. Masling. Hillsdale, NJ: The Analytic Press, pp. 27–48.

Benedek, T. (1973), *Psychoanalytic Investigations.* New York: Quandrangle/New York Times, pp. 322–349.

Deutsch, H. (1924), The menopause. *Internat J. Psychoanal.*, 65:55–62, 1984.

Freud, S. (1894), On the grounds for detaching a particular syndrome from neurasthenia under description "anxiety neurosis." *Standard Edition*, 3:90–117. London: Hogarth Press, 1962.

_____ (1905), Three essays on the theory of sexuality. *Standard Edition*, 7:173–222. London: Hogarth Press, 1953.

_____ (1912), Type of onset of neurosis. *Standard Edition*, 12:229–238. London: Hogarth Press, 1958.

_____ (1917). Introductory lectures on psycho-analysis: Lexture XXV – Anxiety. *Standard Edition*, 16:392–411. London: Hogarth Press, 1963.

_____ (1926), The question of lay analysis. *Standard Edition*, 20:179–258. London: Hogarth Press, 1959.

_____ (1937), Analysis terminable and interminable. *Standard Edition*, 23:211–253. London: Hogarth Press, 1964.

Formanek, R. (1987), Depression and menopause: a socially constructed link. In: *Women and Depression.* ed. R. Formanek & A. Gurian. New York: Springer, pp. 255–271.

Lang, J.A. (1984), Notes toward a psychology of the feminine self. In: *Kohut's Legacy*, ed. P. E. Stepansky & A. Goldberg. Hillsdale, NJ: The Analytic Press, pp. 51–69.

Lax, R. (1982), The expectable depressive climacteric reaction. *Bull. Menninger Clin.*, 46:151–167.

Stern D.N. (1985), *The Interpersonal World of the Infant*, New York: Basic Books.

II

*Psychosocial,
Cross-Cultural, and
Research Perspectives*

4

Psychosocial Influences and Life Events at the Time of the Menopause

J. G. GREENE

In the last quarter of a century a considerable body of empirically based research has grown up on the effect of social and psychological factors on women during the climacteric years and especially at the time of the menopause. This chapter examines this body of research with the purpose of determining the trends that have emerged. All the studies reviewed were carried out in Western societies using research methods that have evolved over the years within the behavioral and social sciences.

The research strategy adopted in most of these studies was to select a sample of women from the general population within the climacteric years and examine the association between putative causal or independent variables (social class, employment status, marital adjustment) and some outcome or dependent variable. The latter was almost invariably a checklist of "nonspecific" symptoms, that is, symptoms commonly reported by women around the time of the menopause and that unlike, for example, vasomotor symptoms, could not be directly attributed to hormonal or metabolic changes. These symptoms consist of a mixture of psychological, psychosomatic, or somatic complaints. In employing this measure, some researchers simply used a total symptom count; others grouped symptoms in an *ad hoc*, or face validity, manner; whereas others used more scientifically based group-

Table 1
Symptoms and groupings agreed by at least two factor analytic studies
(Greene, 1987)

| | | Psychological | |
Vasomotor	Somatic	Anxiety	Depression
Hot flushes	Tiredness	Feeling tense	Feeling unhappy
Night sweats	Muscle and joint pains	Attacks of panic	Loss of interest in things
Vaginal dryness	Parts of body feel numb/tingling	Palpitations	Irritability
	Headaches	Sleep disturbed	Crying spells
	Feeling dizzy or faint	Excitable	
	Breathing difficulties	Difficulty in falling asleep	
	Backaches	Poor memory	
	Loss of feeling in hands/feet	Difficulty in concentration	

ings derived from a factor analysis of symptoms. Table 1 shows the typical symptoms and groupings that have emerged over the years from factor analytic studies (Greene, 1987).

The studies reviewed here can be grouped into three broad categories — those relating to sociodemographic variables, those investigating the role of women's attitudes to the menopause, and those dealing with immediate interpersonal factors. In addition, a small group of studies using research methods derived from life event research has recently been added to the literature. Each of these areas will be reviewed in turn.

SOCIODEMOGRAPHIC FACTORS

It has long been fashionable to regard preoccupation with the menopause as peculiar to the middle and upper classes of society and occurring among women who, having no need to work, have little to do other than be concerned with aging and its physical manifestations. Nothing could be further from the truth, and numerous studies testify to this. For example, no evidence for this was found in a survey of British women by McKinlay and Jeffreys (1974). These authors found that the severity of symptoms in this general population sample was unrelated to social class, educational level, or employment status. Others, however, have found that, if anything, it is women of *low* socioeconomic status (usually defined in terms of occupational level, income, or educational attainment) and/or who are *not* employed who report an excess of symptoms around the time of the menopause. For the moment it is convenient to review the data on socioeconomic and employment status separately.

Socioeconomic Indices

One of the first studies to provide evidence in this respect was that by Jaszmann, Van Lith, and Zatt (1969). In their survey of a general population of Dutch climacteric women, these authors found the number of symptoms to be significantly higher in women of low income and educational level. However, no data were presented in this survey for vasomotor and nonvasomotor symptoms separately so that differential effects of sociodemographic factors on different types of symptoms could not be ascertained. In later studies of the effects of sociodemographic factors on symptoms, such distinctions have been made, with revealing results.

One of these was a study of a general population of Scottish women by Greene and Cooke (1980). In that survey, using two symptom scales derived from a factor analysis (Greene, 1976), nonspecific somatic and psychological symptoms were examined in relation to climacteric status separately from vasomotor symptoms. Information was also gathered at time of interview to allow subjects to be categorized according to socioeconomic status using the British Registrar General's classificatory system. No relationship was found between vasomotor symptoms and social class status, but there was a marked association between the latter and other symptoms. This effect is illustrated in Figure 1 for both the somatic and psychological symptoms scales. There it can be seen that, for both scales, mean symptom scores of women of low socioeconomic status increased more than did those of women of high socioeconomic status during the climacteric (40–55 years) and remained higher into the postclimacteric period. This effect is, however, greater for psychological symptoms, for which

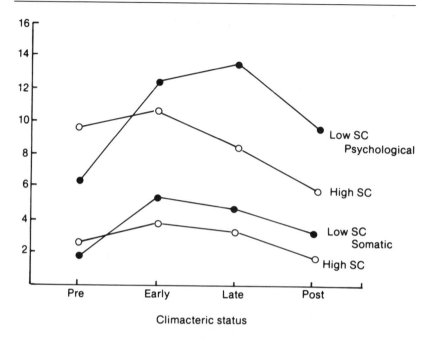

FIG. 1   Mean scores on two symptom scales in relation to social class (SC). (From Greene, 1984.)

the class difference, during the late climacteric, achieves statistical significance.

A similar differential relationship between socioeconomic status and symptoms was found in a study of a general population of Italian women by Campagnoli et al. (1981). In addition to information about their physical and socioeconomic level, these women were also asked about any symptoms they had experienced at the time of the menopause. These were divided into "somatic" (hot flushes and sweating) and "psychic" symptoms (anxiety, feeling depressed, irritability, crying spells), each symptom being rated according to degree of severity. This study found that socioeconomic status was unrelated to vasomotor symptoms, but women of low status tended to report more severe psychological symptoms than did women of high status.

Hunter, Battersby, and Whitehead (1986) reported similar findings in a large-scale survey of climacteric women in the U.K. Using multiple regression analysis, social class was found to predict a variety of categories of complaints (depressed mood, somatic symptoms, cognitive difficulties, anxiety, and sleep problems) but not vasomotor symptoms, derived from a factor analysis. That is, women of low social class showed an excess of all of the foregoing types of nonspecific symptoms. As the authors note, lower social class was associated with many other potentially relevant variables in this survey, such as financial problems, number of children and self-rated poor health, thereby providing clues to the mechanism whereby low social class may produce symptoms in climacteric women.

As in the study by Jaszmann et al. (1969), Polit and Larocco (1980), in a study of a randomly selected group of American climacteric women, found that women of low educational attainment tended to report more symptoms than did those of high attainment. Although the overall relationship was fairly modest, inspection of individual symptoms revealed that where sociodemographic variables were associated with symptoms, these were mainly psychological in nature, and that their effects on such symptons could be fairly substantial. Table 2 illustrates the effect of educational attainment on two such symptoms. Vasomotor symptoms, on the other hand, showed no association with educational level.

Abe and Moritsuka (1986), in a study of 432 Japanese women, also implicated educational level as a factor associated with symptomatology. In this case-control study of a matched clinical and control population, women of low educational level had a high relative risk of experiencing severe symptoms, as did women employed as unskilled laborers, although to a somewhat lesser degree. Like the study by Hunter et al. (1986), this Japanese study suggests that other "psychic" factors such as self-rated health, self-esteem, and life satisfaction may mediate the effects of socioeconomic variables.

In a study of Norwegian women, Holte and Mikkelsen (1982)

Table 2

Percentage of Women Reporting Symptoms in Relation to Educational Attainment (Polit and Larocco, 1980)

Symptom	College Graduates	Non-College Graduates
Depression	19	64
Lack of Energy	24	63
Vasomotor	No differences	

examined six categories of symptoms, also derived from factor analysis, in relation to a number of sociodemographic factors. However, in this particular study, the association between these factors and symptoms was generally negative or low, the only positive relationships being that women whose husbands' income was low tended to report more diffuse somatic symptoms.

The authors account for these generally negative findings by suggesting that because Scandinavian countries are highly developed welfare states relative to other Western industrialized societies, their populations are economically and culturally homogeneous at a high level of income. This is an interesting point because it follows that in those societies with a high standard of living the effects of the climacteric may be relatively benign and that where variation in response does occur, sensitive social and psychological factors may be etiologically more important. Indeed, in this particular study it was found that measures of previous "menstrual coping" (pain, nausea, depression at menstruation) and the quality of a women's social network were more powerful predictors of psychological and general somatic symptoms than were sociodemographic factors.

In all the preceding studies the only outcome measure considered was symptomatology. Evidence for the more extensive consequences that being of low social class may have for women during the climacteric years comes from an earlier general population survey of Swiss women carried out under the auspices of the International Health Foundatiom (I.H.F.) by Van Keep and Kellerhals (1974). Not only was low social class associated with an increase in symptoms at the menopause, it was also associated with a variety of other social and psychological characteristics assessed in this study.

Women of lower social class, throughout the climacteric years, showed poor "subjective adaptation"; they evaluated highly the traditional female role of being dependent and maternal; they tended to have less satisfactory sex lives, and marital and family disharmony tended to be greater; all aspects of their wider social relations – cultural activities, social contacts and social integration – were reduced. Figure 2 shows these effects with respect to subjective adaptation. It illustrates a typical pattern in which women of lower social class – who are low on this characteristic throughout their middle years – undergo a considerable decrease just at the time of the menopause.

The finding in regard to sexual functioning corresponds to the

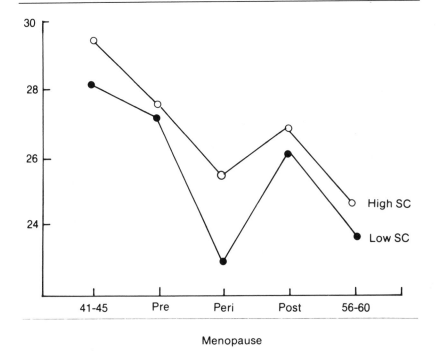

FIG. 2   Index of subjective adaptation in relation to social class (SC). (From Greene, 1984.)

result of two other studies. Hallstrom (1977), noting that various aspects of sexual functioning had begun to decline around the time of the menopause in a group of Swedish women, found this decline to be greater in women of lower social class. Similarly, Garde and Lunde (1980), in a study of Danish women, found that women of lower social class had a considerably higher proportion of sexual problems (48%) than did those of high socioeconomic status (9%).

Nevertheless, the IHF Swiss study is of special importance in that it demonstrates that socioeconomic status is associated with many aspects of a woman's personal and social functioning during the climacteric, apart from symptoms, which may in themselves merely be manifestations of these other concerns.

Employment

It will be recalled that in their survey of British women McKinlay and Jeffreys (1974) found no differences in symptomatology between women who were employed outside the home and those who were not so employed. However, Holte and Mikkelson (1982) found that Norwegian women who were not employed outside the home tended to report more diffuse somatic symptoms. Hunter et al. (1986), on the other hand, found British women in a similar situation to report not only more somatic symptoms, but also anxiety and sleep problems.

In an earlier study of the effects of employment on climacteric women in Germany, Prill (1977) found that 24% of women having no occupation outside the home suffered from "severe climacteric symptoms" as against 8% of those who were working. The author concluded that an important factor contributing to this difference was the woman's reason for working or not working. Prill observes that among women who had to work for financial or other unwelcome reasons, and among those who wanted to work but because of circumstances were not able to do so, symptoms were the most severe. As we shall see from later studies, simple lack of employment per se is probably not the critical factor influencing symptoms.

This conclusion was confirmed in the study of American women by Polit and Larocco (1980), who found, in addition to the effect of social class, that women who were employed outside the home reported fewer symptoms. However, part-time workers tended to resemble nonemployed women more than they resembled full-time employees in their reporting of symptoms. For example, only 18% of women working full time, compared with 52% of part-time workers and 45% of nonemployed women, reported having trouble sleeping. Similar results were obtained with respect to other psychological symptoms. These results confirm Prill's (1977) observation that being employed per se is not the critical factor. What may be more important is that a woman is pursuing a full-time career, rather than working part time perhaps to supplement the family income. Full-time employment would obviously be facilitated by a higher level of educational attainment. Furthermore, it is probable that women of low social class would not be pursuing a career and would therefore not experience the beneficial effect of career-oriented employment. Confirmation for this probability comes from a study by Abe and Moritsuka (1986), who found that the relative risk of symptoms of Japanese women employed as unskilled laborers was greater than for those not employed at all.

That the effect of being employed depends on social class was convincingly demonstrated in the final study to be considered in this section. Severne (1979), in a second study promoted by the International Health Foundation, this time of Belgian women, examined vasomotor symptoms (Circulatory Index) and psychological symptoms (Nervosity Index) separately in relation to social class and employment status. Vasomotor symptoms were unrelated to either of these variables.

A different picture emerged in the case of nervous symptoms. These symptoms were related to both social class and employment status, but in a complex way, in that the effect of being employed depended on the social class of the women. This is illustrated in Figure 3, where the scores on the Nervosity Index of the four subgroups of women is quite disparate at each menopausal stage. It is clear from this figure that, once again, women of lower socioeconomic status had the more

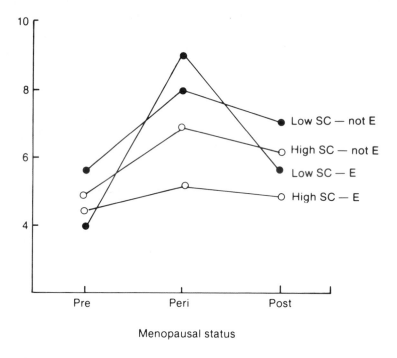

FIG. 3   Mean scores on the nervosity index in relation to employment (E) and social class (SC) (From Greene, 1984.)

severe psychological symptoms at the time of the menopause. However, among these women, those who were employed experienced the
more marked increase in symptoms at that time. In contrast, among
women of higher social class, those employed had the least severe
symptoms. In other words, the effect of employment on symptoms is
reversed depending on the socioeconomic status of the women. Similar relationships were found between social class and employment
and other measures of women's functioning, these measures being the
same as those employed in the Swiss IHF study.

Thus, in these paradoxical relationships, being employed seems to
protect women of higher social class but has no beneficial effect on,
and may even be harmful to those of lower social class. Severne (1979)
accounts for this harmful effect by suggesting that "it might well be
that the combination of a household and a physically demanding job
is for many less privileged women too much at that time" (p. 108). This
observation complements that made earlier in this section in relation
to the studies of Prill (1977) and Polit and Larocco (1980), namely, that
employment is beneficial only if it is intrinsically rewarding, and not if
it is only for the purpose of supplementing the family income, as it is
for many working-class women.

The outcome of studies investigating the effects of sociodemographic variables is shown in Table 3. In summary these studies clearly
demonstrate that it is mainly underprivileged women of low socioeconomic status, low income, low educational level, and with limited
employment satisfaction who suffer most during the climacteric.
These factors exercise their influence mainly on psychological symptoms and probably on other aspects of personal and social adaptation.
While it would be reasonable to assume that such women might be
adversely affected throughout their life span, there is good evidence
for thinking that these adverse effects increase during the climacteric
years and particularly around the time of the menopause.

ATTITUDES TOWARD THE MENOPAUSE

It appears that socioeconomic and other broad sociological factors
underlie, at least in Western societies, the varied manner in which
women in general respond to or experience the menopause. However,

Table 3
Sociodemographic Factors and Climacteric Symptoms

Authors	Low Socio-economic status	Low Income	Low Education	Not Employed	Part-time or unskilled Employment
McKinlay and Jefferys (1974)	0		0	0	
Jaszmann et al. (1969)		+	+		
Greene and Cooke (1980)	+				
Campagnoli et al. (1981)	+				
Hunter et al. (1986)	+			+	
Prill (1966)				+	
Polit and Larocco (1980)		0	+	+	+
Abe and Moritsuka (1986)			+		+
Holte and Mikkelsen (1982)		+	0	+	
Van Keep and Kellerhals (1974)	+				
Severne (1979)	+			+	

+ = Factor found to be associated with symptom frequency or severity
0 = Factor found not to be so associated

for the individual woman an important determinant in mediating the effects of these factors is thought to be the attitudes she has formed to the menopause and her perception of its consequences, real or imagined. Over the past two decades or so there have been a number of empirical studies of women's attitudes to the menopause, most of which have been carried out in the United States.

The first systematic study of women's attitudes to the menopause using a well-constructed measure was carried out by Neugarten et al. (1963). The construction of this scale will be described here in some detail as it has become the most widely used instrument of its kind and has been used in several of the studies to follow. The Attitude-Toward-Menopause (ATM) Checklist consists of 35 statements reflecting a diversity of opinions about the menopause. The checklist was administered to a general population of American women in the age range 21–65 years. The responses of these women, using a 4-point scale of agreement, were then submitted to a factor analysis. This revealed that the 35 statements could be grouped into seven categories, each of which was identified and labeled by the authors as reflecting a different aspect of attitude toward the menopause. These categories are shown in Table 4, together with an example of a statement from each.

Individual women's responses were then analyzed in terms of these

Table 4
Attitude Categories of the Attitude-Toward-Menopause Checklist
(Neugarten et al., 1963)

Category of Attitude
Negative affect
(e.g., menopause is an unpleasant experience)
Postmenopausal recovery
(e.g., women generally feel better after the menopause)
Extent of continuity
(e.g., menopause does not really change a woman in any way)
Control of symptoms
(e.g., women who have trouble are those expecting it)
Psychological change
(e.g., women often get self-centered at the menopause)
Unpredictability
(e.g., menopause is a mysterious thing women do not understand)
Sexuality
(e.g., after the menopause a woman is more interested in sex)

categories. The main finding to emerge from this study was that younger women, with no direct personal experience of the menopause, had more negative attitudes to that event than did those who were currently experiencing or who had passed through that phase of their lives. It appears that women may be more apprehensive about the menopause than they need be and that it does not, in retrospect, have the negative consequences many fear. Although about half of those women who had experienced the menopause agreed that the menopause was to some extent an unpleasant experience, the majority reported a good recovery from the experience with little or no prolonged effect on their basic personality or life style. A common theme in the literature is that one of women's main concerns at the menopause is the loss of reproductive capacity. The authors note that little evidence in support of this speculation emerged from this study. Very few women endorsed this view; more were preoccupied with the consequences of menopause as signs of aging. In short, this empirical study suggests that the common stereotype of the menopause and its consequences dissipates in the light of experience.

Seventeen years later, Eisner and Kelly (1980) carried out an exact replication of the Neugarten et al. (1963) study, also in an urban American population sample. The object in replicating the original study was to determine whether or not there had been any change in women's attitudes as a result of contemporary feminist thinking. The researchers also examined the influence of such other variables as race, socioeconomic status, and level of education on women's attitudes. In their study, as in Neugarten's original research, clear age differences emerged. Once again, younger women (age range 21–44) seemed more negative than older, menopausal and postmenopausal women in their attitudes to the menopause. While similar differences were found between age groups for both black and white women, the attitudes of black women were in general less positive than those of white women. Low income and low educational level were also found to be associated with a negative attitude, which perhaps explains the more negative views of black women.

In comparison with women in the earlier study, those in the Eisner and Kelly (1980) study tended to have slightly more positive attitudes toward the menopause. When, however, racial groups were compared separately, white women's attitudes had changed in a positive way much more than had those of black women. Although the authors conclude that "in general there do not seem to be momentous shifts in the direction of more positive attitudes towards the menopause over the last decade and a half" (p. 8), it seems likely that among women of higher social class there have been some observable shifts. But what is more interesting is that age differences in attitudes still persist, particularly among women of lower social class.

Additional evidence for the influence of socioeconomic status on attitudes, comes from a study by Dege and Gretzinger (1982), who also used the ATM Checklist. This is an unusual study because not only were the attitudes of women themselves examined, but those of their immediate families were also ascertained, the sample consisting of nine American families. The attitude of the sample as a whole tended to be a negative one, with an overall average of 57% negative responses, but within the sample there was wide intergroup variation. Surprisingly, women themselves had the least negative attitude and children the most. Attitudes, however, tended to be similar within families, there being a high level of agreement among women, their husbands, and their children. Consistent with the finding of Neugarten et al. (1963) and Eisner and Kelly (1980), younger women had a more negative image of the menopause than did older women. Perhaps the most significant finding of this study was the presence of what could be interpreted as a strong class influence. When families were divided into two groups according to the woman's educational level, those families in which the woman was of a high educational level shared a consistently more positive attitude toward the menopause. These differences are shown in Table 5.

A similar association between negative attitudes to the menopause and low educational level was observed by Lincoln (1980) in an unpublished doctoral thesis. Severne (1979), in the report on the IHF

Table 5
Percentage of Positive Response in Attitude Towards the Menopause
(Dege and Gretzinger, 1982)

Woman's level of Education	Women	Husbands	Children
High	61	57	45
Low	35	25	35

Swiss survey, also briefly noted that, although about one-third of women expressed a pessimistic view of the climacteric, such women were more often than not of low socioeconomic status and educational level. These class differences were attributed to lack of information about and understanding of the menopause among women of low social status.

Another study using the ATM Checklist is that described in Perlmutter and Bart (1982), of a somewhat selective group, in terms of social class, of urban American women. In brief, while subjects in this study reported an overall positive attitude toward the menopause, they also believed that the menopause was associated with negative moods. In general, sociodemographic variables were found not to be related to attitudes, but older subjects and those who were postmenopausal tended to have more positive attitudes than younger women. The latter finding is, of course, consistent with the findings of Neugarten et al. (1963), Eisner and Kelly (1980), and Dege and Gretzinger (1982). That sociodemographic variables were not related to attitude, a finding that is inconsistent with other work, could be due to the sample's being biased toward the middle to upper social classes, thereby giving a narrow socioeconomic range.

More recently, Leiblum and Swartzmann (1986) carried out a study similar to that of Eisner and Kelly (1980). They reexamined attitudes in the light of the evolution in menopausal treatment and philosophy that has taken place within the last few decades. Their sample consisted of 244 general population American women, many of high educational attainment, within the age range 15–74 years, who completed a brief 10-item Menopause Attitude Questionnaire derived from the more lengthy ATM Checklist.

The main findings were that, while the majority of women felt that the menopause should be viewed as a "medical condition" and treated as such, few regarded it as a particularly serious one. Natural treatments, however, were preferred over hormonal ones, and psychological difficulties were more likely to be attributed to distressing life changes than to hormonal changes, and the idea that sexuality was seriously compromised was strongly rejected. As usual, class differences emerged, with less educated women being more likely to subscribe to a medical model of the menopause. The authors conclude that, although there has been a clear coming together of attitude to the menopause in the past two decades, women are still undecided about whether the menopause should be viewed positively as a "developmental marker" or as a condition requiring medical intervention. Optimistically, Leiblum and Swartzmann express the view that wider dissemination of information about the menopause will result in fewer attitudinal differences among women.

All the studies so far reviewed were carried out in the United States. In the late 1960s however, the International Health Foundation (1969) carried out a large-scale international survey of women's attitudes toward the menopause in five European countries—Belgium, France, Britain, Italy, and West Germany—using a total sample of 2,000 women between 46 and 55 years of age. The main instrument for assessing attitudes was a list of 13 statements expressing common views about the menopause, with which the women were asked to agree or disagree.

In general, the attitudes of women in all five countries were fairly positive. The majority of women did not see menopause as having a major impact on their relations with their spouses, either sexual (55%) or personal (69%), particularly if the couple was happily married (84%), and indeed many women saw advantages, particularly with respect to freedom from menstruation (72%) and risk of pregnancy (72%). Most of the women, however, did see menopause as a time of physical upset (69%) and, to a lesser degree, as a time of psychological stress (57%). As far as national variations were concerned, there were few marked trends apart from the finding that, in general, British women had a consistently more optimistic outlook, perhaps reflecting the stoicism of the average middle-aged British woman of that time. Although a large-scale, large-sample study, this is not a particularly revealing study since no attempt was made to examine the antecedents or consequences of particular attitudes.

We conclude this section by turning to the only attempt to examine systematically the manner in which attitudes toward the menopause may actually influence the response to and feelings of women at the time of the menopause, that of Hunter (1987; see also Greene and Lock, 1987). In this study, a number of questions on beliefs about the menopause were included in the protocol. As in other studies, stereotype proved to be more negative than was later reported experience of the menopause. Negative stereotype nevertheless predicted depressed mood in the perimenopause and postmenopause but was not associated with current mood state. Adopting a cognitive model, Hunter argued that some women may hold negative beliefs about the menopause that are relatively independent of depression. This may lead to negative interpretations of physical change and inappropriate attribution of depressed mood to the menopause. Other women, however, who are depressed both before and after the menopause, may also interpret changes negatively because their depressed state affects their thinking.

Hunter also found women who sought medical help to be characterized by two specific beliefs, namely, that menopause is uncontrollable and that it is psychologically upsetting. Holding such beliefs was also a characteristic that distinguished a clinic sample from a nonclinic sample. The women in the clinic sample tended to report having suffered from premenstrual tension and generally had a negative view of their own health. The cognitive interpretation of these findings is that there is an interplay between the experience of premenstrual tension and the development of certain attitudes about aspects of the menstrual cycle, that is, that it is uncontrollable and is associated with both psychological and physical change. Perceived inability to control events as an etiological factor in psychological disorders derives, of course, from the theoretical and empirical work of Seligman (1980) on learned helplessness.

This model, which is depicted in Figure 4, illustrates the central role of cognitions or attitudes in mediating between causal and outcome variables. In the light of modern cognitive therapy, this model has some direct practical implications. First, Hunter considers that, in attempts to counter negative stereotypes, it may be productive to identify and deal with specific beliefs, for example, those regarding controlability and psychological experiences. Second, helping women cope with menstrual problems before the menopause might in turn help them feel more positive about coping during the menopause itself.

The outcome of the studies of attitudes to the menopause is summarized in Table 6. The main trend running through the studies is that, although some women in Western societies do have an overall negative image of the menopause and its consequences, this view is not as widespread nor as marked as has been thought. Where a negative

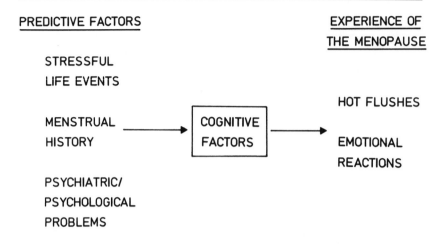

FIG. 4   Model of cognitive factors as mediators. (From Hunter, 1987.)

attitude does exist, it appears to be based in part on a stereotype of the menopause, since it is found to be stronger in younger than in older women. Among women with actual experience of the event, these negative attitudes decline. A major influence on attitude to the menopause is, again, social class, with women of lower socioeconomic status, income and education having more negative expectations. This is, of course, consistent with the adverse effects that sociodemographic factors have on symptoms and other functions during the climacteric and is presumably one of the ways these effects are mediated. Attitudes toward the menopause appear to have become somewhat less negative in the last two decades. This change has occurred largely among women from higher socioeconomic groups; Among women of less privileged status, the negative image has tended to persist, although even there one now finds greater diversity in attitude. This discrepancy may be due to the greater availability of information about the menopause, greater social mobility, and the erosion of traditional working-class attitudes.

INTERPERSONAL FACTORS

A common theme in the literature is that the climacteric occurs just at a time in the life cycle when a number of coincidental changes may be

Table 6
Summary of Studies of Attitudes to the Menopause

Authors	Country	Type of Population	Measure of Attitude	Factors Associated with Negative Attitude
Neugarten et al. (1963)	USA	General	ATM checklist	Younger women
Eisner and Kelly (1980)	USA	General	ATM checklist	Young women, women of low income and education
Dege and Gretzinger (1982)	USA	Personal contacts	ATM checklist	Younger women, women of low education
Perlmutter (1981)	USA	General	ATM checklist	Younger women
International Health Foundation (1969)	5 European countries	General (Random)	13-item questionnaire	Women of low socioeconomic status (Severne, 1979)
Leiblum and Swartzmann (1986)	USA	General	10-item questionnaire	Younger and less educated women
Hunter (1987)	UK	General, Clinic	Attitude questionnaire	Depressed mood, seeking help, premenstrual tension

taking place in the woman's interpersonal and immediate life situation. Regardless of the effects of the menopause, such changes, of which the departure of children from home is the most commonly cited, are seen as altering the woman's social role and status, necessitating some degree of psychological and social readjustment. Should these role changes occur in conjunction with the menopause, then the outcome, it is assumed, may be all the more adverse. In addition, some role changes, such as the loss of reproductive function, may in themselves be a direct consequence of the menopause. Thus, the climacteric woman is seen as passing through a stage of both psychosocial and biological transition, each change of which is intrinsically linked with the other.

Despite these widely held beliefs, it is extremely difficult to obtain empirical evidence that such events per se impinge on women at the menopause to any great degree. The most frequently studied "mid-life event" has been the departure of children from the family home. This event had been examined in two of the studies already referred to in the socioeconomic section.

In the Swiss IHF study, Van Keep and Kellerhals (1974) noted whether women had children living at home or not. In the case of the peri- and postmenopausal women, there was little difference in symptom severity between women with or without children at home. However, during the premenopause, women without children at home had considerably higher symptom scores than did those with children. This the authors refer to as an "anticipated climacteric," implying that the departure of children in the early climacteric, before the actual event of the menopause, may prematurely precipitate symptoms usually experienced later. This is the only study to demonstrate any association between symptoms and the absence or departure of children from home. It suggests that any negative response to the departure of children from home may have little to do with the menopause and may indeed be more distressing should it occur before that event. Furthermore, neither the absence nor the presence of children at home was associated with any of the other measures of social and psychological functioning used in this study.

Likewise, Holte and Mikkelsen (1982), in their Norwegian study, also investigated the effect of having children at home or not on their six factorially derived categories of symptoms. They also included a measure of the quality of a woman's current social network, as reflected in the number of friends and confiding relationships she had. While the symptom factors of mood lability and nervousness were high in women with limited social networks, none of the six categories of symptoms was associated with either the presence or absence of children at home. Thus, pre-existing social factors seemed to affect symptoms, whereas current psychosocial change, in the form of the departure of children from home, had no such effect. The former finding concurs with that of Abe and Moritsuka (1986), who found that, among Japanese women, those with few intimate friends had a higher relative risk of experiencing climacteric symptoms than did those who had many friends.

In a study of a group of British menopausal women, Crawford and Hooper (1973) found no relationship between menopausal status and symptoms and attitude toward two family events: marriage of a child and birth of a grandchild. Women currently experiencing the menopause did not have a more negative attitude than others did to these events, nor did women with a negative attitude toward either event report more symptoms. Furthermore, although as many as 75% of the women felt that the forthcoming marriage was going to mean a change in their way of life, and 52% felt similarly about the coming grandchild, neither menopausal status nor symptoms were related to these views in any way. The most striking feature of this study, therefore, is the lack of association of either of these psychosocial changes to menopausal status or symptoms.

Methodologically Crawford and Hooper's was a poorly designed study, but similar results were reported by Lowenthal and Chiriboga (1972). Using in-depth interviewing and assessment techniques, they looked in some detail at the effect the imminent departure of a child from the home had on a small group of climacteric women. The main measure was a life evaluation chart by means of which the subjects rated different periods of their lives according to the satisfaction they had provided.

For only three women was their present phase of life rated lowest relative to others, and for none of them did these low ratings have anything to do with the impending departure of their youngest child. Furthermore, in response to direct questioning in interview, very few saw the departure of children as a turning point in their lives or as a particular source of frustration. In those instances where such an event was described as a "turning point," the child had departed from home under unhappy circumstances. While several women reported marital difficulties, none indicated that these problems were in any way connected with the impending empty nest. These authors concluded that "neither responses to specific questions about critical periods and problems nor the content of these detailed protocols as a whole convey the impression that the prospects of the departure of the youngest child are in any way threatening for this pre-empty nest sample" (p. 14).

In a later study, the second of these authors further examined the impact of the empty nest on men and women in middle life (Krystal and Chiriboga, 1979). This unique study is the only longitudinal study of its kind in this area. The subjects, 45 middle-aged men and women, most of whom were expected to be exposed to the empty nest process, were followed up over a five-year period as they went through this experience. Each subject was assessed initially, and again after one and a half and then after five years, using the Bradburn Morale Scale, which is similar in content to symptom checklists used in other studies, and an Activity Checklist, designed by one of the authors. At each assessment point, which one of three "empty nest" conditions prevailed was determined for each subject. These were Full (all children still at home), Partial (at least one child had left home but not all) and Empty (all children left home).

The only significant differences to emerge for those experiencing a changing situation were that women changing from a Full or Partial to an Empty nest showed a significant *decrease* in one of the 18 Morale Scales, namely, depression. In general, the pattern of change suggests that women who are well into the transition, or who are fully through it, have reorganized their life styles to accommodate the increase in free time and change of role. None of the findings of this study support a "crisis theory," the authors concluding that "the overall impression obtained was one of positive rather than negative reactions to the empty nest and that the so-called crisis of the empty nest is more a collective myth than an experiential reality" (p. 219).

In a study of a clinical sample of Australian women, Schneider and Brotherton (1979) using the Beck Depression Inventory, examined a number of psychosocial factors, including the departure of children from home, in relation to psychiatric depression. The main findings were that depressed women showed a significantly greater frequency of marital dissatisfaction, economic difficulty, early developmental disturbance, and "role impairment." The last referred to a lack of interest or inability to function adequately either at work or in respect to interpersonal roles. Stress associated with the loss of the reproductive function, the care of aged parents, changes in parental role and such precipitating factors as death or illness of loved ones was not significantly different between the depressed and nondepressed groups. The authors conclude that their results support the view "that premorbid functioning and personality are important predictors of a woman's ability to cope with the stresses of the menopausal period" (p. 157). In short, the significance of this study is that depressive symptoms at the time of the menopause are not precipitated by psychosocial factors thought to be peculiar to that time but are related more to general, chronic, and preexisting problems.

Like Krystal and Chiriboga (1979), Uphold and Susman (1981) also investigated the relationship between symptom severity and stages of childrearing in a group of 185 climacteric women. There were three such stages: prelaunching (all children at home), transitional (some children at home), empty nest (no children at home). Marital adjustment was also assessed with the Dyadic Adjustment Scale. The main finding was that, throughout the climacteric, women low on marital adjustment had more numerous and more severe symptoms than did those who had good marital relations. There was no evidence that child rearing stage was related to symptoms in any way; women low on marital adjustment show the same high frequency and severity of symptoms at all child rearing stages. These effects are illustrated for mean number of symptoms in Table 7 and appear quite convincing.

These findings refer to the sample of women as a whole. When women were subdivided according to menopausal status, menopausal women were found to have many more symptoms than did those who were pre- or postmenopausal. However, this increase in nonspecific symptoms at the menopause occurred largely in those women who had a poor marital relationship. As there was no apparent worsening of this relationship among these women at the time of the menopause, the increase in symptoms at that time is clearly exacerbated by an already existing poor marital situation.

Table 7

Mean Number of Symptoms in Relation to Marital Adjustment and Child Rearing
Stages (Uphold and Susman, 1981)

Child Rearing Stage	Marital Adjustment		
	Low	High	Total
Prelaunching	12.1	9.2	10.6
Transitional	13.3	10.1	11.8
Empty nest	12.5	10.0	11.2
Total	12.9	9.9	

The authors conclude that the quality of a woman's marriage is a potent factor in influencing her reactions during the climacteric. They rightly point out that such a conclusion regarding the marital relationship per se must be tentative as the quality of the relationship may be a reflection of poor emotional adaptation in general. Furthermore, this influence appears to be particularly marked at the perimenopause, suggesting that at that time women experiencing poor marital relationships are particularly vulnerable. Of added interest in this study is, of course, the failure once again to find any association between symptoms and the departure of children from home.

A summary of the outcome of studies reviewed in this section can be found in Table 8. Despite a widespread belief, there is little evidence that the departure of children from home has a serious effect on climacteric women, certainly in terms of contributing to symptomatology. There is, however, some suggestion that when it does have such an effect, the child has either left home in unhappy circumstances or relationships within the family have been overprotective (Levit, 1963; Bart, 1971; Lowenthal and Chiriboga, 1972). It is probable, therefore, that these infrequent instances—mostly occurring perhaps, among clinical groups—have given rise to the widespread idea that loss of maternal role may precipitate adverse reactions in a substantial number of climacteric women.

The evidence, such as it is, indicates that circumstances peculiar to the time of the climacteric, such as the departure of children from home and the loss of reproductive and child-rearing functions are not those which to any great degree make women more susceptible to symptoms at that time of life. On the contrary, such symptoms appear to be associated more with preexisting problems such as marital

Table 8

Summary of Studies Investigating Effects of Interpersonal Factors on Climacteric Women

Authors	Country	Type of Population	Outcome Measures	Factors Not Related to Outcome Measures	Factors Related to Outcome Measures
Van Keep and Kellerhals (1974)	Switzerland	General (Random)	Climacteric index, other functions		Absence of children during premenopause
Holte and Mikkelsen (1982)	Norway	General (Random)	Six symptom factors		Quality of social network
Crawford and Hooper (1973)	England	General, clinic	Self reported symptoms	Absence of children from home; Departure of children, arrival of grandchild, marital adjustment	
Lowenthal and Chiriboga (1972)	USA	Not reported	Life evaluation chart	Pre-empty nest	
Krystal and Chiriboga (1979)	USA	Not reported	Morale scale activity checklist	Stages of child rearing	
Schneider and Brotherton (1979)	Australia	Clinic	Beck depression inventory	Loss of reproductive function, empty nest, aging parents	Marital problems, economic difficulties, problems in adolescence, role impairment
Uphold and Susman (1981)	USA	General, clinic	Symptom questionnaire	Stages of child rearing	Marital adjustment
Abe and Moritsuka (1986)	Japan	General, clinic	Symptom questionnaire		Quality of social network

dissatisfaction, financial difficulties, limited social networks and support systems, and earlier premenstrual difficulties. Although, like poor socioeconomic conditions, these problems may provoke symptoms and complaints in women at any time of life, there is good reason for thinking that women experiencing these adversities may suffer more during their climacteric years,

LIFE EVENTS AND THE MENOPAUSE

A relatively recent development in menopause research has been the application of the methodology of life event research to the investigation of the effect of adverse psychosocial factors on women during the climacteric. Life event research is that field of research concerned with the association between the onset of illness and the occurrence of recent events or changes in the individual's physical and social environment. The idea that the occurrence of discrete life events, particularly stressful ones, may precipitate physical, psychosomatic, or psychiatric conditions is not new. Such ideas have a long history both in popular and scientific thinking. However, it was not until the last two decades that a systematic method of assessing stressful life events and their relation to illness was developed.

Life Event Methodology

Three separate but overlapping methods of measuring life events can be distinguished. Historically, the first was that of Holmes and Rahe (1967), whose pioneering work in the mid-60s in overcoming the inherent circularity of attempting to measure stress by its effects—that is, in terms of illness or symptoms—led to systematic research into life event stress as we now know it.

Their original measure consisted of a checklist of 43 discrete events, the degree of change or adjustment necessitated by each being determined by a method of quantification based on consensus scaling. Consensus scaling was achieved by having a group of normal subjects assign to each event a rating based on the amount of change in the pattern of life that event would require from the average person, irrespective of its desirability. These ratings were expressed in relation to marriage, which was assigned a fixed score of 50. The result is a checklist of events, each given a weight equal to the mean of these ratings.

Subsequently, for any individual, the weights of each event reported are summated to yield a Total Life Change Score based on a population consensus, independent of the individual's own reaction to the event, which is usually the presence of illness or symptoms. In most life event research, events experienced by the subject are recorded in retrospect from within a fixed time period, six months or one year, prior to the onset of the illness or symptoms.

The second method of measuring life events, developed by Eugene Paykel and his colleagues, is similar in general principles to that of Holmes and Rahe. It too is a checklist approach in which the severity of the effect of an event is based on consensually derived judgments. However, there are some important differences. Paykel, Prusoff, and Uhlenhuth (1971) conceive of stress in terms of the degree of upset produced by the event. They argue that unpleasant events and pleasant events will have different effects, although the individuals involved may require the same amount of readjustment according to Holmes and Rahe's criteria. Paykel's method of arriving at weights for different life events also differs from that of Holmes and Rahe in that normal subjects were asked to judge how upsetting each event might be for the average person. Judgment was by means of a 0 (least upsetting) to 20 (most upsetting) equal interval rating procedure with no event fixed. Weights derived in this way have been found to be remarkably consistent and stable across different social and national groups (Paykel, McGuiness, and Gomez, 1976)

Paykel and his colleagues have also devised a system of categorizing life events. In this system events are subdivided in three ways: Area of Activity (e.g., health, family, employment, marital, legal); their Desirability or Undesirability; and the social field of the subject, that is, whether they involve people coming into (Entrances) or leaving (Exits). Using the weights for each life event derived from the consensus scaling procedure, as with the Holmes and Rahe method, a Total Life Stress Score can be calculated for any individual subject. In addition, separate stress scores can be calculated for any individual for each of the foregoing categories of life events using the same weights.

Although similar in principle, Paykel's method of measuring life events is a more refined one than that of Holmes and Rahe.

The third method of assessing life events, that of Brown and Harris (1978), departs from that of other researchers in regarding as the most critical factor the implications of an event for the individual rather than any consensual rating of its importance. The logic of regarding the implications of an event for the individual as important produces a radically different way of eliciting reports of events. In assessing the personal implication of the event for an individual, the context and circumstances surrounding the event must be taken into account. Accordingly, Brown and Harris dispense with the method of eliciting life events through the checklist approach; instead they use lengthy and extensive interviews carried out by specially trained interviewers. In this way details of all the circumstances surrounding any event and the context within which it occurs are obtained. On the basis of this information, rather than by means of consensual weights, the degree of contextual threat of an event for the particular individual is determined.

Despite the marked difference in method, the broad empirical findings of Brown and Harris are remarkably similar to those of Paykel and his co-workers, as Andrews and Tennant (1978) point out, especially in regard to the influence of life events on psychiatric conditions. Indeed, most researchers prefer the checklist method, presumably because of its easy use. However, Brown and Harris's unique contribution has been the development of a theoretical model that uses intervening variables, such as vulnerability, moderating variables, and symptom formation factors, to link life events to psychiatric depression in women (Brown and Harris, 1978). This model, as will be seen shortly, is of some relevance to the subject of the menopause.

Studies of Life Events and the Menopause

Menopause in fact appears as an item on the Paykel checklist, presumably because it is similar to any other event in that it requires a degree of readjustment. The rating it obtains on the consensus scaling in a general population sample places it well down the list, with the rating of British and American samples being very similar (Paykel et al., 1976). The only other study to examine menopause as a life event in any detail is an American study by Kahana, Kiyak, and Liang (1980), who investigated its perceived readjustment value in a group of young women (college students) and older women (over 60 years) and groups of men of a similar age range. For this purpose the Holmes and Rahe (1967) checklist was modified to include the menopause and other items thought relevant to an older population. The method for obtaining consensual judgments was the same as that of Holmes and Rahe.

In general, women rated the menopause as requiring little readjustment when compared with other life events. There were no differences between the ratings of younger and older women, although men, especially older ones, tended to rate it as requiring greater readjustment. Black women, however, were found to rate the menopause as requiring almost twice the degree of readjustment as did white women, a finding the authors attribute to low socioeconomic status along with domestic and family factors.

These findings and conclusions are not unlike those described earlier, in the attitude section of this chapter. Indeed, to some extent, Kahana and her colleagues are using life event methods to assess attitudes of different groups toward the menopause, whereas traditionally life event researchers have been concerned with determining the impact of life events on individuals in terms of symptoms or illness. This approach characterizes the few other life event researchers, who have used the menopause as an intervening variable, or the symptoms thereof as dependent variables. To date there have been only three such studies.

The first of these is by Resnick (1984; see also Severne and Greene, 1986), who reported a study of the relationships between significant life events and sources of stress on the one hand, and chronological age and menopausal status, on the other, in a group of 145 healthy American women in the age range 36–75 years. Life events were assessed using the Holmes and Rahe (1967) Social Readjustment Rating Scale modified for an older female population. Life events were categorized into five groups on the basis of their content: marital, family, work, personal relationships, finance. Total stress scores were found to be related to neither chronological age nor menopausal status. The only significant finding in respect to the subcategories was that stress scores were negatively related to age for both work and finance categories, a not unsurprising finding. Thus, none of the categories of life event stress was greater at the menopause than at any other time.

Resnick suggests that these generally negative results were due to the use of preselected categories of life events with predetermined weights. In an attempt to make the measures more personalized, a method was used by which subjects were asked detailed questions about the most satisfying event, the most difficult event, and so on, that had occurred in the previous year. The most interesting findings to emerge were that, although comments relating to children were not uncommon, women seldom referred to children leaving home as a problem. Frequently mentioned as positive life events were work-related and other types of "mastery" experiences. Events relating to interpersonal relationships also featured highly, with deaths and illness of others being particularly mentioned as areas of concern. These findings, in general, are consistent with those of others using investigative techniques other than the life event one and, as will be seen, anticipate some of the findings from other life event research in this area.

As no measure of symptoms was included in Resnick's (1974) study, it was not possible to determine what relationships, if any, existed between adverse reactions and life events at the climacteric. Several measures of symptomatology as well as life events were included in a life event study of Australian women by Ballinger (1985) in an investigation of the differences between a patient group consisting of 123 women attending a menopause clinic and a control group of 164 women selected from among women at a shopping center. Groups were matched for geographic and socioeconomic variables. Life events were assessed using a questionnaire derived from the 67-item Tennant-Andrews Scale (Tennant and Andrews, 1976), which had been designed for use with an Australian urban population. This instrument yields three measures of life events—total events, change, and distress. Ballinger also included a measure of "coping with stress," using a rating method based on a semistructured interview. Climacteric symptoms were classified according to whether they were hypothalamic, meta-bolic, or psychological.

The main findings were that the patient group was significantly higher on all three measures of life event stress, reported more climacteric symptoms, especially psychological ones, and had poorer coping skills than did the control group. Thus, not only did patients report more life events, they also perceived the same events as causing more distress and change in their lives. Nevertheless, within each group, life event measures and symptom measures were by and large uncorrelated, although the stress coping measure was the one found to be most highly correlated with psychological symptoms.

In the light of these findings, Ballinger concludes that, for the most part, psychological symptoms at the menopause cannot be a direct result of stressful life events. She proposes a model whereby "physical vulnerability, brought on by hormonal changes, interacts with psy-chological vulnerability to life stress so that those with good coping skills are better able to override the effects of hormonal changes and so suffer fewer and less severe psychological symptoms" (p. 326).

Ballinger's resort to the use of the concept of vulnerability is of some interest, for although she does not cite his work, this concept has a central role in the life event model devised by George Brown (Brown and Harris, 1978) to account for why life events provoke psychiatric depression only in certain women. In this model, vulnerability, by definition, does not have an effect in itself but increases the risk or severity of symptoms in the presence of other factors, for example, life events. Brown's model has greatly influenced the present author in the development of a life event vulnerability model of the climacteric (Greene, 1984) into which Brown's other important concept, symptom formation factor, is incorporated. The latter refers to factors that determine the type and nature of the symptoms provoked.

This model was constructed on the basis of relationships between life events and symptoms among women of different ages that had emerged in the study, referred to earlier, of an adult population of Scottish women (Greene and Cooke, 1980; Greene, 1983). In that study, symptoms were assessed by means of two scales, one repre-senting psychological, the other somatic symptoms. These scales, it will be recalled, had been constructed on the basis of a factor analysis (Greene, 1976). Life events were measured by a combination of the

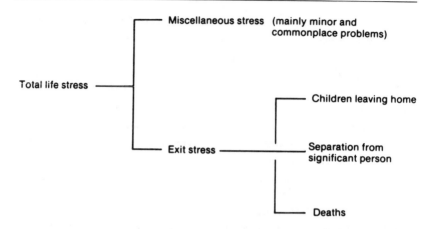

FIG. 5   Breakdown of main categories of life stress during the climacteric. (From Greene, 1984.)

methods of Brown and Paykel in which, in the course of a semistructured interview, events were elicited using the Paykel checklist and scored using his consensually derived weights. In this way, total life stress scores were obtained, as well as stress scores for different categories of events. The two main categories of events found to be of relevance in the study were "Exits" (departures of others from the social field of the subject) and "Miscellaneous" events (what is left after exits are taken out, consisting of a mixed group of everyday problems arising from work, illness, finance, housing, etc.). In this study sample, Exits comprised deaths, departure of children, and departure of significant others, in that order. Figure 5 shows this breakdown of life events.

Climacteric Vulnerability

The concept of climacteric vulnerability is based mainly on differences found between preclimacteric women (in their 30s) and climacteric women (in their 40s), in the relationship between life event stress and psychological symptoms. These differences were as follows:

1. There was no difference between preclimacteric and climacteric women in the severity of miscellaneous life stress.

2. Psychological symptoms, however, were significantly more frequent among climacteric than among preclimacteric women.
3. Among preclimacteric women there was no significant correlation between the severity of miscellaneous life stress and psychological symptoms ($r = 0.12$)
4. Among climacteric women there was a highly significant correlation between the severity of miscellaneous life stress and psychological symptoms ($r = 0.46$; $p < 0.001$).

From this pattern of results it was inferred that women experiencing a high degree of miscellaneous life event stress become less able to cope with such stress as they enter the climacteric and that they express this inability to cope in the form of increased psychological symptoms. Hence the notion of greater vulnerability to life events during the climacteric period of life. The increase in psychological symptoms, therefore, is a response to a nonspecific group of life events.

Symptom Formation

The concept of symptom formation factors, on the other hand, was based on the finding that somatic symptoms were significantly more severe in women who had experienced a more specific type of life event, namely, a recent bereavement, usually due to the death of a close friend or a member of their natal family. Such bereavements were, as might be expected, more common among climacteric than among preclimacteric women. The somatic form of these symptoms was thought to be influenced by those of the deceased or, alternatively, were an exacerbation of existing physical climacteric symptoms. Hence the classification of bereavement as a symptom formation factor. It was also considered that the sensitivity of these women to the death of members of their natal family was due to the close familial ties existing within this particular population and the consequent loss of social support as a result of the death.

This model is illustrated in Figure 6. There certain factors are classified as *provoking agents*—in this case life events, usually capable on their own of producing symptoms or illness. Others are classified as *vulnerability factors*, which do not themselves have an effect but

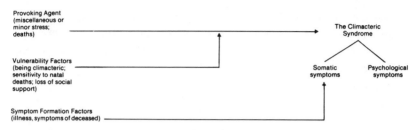

Fig. 6   A life event vulnerability model of the climacteric. (From Greene, 1984.)

increase the risk of illness or the severity of symptoms in the presence of a provoking agent. The climacteric is classified as a vulnerability factor since, as found in the study, life events provoke symptoms to a greater degree at that time of life than they do during the preclimacteric. A third set of factors included in this model are *symptom formation factors*, such as the illness of a deceased person, which can influence the nature of the symptoms experienced or the form the stress reaction takes. In this model, vulnerability and symptom formation factors are viewed as intervening variables that determine respectively the severity and the form of the woman's reactions to life stress during the climacteric.

CONCLUSION

In the foregoing model, the vulnerability of climacteric women to stressful life events is seen as arising from the fact that at that phase of their life span they are passing through a time of physical, psychological, and social transition that requires some degree of readjustment that places demands on their physical and mental resources. Thus, women experiencing stressful life events have additional demands placed on these resources and, for some, these demands are manifested in the form of "illness behavior." This concept of vulnerability can, of course, be applied to encompass the manner in which other psychosocial factors induce adverse reaction among women at that stage in their lives. We have seen, for example, that broad sociodemographic factors are associated with an elevation of symptoms during the climacteric years, especially around the time of the menopause. It has been hypothesized that these factors exercise their effect largely by the extent to which they either impel postmenopausal women to develop personally satisfying or socially significant roles or prevent them from doing so. Concerns regarding one's future role in life would seem natural during this transitional phase of life, in which the menopause acts as a developmental marker. Attitudes of women toward this marker and their expectancies of its consequences would therefore play an important contributory role in the elevation of symptoms and complaints, for instance, illness behavior. Vulnerability would also mediate the symptomatic effects of those other adverse personal and social problems which predate the climacteric, such as an unsatisfactory marital relationship or a limited social network. Finally, climacteric vulnerability could also exacerbate an already present psychological condition or make a former one recur, such as in the case of a woman with a longstanding chronic depressive condition or a recurring anxiety state.

Implicit in the idea of vulnerability is the assumption that neither the climacteric nor the menopause need itself be associated with illness behavior of either a physical or psychological nature. Vulnerability is a potential state that does not by itself provoke symptoms or illness but requires other etiological factors to be present, the effects of which it serves to mediate. We have seen that these factors are many and come from different conceptual domains—cultural, sociological and psychological. A point has been reached where it is not only possible, but also necessary, because of the many etiological factors involved, for researchers to construct clear psychosocial models of the climacteric (Greene and Lock, 1987). These would not only specify the nature and direction of causal relationships, but also provide heuristic hypotheses to guide future research.

REFERENCES

Abe, T. & Moritsuka, T. (1986), A case control study on climacteric symptoms and complaints of Japanese women by symptomatic type for psychological variables. *Maturitas*, 8:255–265.

Andrews, G. & Tennant, C. (1978), Life event stress and psychiatric illness. *Psychol. Med.*, 8:545–549.

Ballinger, S. (1985), Psychosocial stress and symptoms of menopause: a comparative study of menopause clinic patients and non-patients. *Maturitas*, 7:315–327.

Bart, P. (1971), Depression in middle-aged women. In: *Women in Sexist Society*, ed. V. Gornick & B. Moran. New York: Basic Books, pp. 99–117.

Brown, G. & Harris, T. (1978), *The Social Origins of Depression: A Study of Psychiatric Disorder in Women*. London: Tavistock.

Campagnoli, C., Morra, G., Belforte, P., Belforte, L. & Tousijn, L. P. (1981), Climacteric symptoms according to body weight in women of different socio-economic groups. *Maturitas*, 3:279–287.

Crawford, M. & Hooper, D. (1973), Menopause, aging and family. *Soc. Sci. Med.*, 7:469–482.

Dege, K. & Gretzinger, J. (1982), Attitudes of families toward menopause. In: *Changing Perspectives on Menopause*, ed. A. Voda, M. Dinnerstein & S. O'Donnell. Austin: University of Texas Press, pp. 60–69.

Eisner, H. & Kelly, L. (1980), Attitudes of women toward the menopause. Presented at meeting of the American Gerontological Society. San Diego, CA.

Garde, K. & Lunde, I. (1980), Social background and social status: Influence on female sexual behavior. A random sample study of 40-year old Danish women. *Maturitas*, 2:241–246.

Greene, J. G. (1976), A factor analytic study of climacteric symptoms. *J. Psychosom. Res.*, 20:425–430.

———— (1983), Bereavement and social support at the climacteric. *Maturitas*, 5:115–124.

———— (1984), *The Social and Psychological Origins of the Climacteric Syndrome*. Brookfield, VT: Gower.

———— (1987), Factor analyses of climacteric symptoms. Presented at a meeting of the Italian Menopause Society, Rome, Italy.

———— & Cooke, D. J. (1980), Life stress and symptoms at the climacteric. *Brit. J. Psychiat.*, 136:486–491.

Greene, J. G. & Lock, M. (1987), Psychosocial models of the climacteric. In: *The Climacteric and Beyond.*, ed. L. Zichella, M. Whitehead & P. A. van Keep. Park Ridge, NJ: Parthenon, pp. 155–167.

Hallstrom, T. (1977), Sexuality in the climacteric. *Clin. Obstet. Gynaecol.*, 4:227–239.

Holmes, T. H. & Rahe, R. H. (1967), The social readjustment rating scale. *J. Psychosom. Res.*, 11:213–218.

Holte, A. & Mikkelsen, A. (1982), Menstrual coping style, social background and climacteric symptoms. *Psychiat. Soc. Sci.*, 2:41–45.

Hunter, M. (1987), A cognitive-interactional approach to the menopause. Presented at the Fifth International Congress on the Menopause, Sorrento, Italy.

Hunter, M., Battersby, R. & Whitehead, M. (1986), Relationships between psychological symptoms, somatic complaints and menopausal status. *Maturitas*, 8:217–228.

International Health Foundation (1969), *A Study of the Attitudes of Women in Belgium, France, Great Britain, Italy and West Germany*. Brussels: I. H. F.

Jaszmann, L., Van Lith, N. & Zaat, J. (1969), The perimenopausal symptoms: The statistical analysis of a survey. *Med. Gynaecol. Sociol.*, 4:268–277.

Kahana, E., Kiyak, A. & Liang, J. (1980), Menopause in the context of other life events. In: *The Menstrual Cycle.*, ed. A. Dan, E. Graham & C. Beecher. New York: Springer, pp. 167–178.

Krystal, S. & Chiriboga, D. (1979), The empty nest process in mid-life men and women. *Maturitas*, 1:215–222.

Leiblum, S. R. & Swartzmann, L. C. (1986), Woman's attitude towards the menopause: An update. *Maturitas*, 8:47–56.

Levit, L. (1963), Anxiety and the menopause: A study of normal women. Unpublished doctoral dissertation, University of Chicago.

Lincoln, N. L. (1980), Women's attitudes towards menopause as related to self-esteem. Unpublished doctoral dissertation, Yale University.

Lowenthal, M. F. & Chiriboga, D. (1972), Transitions to the empty nest: Crisis, challenge or relief. *Arch. Gen. Psychiat.*, 26:8–14.

McKinlay, S. & Jeffreys, M. (1974), The menopausal syndrome. *Brit. J. Prev. Soc. Med.*, 28:108–115.

Neugarten, B., Wood, V., Kraines, R. & Loomis, B. (1963), Women's attitudes toward the menopause. *Vita Humana*, 6:140–151.

Paykel, E. S., McGuiness, B. & Gomez, J. (1976). An Anglo-American comparison of the scaling of life events. *Brit. J. Med. Psychol.*, 49:237–247.

_____ Prusoff, B. A. & Uhlenhuth, E. H. (1971), Scaling of life events. *Arch. Gen. Psychiat.*, 25:340–347

Perlmutter, E. & Bart, P. B. (1982), Changing views of "the change": A critical review and suggestion for an attributional approach. In: *Changing Perspectives on Menopause*, ed. A. Voda, M. Dinnerstein & S. O'Donnell. Austin: University of Texas Press, pp. 187–199.

Polit, D. & Larocco, S. (1980), Social and psychological correlates of the menopausal symptoms. *Psychosom. Med.*, 42:335–345.

Prill, H. J. (1977), A study of the socio-medical relationship at the climacteric in 2232 women. *Curr. Med. Res. Opin.*, 4:46–51

Resnick, J. (1984), Significant life events and sources of stress in healthy climacteric women. Presented at the Fourth International Congress on the Menopause, Orlando, FL.

Schneider, M. & Brotherton, P. (1979), Physiological, psychological and situational stress in depression during the climacteric. *Maturitas*, 1,153–158.

Seligman, M. E. P. (1980), *Human Helplessness: Theory and Application.* New York: Academic Press.

Severne, L. (1979), Psycho-social aspects of the menopause. In: *Psychosomatics in Peri-Menopause*, ed. A. Haspels & H. Musaph. Lancaster, Eng.: M. T. P. Press, pp. 101–120.

_____ Greene, J. G. (1986), Lifestyles: Coping with life events and stress at the climacteric. In: *The Climacteric in Perspective*, ed. M. Notelovitz & P. van Keep. Lancaster, Eng.: M. T. P. Press, pp. 299–313.

Tennant, C. & Andrews, G. (1976), A scale to measure the stress of life events. *Aust. N. Z. J. Psychiat.*, 10:27–32.

Uphold, C. & Susman, E. (1981), Self reported climacteric symptoms as a function of the relationship between marital adjustment and child rearing stages. *Nursing Res.*, 30:84–88.

Van Keep, P. & Kellerhals, J. (1974), The impact of socio-cultural factors on symptom formation: Some results of a study on aging women in Switzerland. *Psychother. Psychosom.*, 23:251–263.

5

Aging into Transitions

Cross-Cultural Perspectives on Women at Midlife

NANCY DATAN

This chapter examines the implications of findings from a broad-scale study designed to explore the relationship between culture and psychological well-being in middle age. Ethnic identity was used as an approximate measure of the degree of modernity of middle-aged women in five Israeli subcultures: Israel-born Moslem Arabs, and immigrant Jews born in North Africa, Persia, Turkey, and Central Europe. Although all the women were born in the same decade, 1915–1924, each was born into an ethnic group representing a different cultural configuration and a different stage in the process of social change.

This chapter was written after Nancy Datan's death in May 1987. It was constructed by her husband, Dean Rodeheaver, from memories, presentations, and publications: *A Time to Reap: The Middle Age of Women in Five Israeli Subcultures*, written by Nancy Datan, Aaron Antonovsky, and Benjamin Maoz and published in 1981 by the Johns Hopkins University Press, is the complete account of the study described here; "Aging into Transitions: Cross-Cultural Perspectives on Women at Midlife" was presented originally by Nancy Datan at the meetings of the American Psychological Association in 1986; finally, colloquium material presented periodically from 1977 to 1987 is also included. These represent Nancy's most recent thoughts on the research and its implications for women's lives in a changing world.

This chapter is also the product of the encouragement and assistance of Ruth Formanek.

The study was the work of three people—medical sociologist Aaron Antonovsky, psychiatrist Benjamin Maoz, and developmental psychologist Nancy Datan—and originated in Maoz's observation that Israeli women from Near Eastern and North African countries were seldom hospitalized for "involutional depression,"[1] especially when compared with women of European origin. This observation was confirmed by Antonovsky's review of Israeli national health statistics: National incidence of involutional psychosis among women of Near Eastern origin was virtually nil. Given the enormous variations in cultural conditions that Jewish immigrants to Israel represent, Maoz and Antonovsky speculated that the incidence of involutional psychosis reflected cultural differences in stressful or supportive climates for the middle age of women. Specifically, they hypothesized that stress in middle age is a function of modern, youth-oriented European culture and is manifest in both the extreme response of involutional depression in some women and nonpathological distress in normal women. The overvaluation of youth and concomitant devaluation of middle age and old age for women in modern cultures make menopause a transition to a devalued status. In addition, the researchers suggested, the tendency toward active coping among modern women leads to frustration since menopause is an uncontrollable transition. This hypothesis was supported by psychoanalytic views on menopause, exemplified by Helene Deutsch's (1945) claim that menopause represented a "a closing of the gates"; the loss of fertility, an omen of aging and death (p. 478). By contrast, women in traditional cultures, having borne more children, have had the fullest possible expression of their femininity. Menopause ends years of uninterrupted childbearing, brings relief and no regrets, and signals a transition to the elevated status of matriarch.

I joined the study after this hypothesis had been formulated and offered a contradictory view to what I have come to call the Quantitative or Rabbit Theory of Femininity: Stress is a function of culture, but it is lowest among European women, who have roles—inside and outside the home—other than childrearing. These women have already coped with previous developmental tasks, as Neugarten, Wood,

---

[1]Involutional depression refers to the psychological consequences of the climacterium and menopause. Its status as a separate nosological entity is questionable.

Kraines, and Loomis (1963) showed with an American sample. Furthermore, childrearing by these women ended years before menopause. Consequently, the incidence of involutional depression was not a reflection of the end of fertility. By contrast, traditional women experience more stress during menopause because their major roles are childbearing and childrearing. The loss of fertility deprives them of the sole source of prestige available to them in their culture.

In addition to these two contradictory, primary hypotheses, two ancillary explanations were formulated:

1. Stress is not a function of culture but the *expression* of stress is. European women experience more psychiatric symptoms whereas Near Eastern women experience somatic symptoms.

2. Stress is not a function of culture, but the diagnosis of depression is. The difference arises from cultural conditions, leading European women to communicate psychic distress and doctors to observe psychiatric symptoms in these women.

THE FACES OF EVE:
THE FIVE ETHNIC GROUPS

The ethnic groups in this study were chosen to represent broad variations in women's cultural experiences, forming crude approximations to a continuum anchored at one end by the traditional Moslem Arab woman and at the other by the modern Central European woman. As Jews and Moslems, the ethnic groups share a religious heritage: all are subject to laws found in Leviticus and elaborated in the Talmud and the Koran governing the sexual and family life cycle of women. Rituals of separation, sexual proscription, cleanliness, and appearance characterize both religious traditions. The diversity in these women's experiences, though, is suggested by the difference between the traditional woman, who is illiterate, who is devoutly orthodox, whose husband was chosen for her, and who has borne children almost continually since menarche; and the modern woman, who has had at least a high school education, who has moved away from orthodoxy toward secularism, who chose her own husband, and who, having planned her childbearing, has only one or two children.

Table 1 provides a comparison of the five ethnic groups on selected

Table 1
Selected Social Characteristics by Ethnic Group (Percentages)[1]

Item	Central Europeans	Turks	Persians	North Africans	Arabs
Ethnic group					
N =	(287)	(176)	(160)	(239)	(286)
Illiterate	0	29	61	60	96
Married before age 16	0	5	35	37	30
Married at age 21 or older	78	51	15	20	22
Husband selected by family	7	46	75	56	95
Conflict with family over choice of spouse	17	23	42	28	16
Seven or more pregnancies[2]	8	19	64	67	79
One-half or fewer of pregnancies brought to live birth[2]	47	17	6	4	4
Seven or more live births[2]	0	5	53	59	72
No children dead after birth[2]	92	77	52	42	22
Five or more living children	0	14	68	68	76
Five or more children currently living at home	0	3	29	36	53
Children now under age 14	16	30	47	57	56
Total childbearing span less than 7 years	70	35	13	20	10
Satisfied with number of children borne	28	47	39	48	59
Wishing to have borne more children	68	38	35	42	19
Wishing to have borne fewer children	3	16	26	10	22
Grandchildren	32	62	79	76	78
Working outside the home (full or part time, including family business or agriculture)	42	21	29	25	35
Feels "needed" by extended family member	46	60	62	51	17
Husband illiterate	0	25	49	53	66
Husband nonmanual worker	77	36	16	22	12
Currently religiously orthodox	21	30	57	85	98
Currently believe family should choose spouse	1	12	21	19	52

[1]From Datan, Antonovsky, and Maoz (1981, p. 18).
[2]Percentage based on medical subsamples.

social characteristics. The modal Central European woman represents the most modern group in the study (modernity is defined below under Method), a modernity that grew out of a European education and the Reform movement among European Jewry. She was educated to at least secondary school in her native country and, having migrated to Israel before or shortly after World War II, has the problems of relocation behind her. She married late—in her early twenties—and chose her husband, who is now most likely a white-collar worker or a professional. About two-fifths of these women work outside the home, one-half of them full time. Hard economic times during the time Israel gained its independence forced these women to bear few children and to delay having them. Childbearing was planned and the number of children restricted by contraceptives and abortion. Consequently, the modal Central European woman wishes that she had borne more children, and, although she is menopausal, she is unlikely to be a grandmother or living in an "empty nest." Finally, only about one-fifth describe themselves as orthodox—most observe only some or no religious rituals.

The Turkish women in the study may be considered transitional in two ways: They are less modern than the Central European women, and there is considerable variation within this ethnic group. Consequently, it is more difficult to describe the modal Turkish woman. Although she did not progress beyond elementary school, the Turkish woman has received some education and is literate. She married at about the age of twenty, as likely to a husband of her own choosing as to one her family chose for her. She came to Israel as a young adult during World War II or in the 1950s during the mass exodus of Jews from Arab countries. Although she arrived in Israel at about the same time as the Central European woman, the Turkish woman is less well-to-do. Her husband is at best lower middle class and is most likely a laborer or skilled manual worker. She had one or two more children than the European woman and, having married earlier, is already a grandmother; she also still may have school-age children living at home. Modernization of religious and social values has occurred during her lifetime, both under Ataturk and in the urban areas of Israel in which she lives, and she is herself transitional: About one-fifth of the Turkish women work outside the home; most do not believe a girl's family should chose her husband for her, and most observe few religious rituals.

Like the Turks, the Persian women most likely migrated to Israel between 1948 and 1955, following the establishment of the state of Israel. Unlike the Turks, with whom they live side-by-side in a heterogeneous urban area, the Persians have not made transitions toward modernization. The modal Persian woman can neither read nor write. She married early—at about 16 years of age—to a man chosen by her family (sometimes over her opposition) and had a large family, perhaps seven children or more; about half of the Persian women still have children under age 14 living at home. She is most likely also a grandmother. About two-fifths of the Persian women work outside the home, usually as unskilled manual workers, a status shared by their husbands, who are also uneducated, unskilled, and often welfare cases. Although she most likely considers herself orthodox or observes some traditional religious practices, her transitional status is reflected in her belief that a girl should chose her own husband and in her regrets at having borne too many children. Tensions resulting from a traditional personal life style amid societal transitions toward modernity, exacerbated by economic disadvantage, are probably greater for the Persians than for any other ethnic group in the study.

During the exodus of Jews from Arab countries, the upper stratum of North African Jewry migrated to France while the uneducated and unskilled fled to Israel. The modal North African woman was about 35 years old then. She received, at best, an elementary school education and is quite likely to be illiterate. She married early, perhaps before age 16, usually to a man chosen by her family with her approval, is likely to have been pregnant at least seven times and has borne seven or more children. Some of her children, still under age 14, live at home; others have children of their own. About one-fourth of the North African women are employed outside the home, usually at unskilled work. Like the Persians, North African men are likely to be unskilled workers or welfare recipients. Unlike the Persians and the Turks, the North Africans lived in a relatively homogeneous community and have not shifted toward modern values—they remain religiously and socially traditional.

The Moslem Arab woman was born into the traditional village life she still leads—her personal and cultural experiences exhibit the greatest continuity of all the groups. She almost certainly is illiterate, married early (at about 17) to a man chosen by her family and approved by her, and has borne children for a major part of her life. She has lost many children through miscarriage, stillbirth, and death in infancy and childhood but still has borne seven or more children. Although she is a grandmother, at least five of her children are still at home. Over one-third of the Arab women work outside the home, usually at agriculture. In both religious practice and social values she is traditional, believing the family should choose a girl's husband for her and characterizing herself as religiously observant.

In sum, the five ethnic groups share religious traditions regarding the sexual and family life cycle of women, but their observance of those traditions ranges from the reforms of the Central Europeans to the ritual observance of the Moslem Arabs, a diversity that is also reflected in educational, work, and childbearing experiences.

METHOD

The study was carried out in four phases: a pilot study of 55 European, Near Eastern, and Israeli-born Moslem Arab women; a broad-scale survey consisting of face-to-face interviews with 1,148 women from the five ethnic groups just described; a follow-up medical examination to which all the interview respondents were invited (697 agreed to come); and follow-up psychiatric interviews with 160 women representing selected subgroups from each of the five ethnic groups. The findings presented here concern the second and fourth phases of the study: the broad-scale survey and the psychiatric interviews.

To maximize homogeneity within the ethnic groups, selected women were sampled from residential areas in which each group was concentrated. The Central Europeans came from a largely middle-class city near Tel Aviv; the Persians and Turks were selected from two predominantly lower-income divisions of Tel Aviv; the North Africans were drawn from two towns in the foothills of the Judean Mountains between Jerusalem and Tel Aviv; and the Arabs were chosen from two large villages in the Little Triangle in Israel's central plain.

Jews were selected randomly from the lists of the Population Registry, stratified by age (45–54) and ethnicity. Arab women aged 45–54 were selected from lists in regional health center files. Although the Turks were somewhat older and the Europeans somewhat younger than the other groups, the age distribution of the groups was similar.

Interviews with the Jewish groups were conducted by mature women from the staff of the Israel Institute of Applied Social Research. Most of the interviews were conducted in Hebrew, but some were conducted in Moghrabi (the Arabic of North Africa), Persian, Spanish, French, or Yiddish. Occasionally, the interviewers translated into a third language that was not the native tongue of either the interviewer or the respondent. These interviews were reviewed later to ensure against distortions of the interview protocol. Interviews among the Arab women were conducted by Israel-born Moslem Arab high school teachers who spoke both Hebrew and Arabic. Responses were recorded in Hebrew, with the exception of Arab idiom, which was recorded in Arabic and later translated.

Before the interview, most of the women were contacted by mail. Other strategies were used with the most traditional groups. Among the North Africans, a public health nurse acted as liaison, and in the Arab villages the regional health officer contacted the men of the families to ask their permission for their wives' participation. About two-thirds of the Jewish women contacted and four-fifths of the Arab women were eventually interviewed. Nonresponse among the Jewish groups varied by ethnicity; refusal was directly related to modernity, and the most common reason for nonresponse was a failure to locate the respondent. Among the Arab women, the most common reason for nonresponse was failure of the husband to grant permission; almost all the Arab women whose husbands agreed were interviewed.

The interview was based on reviews of the literature and on the pilot study (phase 1). The interview schedule consisted of 157 precoded items and 11 open-ended questions dealing with the menopause, social and family roles, personality, psychological well-being, and life history. Indices of modernity, response to earlier psychosexual events, and response to climacterium were derived from some of the items. The index of modernity was constructed using questions about number of living children, choice of husband, literacy, and orthodoxy. Responses to these items formed a six-point Guttman scale ranging from most traditional (eight or more children, spouse chosen by family, illiterate, and orthodox) to most modern (one to three children, spouse chosen by respondent, literate, and nonreligious). Analyses revealed that the index of modernity, however, was less useful in differentiating psychosexual and climacteric responses than was ethnic group identity. Although the index reflected modernity, it evidently was not sufficient to measure modernity. For example, some women bore few children or chose their own spouses not because they were modern but because they were infertile or had no families to choose their spouses for them. Therefore, the groups themselves are viewed hereafter as representing a range in degree of tradition or modernity. The psychosexual indices were derived from responses to items dealing with four developmental issues: menstruation, marital relationships (both interpersonal and sexual aspects), first childbearing, and subsequent childbearing. Guttman scales were created representing a range from negative to positive responses for each issue. Finally, six indices of response to menopause were constructed. These included a symptomatology index (including hot flushes, headaches, breast pains, and so on) and five attitudinal indices: positive or negative view about cessation of fertility, physical and emotional health, changes in social and family status, and changes in the marital relationship.

Follow-up psychiatric interviews were conducted with subgroups of women in each ethnic group who had been identified in the interviews as either well adjusted or poorly adjusted. These judgments were based on self-reported coping, personality, and menopausal symptomatology. Psychiatrists, who were from the same ethnic groups as the respondents, conducted unstructured interviews; they were not informed of the interview judgments.

The interviews and the psychiatric follow-ups focused on the two core questions of the study:

1. How does the degree of modernity, reflected in ethnic group identity, affect a woman's response to the transitions of middle age?

2. How does a woman's childbearing history (which is, of course, a function of modernity) affect her response to menopause and the loss of fertility—the one developmental invariant of middle age?

These questions reflect the study's general concern with the psychological well-being of women with diverse cultural backgrounds and personal histories. The term "psychological well-being" is inadequate to express, though, the central issue of this study. Life in the Middle East is difficult, encompassing a rhythm of pain and pleasure, of struggle and reward. It is a life expressed best in the Yiddish words *tsoris* and *naches*, anemically translatable as trouble or grief, and joy.

TSORIS AND NACHES: THE CLOSING OF THE GATES

To the researchers' complete astonishment, women across the five cultures unanimously welcomed menopause and the cessation of fertility, despite great differences in childbearing history, and despite differences in attitude toward the size of their families. Two-thirds of the modern European women expressed regret that their families were so small—but, when asked whether they regretted their lost fertility or the loss of the chance to bear additional children, they, along with women in other cultures, emphatically declared that they were pleased to be finished with the business of childbearing and childrearing. In other words, the children they told us they wished they had had were what we might call theoretical children, a theoretical family of four or five instead of the actual one or two—but they did not now want to be pregnant and bearing children.

Although these women anchored the modern end of our continuum, they would be considered quite traditional by most of us: they were married in their twenties, became mothers soon afterward. American women who delay marriage until their thirties and may bear a first child in their forties might respond differently. However, I also want to underscore the unanimity of the women in our study, and to stress the diversity of childbearing experience: the European women, who bore only one or two children, planned their pregnancies and terminated unplanned or unwanted pregnancies with readily available abortions.

A high value was placed on fertility in the other four cultures. At the traditional end of our continuum were Moslem Arab women, some of whom did not know whether they had reached menopause because they had never menstruated: They were pregnant or nursing babies from menarche to menopause.[2] A typical pregnancy history at this extreme might look like this: 25 pregnancies, of them 20 brought to term, of them 15 live births, of these 10 living children. Many of the Moslem Arab village women sought out contraceptives from the public health nurse as they neared their forties and told their husbands they could no longer become pregnant. Like the Europeans, the Arabs welcomed the cessation of fertility.

Midway between tradition and modernity were the transitional Persians, the only women of whom a significant percentage told our interviewers that they wished they had had fewer children. Like the Moslem Arabs, the Persian women had grown up in a culture of tradition, but the establishment of the state of Israel and the subsequent rise of antisemitism across the Middle East led to the expulsion of Jews from many Near Eastern countries and to a wave of involuntary emigration. The Persian women were among these refugee populations, and our sample settled in an impoverished quarter of Tel Aviv. The large families, which might have been an economic advantage in the villages of Persia, crowded the tiny flats of Tel Aviv. The open doors of a modern society were closed to these women, many of whom could not read or write. But at their husbands' insistence they continued to bear children well into middle age and then welcomed the end of a succession of involuntary pregnancies.

The more general question of our study, the effect of modernization on psychological well-being in middle age, showed that the original conflicting hypotheses were each half right. Stress was a function of culture, but it was not a linear function. Psychological well-being followed a curvilinear pattern and was highest at the two extremes, among the most traditional and the most modern women, and lowest among the Persian women, at the midpoint in transition. This suggests that the stability of the cultural context, rather than its content, facilitates adaptation to developmental tasks. The European and Arab women experienced the greatest cultural stability—the European women as immigrants to a society founded on European values; the Arabs within the unchanging context of traditional village life. The transitional groups—the Turks, the Persians, and the North Africans—had been socialized into traditional settings and trans-

---

[2]For further discussion of this point, see also Beyene (1986).

planted into a modern culture where traditional cues and resources no longer served them. Self-reported psychological well-being was especially low among the Persians, who experienced the greatest discontinuity between their traditional upbringing and the modern life context they found in their new homes in Tel Aviv. The freedoms of modernity were not available to these transitional women; the plurality of roles of modern society broadened the horizons of other women, including their daughters.

The balance of gains and losses seen by women was a product of individual life experiences and the resulting personal resources they brought to middle age and of the resources and dominant values provided by their culture. The relationship between modernity and coping, for example, was not a simple linear one. One traditional Moslem Arab woman, when asked how her husband reacted to menopause, replied, "Since when is that his business? He didn't stop the menstruation, God stopped it!" Did she have fears about her marriage? Yes, she was afraid her husband might take a second wife outside Israel. How did she cope with that fear? "Oh, I just keep him at home—I don't let him go to Tel Aviv." And her concerns for her physical health, how did she cope with those? She got hormone shots at the regional health service clinic, visited a gynecologist on the West Bank (partly for the excursion), and sought the advice of a faith healer—not the repertoire of passive coping skills sometimes associated with tradition. One would be equally in error to identify modernity with active coping. One European woman, asked about the end of menstruation, replied, "I don't want menstruation to stop; it stopped in Auschwitz," reminding us that the machinery of modern society can immobilize the human spirit as effectively as any network of ritual and tradition. Finally, cultural transition brings the unknown and, for the transitional women in the study, apprehension. "Don't take me out of my kitchen," said a Persian woman; "I tasted nothing of life," sighed a Turk, both considering the potentials of modernization, incompletely fulfilled for them, with regret and neither personal nor cultural resources for coping with the change.

The first ancillary hypothesis, that stress would be equal across cultures but the expression of symptoms would differ, was partly confirmed. Women's specific concerns about menopause varied by culture: Moslem Arabs feared a decline in marital relations with the loss of their fertility; Near Eastern Jews feared a decline in physical health, expressed best by the Persian woman who complained, "The whole body pains me"; and European women feared a decline in mental health—20% of this group agreed with the assertion "During menopause a woman is likely to go crazy," a statement that found no agreement at all in other groups.

The second ancillary hypothesis, that differential rates of clinical depression were a function of cultural bias in psychiatrists, also found partial confirmation. The results suggest that psychiatrists are more likely to diagnose depression in women from cultures other than their own. The psychiatrists in this study, of the same ethnic origins as the respondents, diagnosed depression at about the same rate in every group. Depression was rare but diagnosed equally in each group.

A TIME TO REAP: AGING INTO TRANSITIONS

Both the hypotheses of this study and the psychoanalytic and psychiatric literature from which they were derived are anchored in themes of loss. The principal finding of the study, however, was not loss but transition and change. We uncovered what Ecclesiastes said long ago: To everything there is a season, a time to sow, and a time to reap. Women from cultures selected for their differences did respond differently to the transitions of middle age, but they were surprising in their similarity: Whether a woman had planned and restricted childbearing to only one or two children or had borne children over most of her fertile years, she welcomed the loss of fertility.

With hindsight we realized that despite the obvious differences between the modern European women and the traditional Moslem Arab women, they shared what Antonovsky (1979) has come to call a "sense of coherence": on the affective, cognitive, and instrumental levels, their worlds made sense to them and they were able to affect their worlds. To put it another way, the magic and ritual of "traditional" cultures is what other people do that *we* realize does not work; comparable practices in our own culture, which we don't yet know don't work, we call science and technology.

The Talmud identifies three major sources of ritual impurity:

corpses, lepers, and menstruating women. The separation of husband and wife during menstruation practiced by religious Jews and Moslems and prohibitions against the menstruating woman's participating in religious observances symbolically link menstruation with death and disease. There is another side to this coin, though. The Talmud also evocatively identifies five colors of menstrual blood: like the blood of a wound, like the color of sediment, the shade of the bright-colored saffron, a color like that of water that has had the earth of the Valley of Beit Kerem stirred into it, and the color of two parts of water mixed with one part of the wine of Sharon. And local customs observed by Moslem women include dressing in old, soiled clothing and not combing their hair or making themselves attractive to men in any other way. These suggest that the menstruating woman is seen not simply as "ritually unclean" but as naturally enticing, powerful, and dangerous.

Such expressions of cultural ambivalence tell us something positive about a culture. Douglas (1966) noted that it is rare to find male dominance "flourishing with ruthless simplicity" (p. 142). The one example she provided of such simplicity is the Walbiri, a culture where, "for the least complaint or neglect of duty [the] women are beaten or speared" (p. 141). Such complete subjection of women is very rare. Douglas suggested that what is more common is tension between overt status inequities between the sexes and countervailing covert cultural forces that promote egalitarianism or protect women from the consequences of formal inequities. This tension finds expression in elaborate beliefs, rituals, and practices surrounding sexual pollution.

American drugstores and convenience marts, catering to the needs of modern career women and men, devote entire aisles to scientific and technological solutions to the "problems" of feminine hygiene. (No comparable products for "masculine hygiene" have been successfully marketed, perhaps because there is no supporting cultural context for the belief that men are dirty.) If I understand these products correctly, they are intended to remedy not only acute menstrual uncleanness but also intermenstrual or chronic female uncleanness. Thus, the modern, secular world also conveys images of female impurity; if they are not as dreadful or as ritualistic as the symbolic linking of menstruation with death and disease, neither are they as evocative and seductive as the Talmudic colors of menstrual blood.

And thus this study of the middle age of women in five Israeli subcultures has modern meanings. We took sexual taboos as our point of departure, suggesting that tradition reflects a life course immersed in childbearing and ritual while progress toward modernity is progress away from a life bound by biology and ritual. Yet liberation from traditional role constraints may not create an easier life course but rather a different one. This study teaches us that liberation, with its attendant consequences of greater autonomy and choice, is not a simple progression toward new freedom and prerogatives. Rather, liberation is the exchange of one set of prerogatives for another. The traditional woman, it seems, has bought certainty at the price of ritual constraint. By contrast, freedom of choice and the liberating transitions of modernization can be accompanied by uncertainty and doubt.

In a sense, we are all in transition, immigrants in middle and old age to a changing world for which we are not prepared. Women are likely to continue to struggle to find the rewards of family, which we associate with tradition, and the prerogatives of paid work, sometimes considered the prize of modernity. Considering the panorama of social change represented by the women in this study and the nature of their responses to the same developmental event, it seems that enduring human values — love and work — which Freud summed up as the mark of the healthy adult, may transcend both tradition and modernization. Perhaps the final message of this study is that the task for future generations of men and women is a liberating translation of the best of human tradition.

REFERENCES

Antonovsky, A. (1979), *Health, Stress, and Coping.* San Francisco, CA: Jossey-Bass.

Beyene, Y. (1986), *Culture, Med. & Psychiat.*, 10:47–71.

Datan, N., Antonovsky, A. & Maoz, B. (1981), *A Time to Reap.* Baltimore, MD: Johns Hopkins University Press.

Deutsch, H. (1945), *The Psychology of Women, Vol. 2.* New York: Bantam, 1979.

Douglas, M. (1966), *Purity and Danger.* London: Ark, 1984.

Neugarten, B. L., Wood, V., Kraines, R. J. & Loomis, B. (1963), Women's attitudes toward the menopause. *Vita Humana*, 6:140–151.

6

The Biomedical Study
of Menopause

MADELEINE J. GOODMAN

Menopause is clearly a biological phenomenon, but one that is perceived privately in the context of a woman's physical and emotional health, culture, and social environment. The cessation of menses may be abrupt, brought about by surgery; it may be gradual, with the progressive extending of the intervals between menses, and thus be noted only retrospectively, months after the last period has occurred; or it may be imperceptible, simply the failure of menstrual periods to resume after a final pregnancy. Because menopause is not uniformly described or experienced, and positive evidence of its actual occurrence is not immediately available, it is difficult to study. Yet the scientific study of menopause is of critical value in four areas: In human biology, menopause forms an important and neglected life cycle milestone marking the closing of the reproductive years. In the study of aging specifically, menopause is a key variable. In epidemiology, the occurrence of menopause and variations in its character have been associated, causally or as concomitants, with a wide variety of diseases and conditions ranging from breast cancer and osteoporosis to depression. Finally, in the general education and self-awareness of the population at large an understanding of menopause and its nature is critical to men and women both to enhance women's understanding of the workings of their bodies in overcoming stereotypes about middle-aged women, and to call attention to the dangers of treating menopause itself as a disease.

DEFINITIONS OF MENOPAUSE

Menopause occurs when the ovary ceases to produce sufficient estrogen to sustain the menstrual cycle. From this purely physiological perspective, all adult women are either premenopausal or postmenopausal. Premenopausal women menstruate regularly, with individual variations in cycle length that may be influenced by health status or environmental factors such as nutrition. Postmenopausal women no longer menstruate. If a woman's ovaries and uterus are surgically removed, menopause is immediate. Under natural circumstances the decline of estrogen levels with aging eventually brings on menopause, usually after a time of increasing menstrual irregularity. To differentiate this interim stage from the true cessation of menses, most investigators have agreed to a standard of 12 months of amenorrhea not obviously attributable to such causes as surgery, before applying the designation of natural menopause (WHO, 1981; Kaufert et al., 1986).

The Postmenopause

The median age at last menses in industrial nations is 51 years, but the normal range is from 41 to 59 years, accounting for some 94% of women who undergo natural menopause (Stanford et al., 1987). In natural menopause, the cessation of menstruation is considered to be an external sign of the endocrinological state of the ovary. After 12 months of amenorrhea it is fairly clear that ovulation has ceased and that hormonal levels within the ovary have stabilized. But the postmenopausal state extends throughout the remainder of a woman's life, and further age-related changes in hormonal levels and target tissue responses call for division of the postmenopausal years into stages: Women who have not menstruated for 1–4 years are often said to be in early postmenopause; late postmenopause begins five years after the last menstruation (Ballinger, Browing, and Smith, 1987). This subdivision facilitates reference to menopausal age in place of strictly chronological age in epidemiological studies, where it can be a serious error to estimate menopausal status from chronological age groupings. Much breast cancer research, for example, uses the age categories 50-and-over and under-50 routinely in grouping screening and incidence data, when in fact some of the women aged, say, 50 have, and others have not, undergone menopause (Barbo, 1987; McKinlay, McKinlay, and Brambilla, 1987a).

The Premenopause and the Perimenopause

All women who have not permanently ceased menstruation can be considered premenopausal. The premenopausal category, however, fails to discriminate between women who are menstruating regularly and those whose menstrual cycles are becoming increasingly irregular as they approach their menopause (Kaufert, Gilbert, and Tate, 1987). The term perimenopausal refers to this transition. A perimenopausal woman is one who has menstruated in the past 12 months but not in the past three months (Kaufert et al., 1987).

Even in applying the trichotomous scheme of premenopause, perimenopause, and postmenopause, researchers often have difficulty in assigning subjects to a single category, since it cannot be determined, except retrospectively, whether or not a given subject has achieved her final menstruation. A measure of hormone levels would be more predictive than a simple report of menstrual history, but repeated blood sampling is necessary to all adjustment for diurnal and cyclical variations in hormone levels.

Recalled menstrual cycle data are typically subject to error, especially in the perimenopausal stage, when periods are irregular (Goodman, Grove, and Gilbert, 1984). Even the classic signs of menopause — hormonal fluctuations and physiological events such as flushing — may occur well within the premenopausal years and are quite consistent with regular menstrual periods (Rannevik et al., 1986; Kaufert et al., 1987).

Menopause as a Dynamic Process

The hormonal events reflected in the menstrual patterns of women as they approach menopause are best revealed in longitudinal studies where regular examinations and blood sampling chronicle the fluctuation of hormonal levels and their stabilization after menopause. Longitudinal studies also allow adjustment for the interindividual variation that may mask the more subtle hormonal changes that take place in a person over time. Such studies reveal a physiological continuum, not a sequence of discrete stages or states. Two longitudinal studies have been especially helpful in demonstrating this phenomenon: the Manitoba study of women's menstrual history patterns by Kaufert et al. (1987) and the Swedish study by Rannevik et al. (1986) of ovarian hormone change over time.

In the Manitoba study, 324 women between 45 and 59 years were interviewed every three months to ascertain changes in their menstrual pattern. They were asked to report whether they were menstruating regularly, were menstruating irregularly, or had not menstruated within the past six months. In the course of six interviews, 131 different combinations of these three possibilities were recorded. Based on these data, probabilities were calculated of menstrual pattern change over six months. It was found that women who were menstruating regularly had a high probability of continuing to do so (70%). Women who reported menstrual irregularity were about as likely to stop menstruating (15%) as they were to resume menstruating regularly (13%). It was also possible, although less likely, for women who had not menstruated for six months to resume. About 5% of the women in the study were found to have this pattern. Thus, current menstrual status did not accurately reveal whether women were perimenopausal, premenopausal, or postmenopausal.

In the Swedish study, Rannevick and colleagues (1986) charted the estrogen levels of thirty Swedish women who were born in 1929 and were not taking exogenous estrogens. Their work confirmed that ovarian estrogens decline as menopause approaches and are maintained at low levels after the last menses. However, during the 12 months following the last menses, some of the women in the study retained their premenopausal estrogen levels. Not until two years after the last menstruation did the levels eventually stabilize at less than 25% of the premenopausal levels. Provided the women did not err in recalling the date of their last menses, menstruation is not a precise marker of the final stage of the hormonal changes associated with menopause, and absence of menses apparently need not mean a profound deficit in circulating estrogen.

If the characterization of women as premenopausal or postmenopausal by menstrual activity is not necessarily reflective of their hormonal profiles, the designation perimenopausal is even more problematic. Given the wide age-range for natural menopause, there is no warrant for defining the perimenopausal state on the basis of chronological age. Reliance on reported vasomotor events, such as hot flashes or night sweats, or psychological symptoms, such as depression or irritability, may also be misleading. Kaufert et al. (1987) and Chakravarti et al. (1979) found that these events do not successfully predict the approach of the final cessation of menses. Perimenopause, then, is more a catch-all category than an independently identifiable phase. Kaufert and her colleagues call it "a methodological artifact," since they do not find here a faithful marker of the transition from regular menstrual cycling to menopause. How, then, can the age at menopause be predicted? What determinants are there of the timing of this event?

The Age at Onset of Natural Menopause

Age at menopause has been studied in populations of women around the world, yet many of the studies were based on self-selected clinical samples rather than cross-sectional, geographically defined epidemiological surveys. Clinical populations, by their very nature, are not likely to be representative of the general population, which includes women who do not seek medical assistance for menopausal problems. Studies of nonclinical sample populations are significantly different from clinical studies in the phenomena they discover (Goodman, Grove, and Gilbert, 1978; McKinlay and McKinlay, 1972).

Two recent large cross-sectional studies of nonpatient populations found that the median age at natural menopause was 51 years and that it has remained constant over time (Stanford et al., 1987; McKinlay, Bifano, & McKinlay, 1985). However, in populations living under extraordinary environmental conditions, such as in the high altitudes of the Himalayan region, it appears that both age at first menstruation and age at natural menopause may be later than in more familiar groups (Kapoor and Kapoor, 1986). Age at menarche, the age at first menstruation, has not been found to correlate with age at natural menopause in large population studies of Western women (Treloar, 1974; Goodman et al., 1978; Stanford et al., 1987).

Evidence is beginning to accrue that reproductive histories may have a statistically significant impact on the timing of natural menopause. Menopause may be delayed in women of high parity. In Stanford et al.'s (1987) study of 1423 naturally menopausal women who participated in a national breast cancer screening project, it was found that women who had never given birth had a median age at menopause 18 months younger than parous women in the survey; and the median age at natural menopause increased with the number of offspring. Women with five or more children had a median age at menopause two full years later than nulliparous women in the study population. In women with a history of menstrual irregularity before age 25, menopause was delayed by as many as 23 months. Height, weight, ethnic group, history of breast cancer, and age at first pregnancy seem to have no significant effect on age at menopause. But the use of exogenous estrogens in perimenopause was found to delay the onset of menopause by about 18 months, and a direct relationship between duration of usage and the delay of menopausal onset was observed. Women who had taken menopausal estrogens for two to four years had a median age at menopause of over 52 years, whereas in women who had taken menopausal estrogens for five or more years, the median age at menopause was 53 years, 10 months. Menopause seems to be hastened by about one and three quarter years in women who smoke, but the effect is not correlated with the extent of the habit (McKinlay et al., 1985), an effect perhaps biologically explained by other research that has demonstrated the toxic effect of smoking on ovarian function (Mattison, 1983).

The effect of delaying or accelerating the age at natural menopause may be as significant to a given woman as in early or delayed menarche. The impact seems to be more a matter of self-perceived body image than health status in any major sense. However, the studies tantalize us by suggesting that the disruption of ovulatory cycles, whether by repeated pregnancies or by administration of exogenous estrogens that override the natural cycles, may delay the end to normal menstrual periods.

The study findings, taken by themselves, do not predict the age at menopause for a given woman. Rather, they describe statistical averages and correlations observed in large populations selected on a basis other than menopausal complaints. It is the fluctuation and decline of ovarian hormones in relation to elevation of the gonadotrophic hormones FSH and LH that gives us the most useful indication of the imminent onset of the menopause.

THE EVENTS OF MENOPAUSE

With the advent of the radioimmunoassay technique in the 1960s and its application to the measurement of minute circulating hormone levels in blood serum, it became possible to study ovarian and other physiologically significant hormone levels in women undergoing menopause and to correlate these blood values with reported "menopausal symptoms" such as flushes, hot flashes, night sweats, insomnia, loss of libido, irritability, and depression. This kind of investigation is critical to testing the hypothesis that menopause is a hormone deficiency disease. Association of hormonal changes with "menopausal symptoms" would justify the prescription of exogenous ovarian hormones like estrogen and progesterone for symptom relief. It would also strengthen the rationale for a pharmacological as opposed to a counseling or a traditional (nonmedical) mode of confronting menopausal complaints.

A recent study by Ballinger and colleagues (1987) in Dundee, Scotland, provides us with a careful evaluation of hormonal changes in a sample of 85 women, aged 40–55, in various menopausal stages, from late premenopause through late postmenopause. The regularly menstruating women were subdivided into early premenopausal (younger than age 45) and late premenopausal (age 45–50) categories. The younger and older premenopausal women did not differ significantly from one another in their levels of estradiol, the main ovarian estrogen, at any given week of their menstrual cycles. However, mean progesterone levels were significantly lower in the luteal phase of the menstrual cycle in the older premenopausal women. The gonadotropic hormone FSH was significantly higher across the cycle in the older premenopausal women, but the other gonadotropin, LH, was not significantly raised. Among postmenopausal women, significant differences in estrogen and gonadotropin levels could be observed between the early and late postmenopause groups. Estrogen levels fell sharply in the early postmenopause and then increased somewhat as time since menopause elapsed. Both FSH and LH significantly declined with years since menopause, and the androgen testosterone increased somewhat in the late postmenopausal group.

The most interesting feature of this systematic hormone assay investigation was the finding of uniform patterns of hormonal levels among women within the premenopausal group. Seven out of 25 late premenopausal women displayed a particular hormonal profile of elevated gonadotropin levels while maintaining the normal estrogen levels of cycling premenopausal women. The progesterone levels in these seven women were also distinctive in that they were significantly lower in weeks three and four of the menstrual cycle than in the other 18 late premenopausal women. No differences were found for androgen or thyroid hormones in these women, and it is unclear whether this pattern is an obligatory stage in the transition from regular menstrual cycling to the onset of irregular menses leading to complete amenorrhea, or whether it is one of several possible routes leading to menopause. The correlations between these hormonal patterns and characteristics of menstrual flow are weak. Among the late premenopausal group, a marginally significant elevation of estradiol in week four of the menstrual cycle was detected in those women who reported menorrhagia, or heavy flow. It was hypothesized by the researchers that higher estradiol levels in week four might indicate an anovulatory cycle with extra buildup of the endometrial lining of the uterus causing heavier menstrual flow. In early premenopausal women, no significant differences in hormonal patterns were found among women who reported excessively heavy menses.

For many women, the events of menopause are describable in a collection of "symptoms," which may include such phenomena as hot flashes, sweating, sleep disturbance, depression, and lessening or loss of libido. The reported incidence of these events among women in the premenopausal, perimenopausal and postmenopausal categories varies from population to population and from one "symptom" to another (Goodman, 1980; McKinlay et al., 1987b; Kaufert et al., 1987). Hot flashes, night sweats, and insomnia are not universal concomitants of the menopausal experience. A cross-sectional study of 1746 Swedish women aged 40–66 randomly selected from a Census Register in Goteborg provides a representative population for an epidemiological study of the incidence of these complaints. The authors (Hagstad and Janson, 1986) found that hot flashes and sweating were reported in all three categories of women: pre-, peri-, and postmenopausal. But the incidence was 60% in naturally postmenopausal women and 58% in perimenopausal women. In regularly menstruating premenopausal women, some 18% had already reported flushing. Thus, among naturally postmenopausal women, 40% reported that flushing was "nonexistent". It is unknown why some women experience flushing and others do not and what factors affect the perceived severity of the vasomotor event. Sweating was significantly associated with flushing in naturally postmenopausal women, but half of this group reported "no appreciable complaints." The physiology of the flush is well studied. Decreases in skin resistance, a decrease in core temperature, and elevations in finger temperature, in LH secretion, and in adrenocorticotropic hormone and cortisol release are objective physiological measures of the body's reactions during menopausal flushes (Casper and Yen, 1985). Yet, as Ballinger et al. (1987), conclude "There is clearly no simple relationship between circulating levels of hormones such as oestradiol and the frequency of complaints about flushes and sweats which are commonly attributed to the menopause" (p. 249).

The association of changes in behavior and mood with hormonal changes over the pre-, peri-, and postmenopausal periods is even more ephemeral and difficult to verify. Are these changes attributable to hormonal changes, or are they culturally modulated responses to the self-perception of the onset of menopause? Are they, perhaps, effects of an artifact of the mode of ascertainment of the subjects under study? Socioeconomic factors and patterns of utilization of health care facilities may contribute to the widespread clinical impression that menopause itself is associated with certain emotional "symptoms." In southern California in 1982, 63 of the first 100 clients at a menopause clinic listed emotional symptoms as the "primary reason" for attending the clinic (Anderson et al., 1987). Of these first 100 women to enter the clinic, 77% reported insomnia, 93% irritability and 86% depression. Of these women 51 who had not had hysterectomies took the Zung self-rating depression scale, and 45% were found to have mild to severe depression scores. Only 40% of the clinic women were satisfied with their sex lives. Are these emotional symptoms coincidental to menopause, or are they outcomes? Anderson and colleagues reported that the clinic patients had not achieved any improvement in satisfaction with their sex lives after six months' counseling, and exogenous estrogen therapy, or both. Yet the researchers continue to maintain that a "large number of menopausal women suffer from a variety of physical and emotional problems unique to the menopause" (p. 428). Without sampling strategies that assemble representative populations and without correlations of psychological instruments with hormone levels and controls for age and socioeconomic factors, it is unlikely that biologically significant explanations for emotional symptoms can be found.

Ballinger et al. (1987), who interviewed 48 women attending a gynecological clinic, found no differences in estrogen, progesterone, FSH, or LH levels between depressed and nondepressed women, regardless of menopausal status. In a Greek study of age-matched postmenopausal women, half of whom were given controlled dosages of estrogen and half of whom were not treated, no improvements in reported depression or anxiety were observed over six months in either the treatment or the control group (Iatrakis et al., 1986). As Ballinger et al. (1987) conclude, "Levels of psychiatric morbidity . . . are affected by a large variety of psychological factors, so it is hardly surprising that the relatively small amount of variance, if any, associated with the hormonal changes of the menopause is hard to detect against this 'background noise' " (p. 249).

METHODOLOGICAL ISSUES

Investigations into the relationship between the physiological aspects of menopause and emotional problems such as depression that do not take into account the socioeconomic context, the status of the woman's health, the effects of age, and the cultural and personal meanings of the experience of "menopause" or "depression" are scientifically empty and socially valueless. All women are born into a cohort that lives through a common set of climatic, environmental, and historical circumstances. The diversity of their experiences is set against that background. The women may live within urban or rural communities, assimilate various ethnic and cultural values, work, and form families. They may experience illness, wealth, poverty, social dislocations, or geographical relocations. The decisions that women make over the course of their lives about their futures, their fertility, their education, and their living circumstances create individual patterns. These can be of decisive significance, but with reference to the principal study variables of scientific menopause research they may well show up as mere statistical "variance" or "background noise."

Social science methodology is now adequate to adjust for the effects of education, marital status, major socioeconomic factors, age, and birth cohort. But if the right questions are not asked and the appropriate variables are not measured, research results become uninterpretable, ungeneralizable, or misleading.

Asking the Right Questions

A decline in sexual activity is often reported in many cultures as an event correlated with menopause (Maoz et al., 1977; Davidson and Davidson, 1980; Davidson, 1985). Is this decline attributable to menopause or to the effects of aging and the unavailability of partners? Bachman (1984) and Leiblum and Swartzman (1986) found that many women report a decrease in coital activity but not in sexual interest. Sexual activity is affected not only by the availability, interest and sexual competency of a partner, but also by cultural expectations and norms about behavior in the postmenopausal years. If we are to attempt to relate women's sexuality to menopause, we must adjust for these situational factors.

Reporting and Self-Reporting

Many studies are based on self-reporting of "menopausal symptoms" and on information concerning the regularity, duration, and heaviness of menses (Goodman et al., 1984). Yet notions of "heavy" or "light" flow are not uniform. In women of diverse ethnic and cultural backgrounds reported variation can reflect differences in available containment and sanitary facilities. Personal experience is subjective and limited. Recollection of the date of last menses may become vague as it recedes into the past months and years.

Fatigue, depression, loss of libido—common symptoms according to our literature—are descriptors that carry a cultural and contemporary bias. Women in the nineteenth century might have described their emotional distress in different terms than do women today; and women from different cultures may have different attitudes about the terms in which menstruation and its cessation should be described and about the ways they would like to be seen as encountering it— some minimizing, others maximizing its significance or divergently locating that significance in the sexual, reproductive, personal, psychological, clinical, vocational, or religious realm.

In a study of Mayan women, Beyene (1986) found a complete absence of the menopausal symptoms usually reported in Western cultures. The women she interviewed did not even have an equivalent term for the hot flash in their vocabulary. They perceived menopause solely as the cessation of menses and an end to the sequence of pregnancies. They did report occasional headaches or dizziness, but this they associated with anemia due to frequent childbearing. Beyene found that Mayan women "welcomed" menopause and looked forward to its onset to free them from the ordeals of repeated pregnancies and childbearing. The women reported that after menopause, with "the risk of pregnancy no longer present they felt more relaxed about sexual activities and relieved from the anxiety of unwanted pregnancies" (pp. 62–63). Were these women experiencing a qualitatively different physiological phenomenon or were they minimizing or discounting symptoms because of the positive attitudes they held toward the menopause? What roles did diet and the vigorous exercise of their peasant way of life play in the perception or actuality of menopausal symptoms in this population?

Lock's (1986) work with gynecologists and with menopausal women in Japan focuses on the widespread medical belief in Japan that menopausal symptoms reflect personality characteristics, individual genetic propensities, difficult childbirths, or even guilt over past abortions. Nervous, pessimistic, withdrawn, and lonely women are considered most likely to suffer from menopausal complaints. The physical symptoms of menopause are not expected for all Japanese women, nor are they ubiquitous among the general population of menopausal women in Japan. The prevalence of the classical physical symptoms of menopause in the population Lock studied was very low compared with Kaufert et al.'s (1987) companion work on women in Manitoba. In Manitoba, some 40% of perimenopausal women reported hot flashes, but only 13% of Lock's Japanese population did. Among the Canadian women, 27% of the perimenopausal women experienced night sweats, but only 4% of the Japanese reported this symptom. Only 20% of Lock's Japanese population reported ever having experienced a hot flash, a percentage similar to that found in Japanese women of comparable age living in Hawaii (Goodman, Stewart, and Gilbert, 1977); in Manitoba, 69% of the women studied had at some time experienced hot flashes. The standard clinical studies assume an incidence ranging from 75–85% (McKinlay and Jeffreys, 1974; Mulley and Mitchell, 1976). On the other hand, over 50% of Lock's Japanese sample reported headaches and shoulder stiffness—often a local euphemism for stress.

These variations in reporting symptoms show us how precarious universal generalizations about menopausal events can be and how sensitive the collection of data is to the cultural context of the subjects studied. Lack of a uniform vocabulary to describe the events of menopause and modesty in revealing embarrassing physical details such as hot flashes or sweating may cause under-reporting. Subsuming menopausal symptoms under overly general or unspecific somatic complaints blurs the distinction between menopausally associated symptoms and those related to general health and aging.

Measurement of Variables

Standardized instruments developed to capture relevant information about attitudes, behaviors, and beliefs are often used in an effort to correlate these psychological characteristics with such biological variables as age at menopause, incidence and frequency of hot flashes, night sweats, or menstrual pattern change. The more qualitative anthropological methods of participant observation and ethnography are sometimes discounted as imprecise (Greene, 1984). Many social scientists who study menopause prefer to apply conventional and familiar standardized questionnaires, indices, and scales. But these have been "validated" largely on white American populations, and their applicability to women of other ethnic and cultural backgrounds is problematic. Davis (1986) described with considerable skill how the menopausal women she studied in a Newfoundland fishing village confounded the aims of the Sociocultural Patterns and Involutional Crisis (SPIC) interview schedule (developed by the Datan Consortium) and the Neugarten Attitudes Towards Menopause (ATM) checklist by consistently choosing answers with higher numerical scores because they saw the questionnaires as intelligence tests for "those who think big." The women found the options offered on the multiple choice questions from these instruments hard to relate to the context of their life experience. They were also offended by direct personal questions concerning their reproductive history; they found these excessively prying. Only in answers to open-ended questions did the attitudes, beliefs, and behaviors of this group of women emerge. Their vocabulary, their social and familial relationships, and their perceptions of gender roles framed a context in which the women's individual assessments and responses could be understood. But without the investigator's observations, without this ethnographic roadmap, the measurement of psychological variables and their correlations with biological events would have been meaningless.

It is not social science methodologies alone that are prone to such inaccuracies of measurement. The lack of adjustment for cycle phase in women who still menstruate poses a similar contextual problem on a biological plane for studies seeking to correlate psychological variables with hormone levels. Unless weekly blood sampling is undertaken, investigators need to collect menstrual calendars containing the dates of menstruation prior to and subsequent to blood sampling. This is essential to establish the duration of each woman's cycle and the cycle phase in which the hormones were sampled. Where mood or behavior are assumed to be correlated with menstrual cycle phase, then appropriate statistical adjustment is necessary to control for cycle phase when comparing pre- with postmenopausal women to establish the emotional or behavioral correlates of menopause.

The Study Population

There is no perfect or complete study population. All have limitations of one kind or another. The large, nonclinical, cross-sectional populations that appear to be most representative of the general population make logistical demands that in effect require surveys conducted from standardized questionnaires as the main means of gathering data. Taking blood samples from very large groups is prohibitively costly, and in-depth inquiry of the more intimate type of anthropological investigation is obviously not possible. In practice, large population studies typically limit the investigation of cultural factors to a single question asking respondents to self-identify with one or two or a few ethnic categories. Some large-scale investigations extract information from large data bases collected for other purposes. The analysis by Stanford and colleagues (1987) of Breast Cancer Detection Demonstration Project (BCDDP) data collected in the 1970s is such a study. The investigators overcame some of the bias of clinical populations. But women who did not volunteer for experimental mammographic screening as part of an ACS/NCI (American Cancer Society/ National Cancer Institute) program were unsampled in this data set. Women who do not seek and use medical facilities are underrepresented in this kind of study. And, of course, retrospective analysis of a data base is limited to the data collected, the questions that actually were asked. There is no information, for example, on diet or exercise in the BCDDP data, and the size and fluidity of the study population and the conditions surrounding the original study make it impracticable after a certain point to return to the same subjects for further information.

Small ethnographic studies, for their part, have been criticized as idiosyncratic and unstandardized, thus not easily replicated or compared. The large, longitudinal study design seems to combine the virtues of size and depth. But here too problems of self-reporting and measurement must be overcome. And the issues of compatibility across cultures and over time remain. Clearly, not all researchable questions will yield to a single, standard study design. The extent of normal human variation in the physiological, psychological, and social dimensions of menopause calls for the simultaneous application of cross-sectional, longitudinal, and in-depth cross-cultural research approaches. Through careful cross-checking of all these types of study confidence about our understanding of menopause will be enhanced.

MENOPAUSE AND DISEASE

The relationship between menopause and disease has been depicted in three ways. First, menopause itself has been viewed *as a disease* requiring medical management. Second, menopause has been considered to be a *cause* of illness, a risk factor for the development of osteoporosis, for example, and thus deserving of medical attention to mitigate its putative pathogenic effects. Third, menopause has been studied as a *biological marker*, a factor concomitant with the onset or prognosis of serious illness, such as heart disease and breast cancer. What is the evidence for these three models, and how does the connection of menopause with disease affect our ability to investigate menopause itself?

Menopause as Disease

The view that menopause itself is a disease, with the consequent "medicalization" of menopause as Kaufert and Gilbert (1986) and Bell (this volume) call it, has remained intact in some medical circles since the publication of Wilson's *Feminine Forever* in 1966. Utian (1987) and other gynecologists emphasize that the decline of estrogen production associated with menopause is sufficient evidence "to define the climacteric as an endocrinopathy in which changes in hormonal profile are associated with extensive pelvic and extrapelvic target tissue effects" (p. 10). Utian infers that "the longer these effects are allowed to continue without corrective therapy, the more likely there is to be expression of a pathologic process and clinical symptom" (p. 10).

As Kaufert and Gilbert (1986) point out, only those "symptoms" that can be demonstrated to be ameliorated by the administration of estrogen supplements qualify for inclusion as part of the menopausal syndrome. Hot flashes, night sweats, and osteoporosis, which appear to respond to hormonal therapy, therefore become bona fide attributes of the disease. But hormone treatments do not restore ovulation, so the cessation of ovulation is not included as part of the "disease"—since it cannot be "treated." Psychological symptoms that have proved less tractable to administered exogenous estrogens than have somatic signs of menopause can now, by the same reasoning, be excluded from the menopausal profile.

Much has been written in support of the medical model (Van Keep, 1983; Utian, 1986) and against it (Goodman, 1980; Kaufert and Gilbert, 1986; McKinlay et al. 1987a). But, from a strictly empirical perspective the onus of proof that menopause is a disease requires more than a demonstration of declining estrogen levels. It requires the demonstration of a causal relationship between the hormonal changes and clinical symptoms, a demonstration that Utian (1986) himself admits is lacking: "Proof of direct relationship is generally lacking between climacteric-related hormone changes and the development of any particular metabolic derangement or degenerative process" (p. 2). On the contrary, the only significant correlates of menopause, when we control for age and the aging process, are recourse to medicine and surgery—both artifacts of the medical model (Goodman et al., 1977; McKinlay et al., 1987a). Changes in circulating hormone levels are also observed at puberty, in pregnancy, and after parturition. And physical and psychological changes are often observed in conjunction with these hormonal changes. Yet puberty and childbirth are not thought of as endocrinopathies but rather as normal lifecycle events. Nor is the decline of testosterone in men usually thought of as a disease or treated as one—although there have been some efforts to do both.

In adopting a disease perspective toward menopause and by prescribing exogenous estrogen therapy, despite the lack of biological evidence for the way in which this therapy works to eliminate the manifestations of menopause, we attempt to override natural aging without a full understanding of the general health implications of this decision. The iatrogenic effects of estrogen replacement therapy (ERT) on the development of uterine cancer afford one well-documented instance of the costs of this type of medical management and decision making. As Jick and colleagues (1980) wrote, in the United States "over 15,000 cases of endometrial cancer were caused by replacement estrogens during the five-year period 1971–1975 alone. . . . "This represents one of the largest epidemics of serious iatrogenic disease that has ever occurred in this country" (p. 264).

Menopause as a Risk Factor

The question remains whether menopause is a detriment to the health of women. Does menopause, if not itself a disease, contribute to the development of osteoporosis, depression, or breast cancer among women in their middle years?

With regard to osteoporosis, it has been shown that removal of the ovaries or menopausal decline in estrogen production is accompanied by a rise in calcium excretion in the plasma and the urine, an indirect indication of the resorption of bone (Nordin et al., 1975). With estrogen therapy, urinary excretion of calcium does decline, indicating that the bone resorption is arrested. Yet not every woman who goes through menopause is at high risk for pathological bone fragility leading to fractures. Low calcium intake, malabsorption of calcium, and low estrogen levels combine in the high risk profile (Marshall, Horsman, and Nordin, 1977). Bone density and age-related bone loss are more proximate indications of an osteoporotic tendency. Yet the clinical emphasis is on a "premenopausal prevention strategy" (Brody, Farmer, and White, 1984), which starts women on a long-term treatment protocol even before there is laboratory confirmation of a decline in natural ovarian estrogen levels. The actual probability of fractures associated with osteoporosis over 25 years for women at standard risk is 9% and for those women in the 'high risk' profile, 23%. Estrogen therapy taken for at least five years reduces the risk of fracture by half (Weiss et al., 1980). While menopause is a significant risk factor for the development of osteoporosis, prudent clinicians and women should evaluate its contribution relative to other measurable factors of a more authentically symptomatic character before embarking on long-term estrogen therapy. Here, population-based cross-sectional and longitudinal studies provide us with more broadly anchored estimates of risk in nonclinical populations that need to be considered in medical decision making by asymptomatic women.

The relationship between menopause and depression has been problematic because few studies have used more than self-reported or subjective identification of "depressed mood" or have adequately adjusted for the confounding effects of age and other factors such as prior history of depression. Applying the Women's Health Questionnaire to 682 women attending an ovarian screening program, Hunter and colleagues (1986) found a significant increase in self-reported "depressed mood" in peri- and postmenopausal women in comparison with premenopausal subjects. But the prevalence of depressed mood among the women surveyed, some 25–30%, did not exceed reported rates in general population studies (Dennerstein, 1987). Furthermore, the probability of admission to psychiatric units is not significantly higher in women in their menopausal years than it is for women of other ages (Winokur, 1973).

There is no biological evidence of a relationship between decreased estrogen levels at menopause and the advent of depression. After adjusting for menopausal status, Ballinger and colleagues (1987) found no significant difference in ovarian hormone profiles between women scoring three or four on the standard psychiatric depression scale and those scoring two or less. Clinical trials tend to confirm this finding; administration of exogenous estrogen did not improve depressed mood more than did a placebo, although vasomotor symptoms did respond to the estrogen (Paterson, 1982; Iatrakis et al., 1986). Compelling evidence comes from the McKinlays' (1987b) 27-month follow-up study of a randomly selected cohort of 2500 middle-aged Massachusetts women (McKinlay et al., 1987b). Applying a standard Center for Epidemiological Studies Depression (CES-D) scale and systematically adjusting for the impact of sociodemographic status, prior health status and health care utilization patterns, the McKinlays found that worry over a family member, friend, or work-related individual was significantly correlated with increased depression; "menstrual change associated with the menopause appears to have no significant effect on depression" (p. 355). This result was echoed in a survey of women's attitudes toward menopause conducted by Leiblum and Swartzman (1986), who found that in their sample of 244 menopausal women, respondents "were more apt to attribute psychological difficulties that occurred around the menopause to distressing life changes than to hormonal fluctuations" (p. 54). Thus, the evidence is that the superficial association of menopause with depression is more coincidental than causal. Situational factors, health status, and health care utilization, not hormonal changes, are the appropriate measures of risk for the development of depression in this age group.

In a review of published studies of the relationship of menopause to breast cancer, Alexander and Roberts (1987) found a clear consensus that there is a higher risk of developing breast cancer among women aged 50–54 who are still menstruating and a lower risk of breast cancer among women who underwent menopause earlier than age 45. After adjustment for age and other confounding factors, the relative risk of developing breast cancer is three times as high in postmenopausal women as in premenopausal women. It has also been found clinically that breast tumors detected in perimenopausal women are harder to treat and have a poorer prognosis for nonrecurrence than those of pre- or postmenopausal women (Langlands et al., 1979; Gentili et al., 1981). Alexander and Roberts (1987) hypothesize that high levels of unopposed estrogen during anovulatory cycles in the perimenopausal period may stimulate tumor growth. Whether or not this can be demonstrated, the association of late age at menopause with increased breast cancer risk is an empirical finding that is clinically useful in determining the frequency of recommended mammographic screening for breast cancer. But of course at our present state of knowledge, the identification of a risk factor of this kind serves more as a marker than as a target for treatment.

The study of menopause continues to be a key to our understanding of the biology of aging in women and to the chronic diseases that affect them as they age. It is impossible to study menopause in isolation from the context of the life circumstances and health status of the individual. Whether menopause itself is the primary subject of investigation or a concomitant factor in the study of social roles, aging, or health, it is necessary to support such research with careful definition of terms, appropriate selection and precise measurement of variables, choice of an appropriate study population, and the design and application of adequate analytical tools. Only then will an unbiased depiction of menopause emerge.

REFERENCES

Alexander, F. & Roberts, M. (1987), The menopause and breast cancer. *J. Epidemiol. Comty. Health*, 41:94–100.

Anderson, E., Hamburger, S., Liu, J. & Rebar, R. (1987), Characteristics of menopausal women seeking assistance. *Amer. J. Obs. Gyn.*, 156:428–433.

Bachman, G. (1984), Evaluation of the climacteric women—an overview. *Midpoint*, 1:9–13.

Ballinger, C.B., Browning, M.C.K. & Smith, A.H.W. (1987), Hormone profiles and psychological symptoms in peri-menopausal women. *Maturitas*, 235–251.

Barbo, D. (1987), The physiology of the menopause. *Med. Clin. N. Amer.*, 71:11–22.

Beyene, Y. (1986), Cultural significance and physiological manifestations of menopause a biocultural analysis. *Cult. Med. Psychiat.*, 10:47–71.

Brody, J., Farmer, M. & White, L. (1984), Absence of menopausal effect on hip fracture occurence in white females. *Amer. J. Pub. Health*, 74:1397–1400.

Casper, R.F. & Yen, S.S.C. (1985), Neuroendocrinology of menopausal flushes: An hypothesis of flush mechanism. *Clin. Endocrinol.*, 22:293.

Chakravarti, S., Collins, W.P., Thom, M.H. & Studd, J.W.W. (1979), Relation between plasma hormone profiles, symptoms and response to oestrogen treatment in women approaching the menopause. *Brit. Med. J.*, 1:983–985.

Davidson, J.M. (1985), The psychobiology of sexual experience. *Maturitas*, 7:193–201.

Davidson, J.M. & Davidson, R.J., ed. (1980), *The Psychobiology of Consciousness.* New York: Plenum Press, pp. 271–282.

Davis, D. (1986), The meaning of menopause in a Newfoundland fishing village. *Cult. Med. Psychiat.*, 10:73–94.

Dennerstein, L. (1987), Depression in the menopause. *Obs. Gyn. Clin. N. Amer.*, 4:33–48.

Gentili, C., Sanfilippo, O. & Silvestrini, R. (1981), Cell proliferation and its relationship to clinical features and relapse in breast cancers. *Cancer*, 48:974–979.

Goodman, M.J. (1980), Toward a biology of menopause. *Signs*, 5:739–753.

Goodman, M.J., Grove, J. & Gilbert, F. (1978), Age at menopause in relation to reproductive history in Japanese, Caucasian, Chinese and Hawaiian women living in Hawaii. *J. Gerontol.*, 33:688–694.

Goodman, M.J., Grove, J. & Gilbert, F. (1984), Recalled characteristics of menstruation in relation to reproductive history among Caucasian, Japanese and Chinese women living in Hawaii. *Annals Human Biol.*, 11:235–242.

Goodman, M.J., Stewart, C. & Gilbert, F. (1977), Patterns of menopause: a study of certain medical and physiological variables among Caucasian and Japanese women living in Hawaii. *J. Gerontol.*, 32:291–298.

Greene, J. (1984), *The Social and Psychological Origins of the Climacteric Syndrome.* Adershot, VT: Gower.

Hagstad, A. & Janson, P. (1986), The epidemiology of climacteric symptoms. *Acta Obs. Gyn. Scand.* [Suppl.], 134:59–65.

Hunter, M., Battersby, R. & Whitehead, M. (1986), Relationships between psychological symptoms, somatic complaints and menopausal status. *Maturitas*, 8:217–228.

Iatrakis, G., Haronis, N., Sakellaropoulos, G., Kourkoubas, A. & Gallos, M. (1986), Psychosomatic symptoms of postmenopausal women with or without hormonal treatment. *Psychother. Psychosom.*, 46:116–121.

Jick, H., Walker, A.M. & Rothman, K.J. (1980), The epidemic of endometrial cancer: a commentary. *Amer. J. Pub. Health*, 70.3:264–267.

Kapoor, A. & Kapoor S. (1986), The effects of high altitude on age at menarche and menopause. *Internat. J. Biometeor.*, 30:21–26.

Kaufert, P. & Gilbert, P. (1986), Women, menopause, and medicalization. *Cult. Med. Psychiat.*, 10:7–21.

Kaufert, P., Gilbert, P. & Tate, R. (1987), Defining menopausal status: The impact of longitudinal data. *Maturitas*, 9:217–226.

Kaufert, P., Lock, M., McKinlay, S., Beyenne, Y., Coope, J., Davis, D., Eliasson, M., Gognalons-Nicolet, M., Goodman, M. & Holte, A. (1986), Menopause research: The korpilampi workshop. *Soc. Sci. Med.*, 22:1285–1289.

Langlands, A.O., Pocock, S.J., Kerr, G.R. & Gore, S.M. (1979), Long-term survival of patients with breast cancer: A study of the curability of the disease. *Brit. Med. J.*, 2:1247–1251.

Leiblum, S. & Swartzman, L. (1986), Women's attitudes toward the menopause: An update. *Maturitas*, 8:47–56.

Lock, M. (1986), Ambiguities of aging: Japanese experience and perceptions of menopause. *Cult. Med. Psychiat.*, 10:23–46.

Marshall, D.H., Horsman, A. & Nordin, B.E.C. (1977), The prevention and management of postmenopausal osteoporosis. *Acta Obs. Gyn. Scand.* [Suppl], 65:49.

Maoz, B., Antonovsky, A., Apter, A., Wijsenbeck, H. Datan, N. (1977), The perception of menopause in five ethnic groups in Israel. *Acta Obs. Gyn. Scand.* [Suppl.], 65:69–76.

Mattison, D. (1983), The mechanisms of action of reproductive toxins. In: *Reproductive Toxicology*, ed. D. Mattison. New York: Alan R. Liss, pp. 65–79.

McKinlay, J., McKinlay, S. & Brambilla, D. (1987a), Health status and utilization behavior associated with menopause. *Amer. J. Epidemiol.*, 125:110–121.

———— ———— ———— (1987b), The relative contributions of endocrine changes and social circumstances to depression in mid-aged women. *J. Health Soc. Beh.*, 28:345–363.

McKinlay, S., Bifano, N. & McKinlay, J. (1985), Smoking and age at menopause in women. *Annals Int. Med.*, 103:350–356.

———— & Jeffreys, M. (1974), The menopause syndrome. *Brit. J. Med.*, 28:108–115.

———— & McKinlay, J. (1973), Selected studies of the menopause. *J. Biosoc. Sci.*, 5:533–55.

———— Jeffreys, M., and Thompson B. (1972), An investigation of the age at menopause. *J. Biosoc. Sci.*, 4:161–173.

Mulley, G. & Mitchell, J. (1976), Menopausal flushing: Does estrogen therapy make sense? *Lancet*, i:1397–1399.

Nordin, B.E.C., Gallagher, J.C., Aaron, J.E. & Horsman, A. (1975), Postmenopausal osteopenia and osteoporosis. *Front. Horm. Res.*, 3:131.

Paterson, M. (1982), A randomised, double-blind, cross-over study into the effect of sequential mestranol and norethisterone on climacteric symptoms and biochemical parameters. *Maturitas*, 4:83–94.

Rannevik, G., Carlstrom, K., Jeppsson, S., Bjerre, B. & Svanberg, L. (1986), A prospective long-term study in women from pre-menopause to post-menopause: Changing profiles of gonadotrophins, oestrogens and androgens. *Maturitas*, 8:297–307.

Stanford, J., Hartge, P., Brinton, L., Hoover, R. & Brookmeyer, R. (1987), Factors influencing the age at natural menopause. *J. Chron. Dis.*, 40:995–1002.

Treloar, A. (1974), Menarche, menopause, and intervening fecundability. *Human Biol.*, 46:89–107.

Utian, W. (1987), The fate of the untreated menopause. *Obs. Gyn. Clin. N. Amer.*, 14:1–11.

Van Keep, P. (1983), The menopause, part b: Psychosomatic aspects of the menopause. In: *Handbook of Psychosomatic Obstetrics and Gynaecology*, ed. L. Dennerstein & G. Burrows. New York: Elsevier, pp. 483–490.

Weiss, N., Ure, C., Ballard, J., Williams, A. Daling, J. (1980), Decreased risk of fractures of the hip and lower forearm with postmenopausal use of estrogen. *N. Eng. J. Med.*, 303:1195–1198.

Wilson, R. A. (1966), *Feminine Forever*. New York: M. Evans.

Winokur, G. (1973), Depression in the menopause. *American Journal of Psychiatry*, 130:92–93.

World Health Organization (1981), Research on the menopause. *Technical Report Series*, No. 670.

7

The Menopausal Experience

Sociocultural Influences and Theoretical Models

CHERYL L. BOWLES

MENOPAUSE IN THE CONTEXT OF MIDLIFE

Today the middle years for both men and women are no longer viewed as a time of instability and decline, but rather as a time of development and change (Barnett and Baruch, 1978). Yet, despite the change in viewpoints, the middle years are a "largely unexplored phase of human development" (Brim and Abeles, 1975).

This lack of knowledge of the middle years applies particularly to women. Theoretical work in this area is in its infancy, and empirical findings are scattered and noncumulative. Barnett and Baruch (1978) point to the urgent need for up-to-date knowledge about women, whose longer life span, increasing educational attainments, and participation in the labor force have rendered previous research and theory obsolete.

Barnett and Baruch state that underlying many studies of women in the middle years is a belief in the biological determination of feminine behavior. Because of this belief, a woman's life is often seen only in terms of her reproductive role. Thus, menopause and the "empty nest" become identified as major events of the middle years, just as marriage and children are seen as an essential part of a woman's well-being in earlier years. But while the clinical literature on menopause is problem oriented, empirical studies suggest that this stage of the life cycle presents few difficulties for most women (Neugarten, Wood, Kraines, and Loomis, 1963; Neugarten and Kraines, 1965; Bart and Grossman, 1976; Millete, 1981; Muhlenkamp, Waller, and Bourne, 1983; Voda and George, 1986; Barbo, 1987; Raymond, 1988).

MENOPAUSE AS A DISEASE

In the past, menopause was regarded as a disease, fostering studies that reinforce stereotypic assumptions about middle-aged women. These studies focused on the treatment, elaboration, description, and classification of symptoms and on the physician-seeking behaviors of menopausal-age women. This emphasis has promoted the view that changes occurring during menopause are abnormal and should be treated as such (Greenblatt, 1955; Kerr, 1968; Utian, 1987). The term "change of life" implies that a woman may not be able to live the same life she lived before menopause (Koboso-Munro, 1977; Frey, 1981). The belief that menopause is an abnormal state is still prevalent today. Utian (1987), at a symposium supported by CIBA Pharmaceutical Company on the menopausal and postmenopausal patient, stated that "more than enough evidence exists to define the climacteric as an endocrinopathy. The longer these effects are allowed to continue without corrective therapy, the more likely there is to be expression of a pathologic process and clinical symptoms" (p. 1283).

In the medical community, menopause has been viewed as a deficiency disease associated with decreased production of sex hormones, and it has therefore been studied from an endocrinological and gynecological point of view. Much of the literature associated with menopause has come from clinicians who treated menopausal women with a variety of complaints. The descriptions of groups of symptoms associated with menopause have been accumulated from this data base and have contributed to the myths and stereotypes perpetuated in Western societies (Voda, 1981a). A recent example of this problem can be found in the report of a survey of middle-aged women done by Gath et al. (1987) on psychiatric disorders and gynecological symptoms. The researchers introduce the study by stating that some gynecologists and psychiatrists believe that gyneco-logical symptoms are commonly linked with psychiatric disorders. The implications and conclusions presented in the study are based on insufficient data and do not emerge from the results presented. Yet, the authors state, "Our findings have certain implications for general practice. Thus if a woman presents with a gynecological complaint, particularly with a menstrual complaint, it is advisable to look for any associated psychiatric disorder" (p. 218).

Severne (1979) wonders whether many problems that have been associated with menopause might be generated by negative social attitudes about menstruation and menopause, as well as those toward aging in general and toward the aging female specifically. The perpet-uation of these myths and stereotypes in the literature has been damaging, both in determining the expectations for the approaching menopause and in the way women experience menopausal symptoms (Wilbush, 1981; Voda, 1981a; Brooks-Gunn, 1982; Kaufert, 1982).

This focus on symptoms, both psychological and physical, in menopause research has resulted in a neglect of other factors that may be more relevant. Moreover, it has allowed menopause to become a scapegoat for a variety of complaints (Ballinger, 1981). The focus on symptoms has produced an excessive use of estrogens, which are seen as the specific treatment for the "deficiency state" identified as meno-pause as well as all the symptoms that have been attached to meno-pause (Voda, 1981a).

Dan and colleagues (1980) pointed out that research orginating in medical and psychiatric settings has two serious problems limiting its usefulness. First, the orientation and method of such clinical investi-gations have excluded normal or positive experiences. Second, the clinical samples used in most studies are notoriously unrepresentative of menopausal-age women in general, so that the results cannot be generalized to all such women.

Thus, the results of these clinical studies cannot be relied on as a basis for understanding the normal menopausal experience. More-over, Dan et al. (1980) pointed out that too many studies are devoted to demonstrating physical or emotional symptoms or problems in menopausal age women and too few to understanding and alleviating these reported symptoms or problems.

MENOPAUSE FROM A MALE POINT OF VIEW

Rohrbaugh (1979) suggested that another factor strongly affected past research on menopausal experiences and symptoms. Most clinical researchers in the past were male and thus brought a singularly male point of view to both the conduct and the interpretation of research. Older research, as well as developmental and personality theories, use the male as a norm with whom the female is compared, and any differences are seen as deficiencies or deviancies. These theories fail to take into account the varying role patterns women may occupy, which include combinations of marriage, career, childbearing, motherhood, and caregiving for aging parents or other relatives.

Voda and Eliasson (1985) refer to a growing body of literature that presents a changing perspective on menopause. Written by feminist researchers, the findings are not appended to existing literature, nor do they adhere to existing conceptual or theoretical frameworks to guide their studies. This new effort criticizes existing theories and generates new literature, with women's experiences as the center of investigation.

There is an urgent need for empirically based information on how women experience their sexuality, pregnancy, childbirth, and menopause, and their roles as worker, wife, and mother.

PHILOSOPHICAL AND SEMANTIC ISSUES

The basic philosophy of our Western medical model identifies the *symptom* as the prerequisite for seeking medical consultation. If we do not have well-defined symptoms, we must wait until they become bad enough to permit definition. Thus, investigations that deal with menopause confine themselves to a small percentage of women who have well-defined symptoms. Those with poorly defined symptoms or no symptoms at all are not included. Western medicine's proclivity for prevention seems to have had a negative influence on menopause, because prevention means devising new methods for stopping menopause from occurring, or at least delaying it. This emphasis on prevention has led to the extensive use of ERT.

Another problem in the study of menopause concerns the difference between the terms, *experience* and *symptom*. A woman may have experiences she perceives as not being bothersome. Another woman may have similar experiences and perceive them as unpleasant and decide that they need medical intervention. The woman herself usually determines what experiences are defined as symptoms, although she is frequently helped by friends, family, lay and medical literature, and the mass media. Yet menopause is part of the normal process of a woman's life, not a disease, although symptoms of disease can arise and affect the normal menopausal process.

SOCIOCULTURAL INFLUENCES

It has been postulated that menopause may have different meanings for women of different cultural backgrounds. In some cultures, such as the Chinese, age is respected and status and prestige increased. In such a culture, menopause may be seen as a transition to higher status. In the United States, where youth and sex are highly valued, menopause, as well as aging, are frequently viewed with apprehension, and middle-aged women may be treated with less respect (Frey, 1981).

Cultural attitudes toward sex and childbearing affect women's attitudes and expectations about menopause and, therefore, their experiences during this period (Galloway, 1975). Women in our society are valued for their reproductive ability and mother role; menopause brings a loss of these functions. Bart (1969), in a study of cultural values and women's status, found that in any given culture the status and activities dictated by societal norms as constituting the woman's role during her fertile years become reversed at menopause. Neugarten et al. (1963) and Bowles (1986), in studies of attitudes toward menopause of different age groups, found that younger women viewed menopause as both more important and more negative than did middle-aged and older women.

Brooks-Gunn (1982) has suggested that menopause and menarche have a good deal in common: (1) both are more than physiological events; (2) both are sociocultural events that are given special meaning; (3) both are clouded by contradictory and negative attitudes and beliefs.

Menarche is thought to be traumatic but is also a sign of sexual maturity and womanhood. The literature available to adolescent females from such sources as health classes in junior high and high school often conveys hidden sociocultural messages. In an unpublished study of literature provided to high school girls by the school nurse and health classes, Bowles (1974) found that such literature was most frequently provided and published by the corporations that produce sanitary napkins and tampons. The information on menstruation was presented in a condescending rather than a straightforward, factual manner, with frequent double messages about menarche and menstruation. For example, one source told the reader that the beginning of menstruation was a wonderful, joyous experience that signaled the beginning of womanhood and it should be a time of celebration. However, when it occurred, only her mother or the school nurse should be informed!

The same double messages and "good news-bad news" type of communication are often found concerning menopause. Menopause is seen as the end of sexuality and physical attractiveness, yet it is also a symbol of freedom from the parental role, menstrual periods, and fear of pregnancy. Researchers are influenced both by double messages and by old assumptions, and recent menstrual cycle research points to the importance of cultural attitudes and beliefs in the study of both menstruation and menopause (Parlee, 1981). These attitudes and beliefs, although biased and erroneous, continue to be taken as fact and seem to affect women's attitudes and expectations regarding menopausal experiences (Brooks-Gunn, 1982). Sommer (1981) has pointed to the need for research on the role of expectation in symptom formation.

Kahana (1976), in an attempt to determine the attitudes of college students toward menopause, asked them to describe changes they perceived in their parents between ages 35 and 55. Menopause was not mentioned by any of the 143 students. Yet when specifically asked about their parents' reaction to the mother's menopause, the majority of students reported negative reactions.

In another study, by Kahana, Kiyak, and Liang (1980), negative stereotypes of the menopause were found to be less prevalent among women than among men. Men, especially older men, viewed menopause as a major life change. Bowles (1986a, b) studied the attitudes of 180 middle-aged men toward menopause and found that these men viewed it negatively. A significant difference was found between the average attitude score of this male sample and a sample of women who ranged in age from 18 to 86 years. The men's attitude was considerably more negative than the attitude even of the young women.

WOMEN'S MENOPAUSAL EXPERIENCES

The discussion that follows contains information obtained from the few investigations undertaken on women's menopausal experiences. Often the woman was asked to describe her symptoms; the researchers then looked for associations between particular variables in the woman's life and her symptoms. Thus, the research was conducted from a negative perspective rather than one geared to learning what women actually experience as they move into and through the menopausal phase of their lives.

Weg (1987) discusses the fact that menopause is both a subjective and an objective experience. Objectively, menopause is a series of events that can be analyzed and measured by one means or another. Menopause is also a unique experience influenced by a woman's physical and psychosocial environment. Several studies have investigated women's discussions with physicians of menopausal symptoms or problems. The women were perfectly willing to discuss their menopausal status and ask questions about menopausal changes but did not really see these discussions as abnormal or having to do with problems. One study, by Kaufert (1986), distinguished between *discussion* of menopausal status with a physician and *reporting* menopausal problems to a physician. The sample was made up of 503 women who had menstruated within the past three months but reported changes in regularity and flow (transitional), and 104 women who had not menstruated in the past three months but had done so within the previous 12 months (perimenopausal). Sixty percent of the transitional group and 71% of the perimenopausal group had *discussed* their menopausal status with physicians, whereas only 38% of the transitional and 36% of the perimenopausal groups had *reported* menstrual problems. It thus appears that the women in this study did not view their changing menstrual experiences as problems and, moreover, did not equate having discussed menopausal status with having reported a menstrual problem. Clearly, investigations of menopausal experiences must address the personal definitions and perceptions of the women themselves in contrast to the definitions and perceptions of medical professionals, who often determine whether a woman is experiencing menopausal problems or symptoms. Without input from the women themselves, we depend on an unbalanced data base that reveals only observed objective aspects but omits the subjective. The objective aspects are slanted as well by the predominant view of medical professionals that menopause is a disease.

The empirical investigation of biologic and psychosocial changes during menopause has also been hampered by the lack of standard definitions of terms (el-Guebaly, Atchison, and Hay, 1984). The terms lacking consistent definitions in the various investigations of menopause include climacterium, premenopause, menopause, and postmenopause. Some investigations use the woman's own definition of her menopausal status, while others assign women to premenopausal, menopausal, or postmenopausal categories on the basis of certain criteria; still other studies make no distinction between the various experiental phases of menopause. The same definitions and criteria are inconsistently used across investigations, and comparisons between studies are therefore difficult, if not impossible, to make.

One difficulty associated with the interpretation of research findings and comparison of findings across studies of symptoms is the lack of reliable and valid measures of menopausal symptoms. The symptom checklist approaches the experience of menopause from a negative standpoint. Wilbush (1981) pointed out that symptoms are means of communication, not data, and yet objectification of symptoms as data has already led to difficulties in research and in the interpretation of findings. McKinlay and Jeffreys (1974) have suggested that a symptom checklist leads to overreporting of those specified on the list.

The most frequently reported characteristic of the menopause is the hot flash, or flush. Approximately 50% to 85% of menopausal women experience the hot flash with varying degrees of frequency, intensity, and duration (Tulandi and Lal, 1985b). Many studies of hot flashes focus on the physiological and biochemical aspects and describe physical symptoms and biochemical changes (Bohler and Greenblatt, 1974; Tataryn et al., 1981). Recently, researchers have emphasized treatment of the hot flash, usually by ERT (Coope, Thomson, and

Poller, 1975; Dennerstein, Burrows, Hyman, and Wood, 1978; Tulandi et al., 1985a).

Voda (1981b) conducted a study of the menopausal hot flash based on the assumption that the biomedical paradigm presenting the hot flash as a symptom of disease could not be supported by the existing data base. The study was descriptive in nature, and information was obtained from reports by 67 menopausal women concerning their hot flash experiences over a six-month period. Voda concluded that these women did not view the hot flash as a symptom of disease, and several other studies have supported this conclusion (Kay et al., 1982; Muhlenkamp et al., 1983). A significant outcome of the Voda study was that it provided the initial data for improved understanding of women's experiences of the hot flash as well as the meanings individual women attached to their experiences.

Investigation of the relationship of psychosocial variables and menopausal experience has been scanty. However, several studies have offered some indication that certain variables affect how women experience the menopausal period and symptoms women attribute to menopause. Patrick (1970), in a study of expectations about menopause found a positive correlation between the number of symptoms anticipated and the number reported by white, middle-class women, but not by black, lower-class women. Meltzer (1974) found that women with more positive attitudes toward femininity reported less distress in relation to menopause. Maoz, Dowty, Antonovsky, and Wijsenbeck (1970), in a survey of menopausal women, found a more positive response to menopause in women who did not want to have more children (see Datan, this volume).

Findings from several studies have shown that well-being is higher and depression is lower in women whose children have left home than in women living with young children. The presence or absence of children in the home may well influence attitudes toward, and expectations of, menopause (Lowenthal, 1975; Campbell, Converse, and Rogers, 1976).

Frey (1981) concluded from a study of middle-aged women that career orientation and type of occupation may have a significant influence on the expectations and experiences associated with menopause. Birnbaum (1975) in a study of satisfaction and self-esteem at midlife compared groups of professional women who were married, single, and with or without children, to "homemakers" who had not worked since the birth of their first child. The groups of professional women demonstrated more satisfaction and higher self-esteem than did the group of women with traditional women's roles. These studies have identified factors bound to affect women's expectations and experiences of menopause. However, comprehensive investigations focusing on the identification and explanation of factors that influence women's expectations and experiences of menopause are not found in the older literature and have only recently begun (see Goodman, this volume).

THEORETICAL MODELS OF MENOPAUSAL SYMPTOM/EXPERIENCE ETIOLOGY

Gannon (1985) notes that various theoretical models have been proposed to explain the etiology of menopausal symptoms. The primary model has been a *biomedical one*, which states that both psychological and physical symptoms result from estrogen depletion. Studies done to date do not strongly support this model, but as pointed out previously, the small number of studies that exist, as well as lack of valid measures of menopausal symptoms, limit the ability to draw definitive conclusions at present.

A second model relates to the *premorbid personality* of the woman and views menopausal symptoms as due to a history of poor adjustment rather than to the menopause. Donovan (1951), in a study of 110 women who reported psychological complaints with menopause, found that the majority of women had similar complaints prior to the menopausal period. Polit and LaRocco (1980) found that psychological symptoms during menopause were significantly associated with poor premorbid adjustment, while weight gain and vasomotor symptoms seemed less affected by psychological variables. Bart and Grossman (1976) discussed an unpublished study by Kraines that found that those women experiencing more difficulty with menopause also had low self-esteem and low levels of life satisfaction.

A third model is concerned with *coincidental stress*. Several investigations have indicated that stressful life events that occur during the menopausal period significantly increase the incidence and severity of psychological and physical symptoms. A survey of 408 menopausal-age women found that life stress was significant for women who reported psychological and somatic symptoms, and the relationship between symptoms and stress was greater for younger women in the group (Greene and Cooke, 1980). The stressful life events reported in the study were further divided into those associated with "exit" events, such as death or a child's leaving home. Women between the ages of 35 and 54 experienced the greatest amount of stress, which was related almost exclusively to "exit" events, particularly death (Cooke and Greene, 1981; see Greene, this volume). These results suggest that stress may be a major variable in the experience of psychological and physical symptoms for menopausal women.

A fourth model is Koeske's (1982) *cultural relativist* model, which identifies various societal values and social, political, or economic factors influencing cultural stereotypes of the menopause. Women in the United States are placed in culturally defined roles that are primarily biological in nature. Women are evaluated based on their biological capacity for being attractive and bearing and raising children; whereas for men, performance and intelligence are more important than biology. Women with these culturally defined roles experience the effects of menopause as a loss of their ability to fulfill these roles. Thus menopause for them has negative psychological consequences.

Several assumptions are implicit in the cultural model:

(1) There is a correlation between cultural attitudes toward menopause and symptoms of menopause. In a cross-cultural comparison, Vara (1970) found that Finnish women experienced fewer menopausal symptoms than did American women. This discrepancy was attributed to Finnish women's viewing menopause as a natural process, while American women viewed it as an unavoidable illness. According to Lock (1986a, b), cross-cultural research points up some contradictory results. Mayan Indians (Beyene, 1986), North Africans resident in Israel (Walfish, Antonovsky, and Maoz, 1984), the Rajput of India (Flint, 1974), and the Japanese (Lock, 1986b) reported few or no somatic symptoms. Wright (1983), on the other hand, found a similar incidence of hot flashes among Navaho and "Anglos," although their frequency is different: 65–70% of Anglos reported hot flashes each day, but only 17% of Navahos did. Symptom reporting

was much higher in the North American and European population. In addition, two other studies elicited much higher somatic symptom reporting, one in Zimbabwe (Moore, 1981) and one in Varanasi, India (Sharma and Saxena, 1981). It is unclear, according to Lock (1986a), whether these contradictory findings represent real differences or whether they are artifacts of research design and administration.

(2) Attitudes and symptoms vary across cultures. In a study by Flint (1975), 483 Indian women exhibited few menopausal problems and had no complaints of depression or incapacitation. They were from a society where premenopausal women were considered contaminated and severely limited in their activities, while menopausal and postmenopausal women were given much more freedom. Studies in this area suggest that when menopause is associated with loss of significant roles and reduction of freedom or power, the societal attitude toward menopause is negative. This negative societal attitude will affect the psychological well-being of menopausal women.

(3) Attitudes toward menopause and symptoms vary among distinct subgroups within the culture—for example, employment outside the home—as well as with socioeconomic class and education level. That employed women are less likely to suffer from menopausal depression has been supported by several studies (Polit and LaRocco, 1980; Frey, 1981). In a study by Dege and Gretzinger (1982), attitudes toward menopause were assessed in men and women with varying levels of education. Those men and women who were more educated had more positive attitudes toward menopause than did those who had less education. These results are in agreement with the cultural relativist model, which predicts that women who are employed and/ or educated will rely for self-esteem less on biological roles than on roles related to occupation and education.

Koeske (1982) suggests that this model, in which cultural factors are part of the etiology of menopausal symptoms, cannot stand alone. Rather it must consider other factors and influences. These include physical and biological variables, emotional stress, experience and behavior patterns, and environmental stresses.

Bowles (1984, 1986) has proposed a conceptual model related to menopausal attitude formation and its influence on menopausal experience. This model is based on a combination of several models, including that proposed by Koeske (1982), Fishbein and Ajzen's (1975) model of attitude formation, and Kaufert's (1982) conceptual model regarding the relationship between menopausal symptoms and life events (see Figure 1).

Fishbein and Ajzen (1975) conceptualized attitude as a person's feelings toward, and evaluation of, some object or event. Attitude can be measured by locating the person on a bipolar affective or evaluative dimension with regard to the object or event under study. Beliefs are considered to be the fundamental building blocks for attitude formation; they represent accumulated information about an object or event, either from direct observation, from other information sources, or by way of inference.

Thus a woman learns or forms beliefs about menopause. Her attitude toward menopause is determined by her beliefs that menopause has certain attributes and by her evaluation of these attributes. Beliefs may consist of expectations that menopause is associated with, or follows from, another event, for example, the expectation that the hot flash comes with menopause. Beliefs may also be of a normative nature due to the influence of sociocultural factors.

Kaufert (1982) proposed a conceptual model that considers the relationship between menopausal symptoms and life events coinciding with the menopause. It is not the life events themselves, but their impact on the woman's self esteem, that will determine their meanings. The impact on self-esteem will in turn depend on the definition of the event within the sociocultural context in which it occurs. She suggested that there are social implications to becoming menopausal that vary from one society to another. The definition of the menopause of any social group will be formed from the meaning and consequence of the menopause for the position of women in the structure of that society. This definition forms a stereotype of the menopause experience and is accessible to all members of the society. On its basis, people will develop expectations and beliefs that influence attitudes and interaction patterns of these people with the menopausal woman. The menopausal woman herself will draw from this same stereotype, it will act as a filter through which physiological and psychological experiences are interpreted.

This menopausal stereotype can present either a positive or negative picture of the menopausal experience. When the stereotype is negative, there is a threat to the self-esteem of women as they

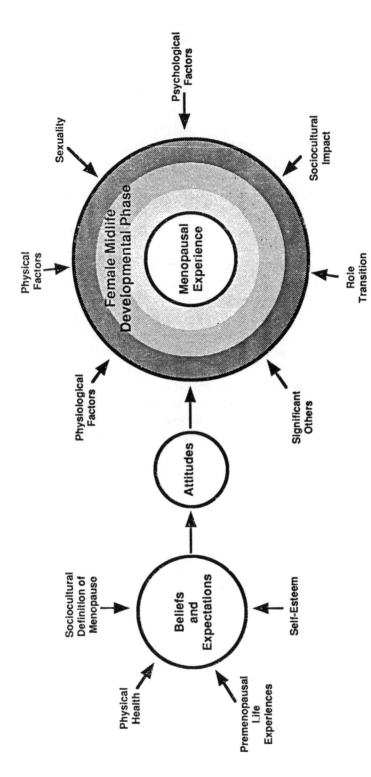

FIG. 1. Conceptual Model of Menopause Attitude Formation and Influence on Menopausal Experience.

approach menopause. When it is positive, it has a more rewarding effect on self-esteem. From this framework, it can then be hypothesized that a woman who initially has low self-esteem will be more vulnerable to a negative stereotype of menopause and will experience more symptoms during menopause. This model certainly suggests the importance of investigating the menopause from a multivariate approach. But the model also makes a case for the importance of assessment of attitudes toward the menopause of women of various ages as well as attitudes of others in the society.

The conceptual model in Figure 1 depicts menopause attitude formation and its influence on menopausal experience and identifies some of the factors associated with the formation of beliefs and expectations about menopause, such as self-esteem, physical health, premenopausal life experiences, and sociocultural definition.

The model presents menopause as only one aspect of the female midlife developmental period and demonstrates how the study of menopause must explore the interaction of many factors. It can serve as a guide to the study of menopausal women and will allow for the inclusion of the most important variables influencing women.

This chapter as well as the most current literature on menopause has emphasized that we do not have accurate data on menopausal women and their experiences. It is the task of researchers who focus on the menstrual cycle, and more particularly on women's experiences of the menopausal transition of that cycle, to provide new and more complete information.

REFERENCES

Ballinger, B. (1981), The menopause and its syndromes. In: *Modern Perspectives in the Psychiatry of Middle Age*, ed. J. Howells. New York: Brunner/Mazel, pp. 279–303.

Barbo, D. (1987), The physiology of the menopause. *Med. Clin. N. Amer.*, 11:11–22.

Barnett, R. & Baruch, G. (1978), Women in the middle years: A critique of research theory. *Psychol. Women Quart.*, 3:187–195.

Bart, P.B. (1969), Why women's status changes in middle age: The turns of the social ferris wheel. *Sociol. Sympos.*, Fall:1–14.

_____ Grossman, M. (1976), Menopause. *Women & Health*, 1:3–11.

Beyene, Y. (1986), Cultural significance and physiological manifestations of menopause: A biocultural analysis. *Cult., Med. Psychiat.*, 10:47–72.

Birnbaum, J. (1975), Life patterns and self-esteem in gifted family-oriented and career committed women. In: *Women and Achievement: Social and Motivational Analysis*, ed. M. Mednick, S. Tangri & L. Hoffman. New York: Wiley, pp. 176–188.

Bohler, C. & Greenblatt, R. (1974), The pathophysiology of the hot flush. In: *The Menopausal Syndrome*, ed. R. Greenblatt, B. Mahesh & G. McDonough. New York: Medicom Press, pp. 29–48.

Bowles, C.L. (1974), An analysis of printed information on the menstrual cycle provided to high school females. Unpublished paper, University of Illinois.

_____ (1984), Measure of attitude toward menopause using the semantic differential model. Unpublished doctoral dissertation, Northern Illinois University.

_____ (1986a), Measure of attitude toward menopause using the semantic differential model. *Nurs. Res.*, 35:81–85.

_____ (1986b), Men's attitudes toward menopause: A preliminary study. Unpublished manuscript.

Brim, O. G. & Abeles, R.P. (1975), Work and personality in the middle years.*Items*, 29:5–16.

Brooks-Gunn, J. (1982), A sociocultural approach. In: A. Voda, M. *Changing Perspectives on Menopause*, ed. A. Voda, M. Dinnerstein & S. O'Donnell. Austin: University of Texas Press, pp. 203–207.

Campbell, A., Converse, P., & Rogers, W. (1976), *The Quality of American life*. New York: Russell Sage Foundation.

Cooke, D.J. & Greene, J.G. (1981), Types of life events in relation to symptoms at the climacterium. *J. Psychosomat. Res.*, 25:5–11.

Coope, J., Thomson, J. & Poller, L. (1975), Effects of "natural oestrogen" replacement on menopausal symptoms and blood clotting. *Brit. Med. J.*, 4:139.

Dan, A., Graham, E., Beecher, C., Bart, P., Komnenich, P., Krueger, J., Pitel, M. Ruble, D. (1980), Synthesis and new directions. In: *The Menstrual Cycle, Vol. I*, ed. A. Dan, E. Graham & C. Beecher. New York: Springer, pp. 339–345.

Dege, K. & Gretzinger, J. (1982) Attitudes of families toward menopause. In: *Changing Perspectives on Menopause*, ed. A.M. Voda, M. Dinnerstein & S.R. O'Donnell. Austin: University of Texas Press, pp. 60–69.

Dennerstein, L., Burrows, G., Hyman, G. & Wood, C. (1978), Menopausal hot flushes: A double blind comparison of placebo, ethinyl oestradiol and norgestrel. *Brit. J. Obs. Gyn.*, 85:852–854.

Donovan, J. C. (1951), The menopausal syndrome: A study of case histories. *Amer. J. Obs. Gyn.*, 62:1281–91.

el-Guebaly, N., Atchison, B. & Hay, W. (1984), The menopause: Stressors and facilitators. *Can. Med. Assn. J.*, 131:865–869.

Fishbein, M. & Ajzen, I. (1975), *Belief, Attitude, Intention and Behavior*. Menlo Park, Ca.: Addison-Wesley.

Flint, M. (1974), Menarche and menopause of Rajput women. Unpublished doctoral dissertation, the City University of New York.

_____ (1975). The menopause:Reward or punishment? *Psychosom.*, 16:161–63.

Frey, K. (1981), Middle-aged women's experience and perceptions of menopause. *Women & Health*, 6:25–36.

Galloway, K. (1975), The change of life. *Amer. J. Nurs.* 75:1006–1011.

Gannon. L. (1985). *Menstrual Disorders and Menopause.* New York: Praeger.

Gath, D., Osborn, M., Bungay, G., Iles, S., Day, A., Bond, A. & Passingham, C. (1987), Psychiatric disorder and gynecological symptoms in middle aged women: A community survey. *Brit. Med. J.*, 294:213–218.

Greenblatt, R. (1955), Metabolic and psychosomatic disorders in menopausal women. *Geriat.*, 10:165.

Greene, J.G. & Cooke, D.J. (1980), Life stress and symptoms at the climacterium. *Brit. J. Psychiat.*, 136:486–491.

Kahana, B. (1976), A life events approach to the study of middle-age changes: Perspectives of parents and adult children. Presented at meeting of the American Psychological Association, Washington, DC

Kahana, E., Kiyak, A. & Liang, J. (1980). Menopause in the context of other life events. In: *The Menstrual Cycle, Vol. I*, ed. A. Dan, E. Graham & C. Beecher. New York: Springer, pp. 167–179.

Kaufert, P. (1982), Anthropology and menopause: The development of a theoretical framework. *Maturitas*, 4:181–193.

_____ (1986), Menstruation and menstrual change: Women in midlife. *Health Care of Women Internat.*, 7:63–76.

Kay, M., Voda, A., Olivas, G., Rios, F. & Imle, M. (1982), Ethnography of the menopause-related hot flash. *Maturitas*, 4:217–227.

Kerr, M. (1968), Psychohormonal approach to the menopause. *Mod. Treatment*, 5:587.

Koboso-Munro, L. (1977), Sexuality in the aging woman. *Health & Soc. Work*, 2:71–86.

Koeske, R. (1982), Toward a biosocial paradigm for menopausal research: Lessons and contributions from behavioral sciences. In: *Changing Perspectives on Menopause*, ed. A. Voda, M. Dinnerstein & S.R. O'Connell. Austin: University of Texas Press, pp. 3–23.

Lock, M. (1986a), Introduction, *Cult., Med. Psychiat.*, 10:1–5.

_____ (1986b), Ambiguities of aging. *Cult., Med. Psychiat.*, 10:23–46.

Lowenthal, M. (1975), Psychological variations across the adult life course: Frontiers for research and policy. *Geronotolgist*, 15:6–12.

McKinlay, S. & Jeffreys, M. (1974), The menopausal syndrome. *Brit. J. Prevent. Soc. Med.*, 28:108–115.

Meltzer, L. (1974), The aging female: A study of attitudes toward aging and self concept held by premenopausal, menopausal and postmenopausal women. *Dissertation Abstracts International*, 35:1055-B.

Millette, B. (1981), Menopause: A survey of attitudes and knowledge. *Issues in Health Care of Women*, 3:263–276.

Maoz, B., Dowty, N., Antonovsky, A. & Wijsenbeck, H. (1970), Female attitudes to the menopause. *Soc. Psychiat.*, 5:35–40.

Moore, B. (1981), Climacteric symptoms in an African community. *Maturitas* 3:25–29.

Muhlenkamp, A., Waller, M. & Bourne, A. (1983), Attitudes toward women in menopause: A vignette approach. *Nurs. Res.*, 32:20–23.

Neugarten, B., Wood, V., Kraines, R. & Loomis, B. (1963), Women's attitudes toward the menopause. *Vita Humana*, 6:140–151.

———— Kraines, R. (1965), Menopausal symptoms in women of various ages. *Psychosom. Med.*, 27:266–273.

Parlee, M. (1981), Gaps in behavioral research on the menstrual cycle. In: *The Menstrual Cycle, Vol. II*, ed. P. Komnenich, M. McSweeney, J. Noack & N. Elder. New York: Springer, pp. 45–53.

Patrick, M. (1970), A study of middle-aged women and menopause. Unpublished doctoral dissertation. University of California, Los Angeles.

Polit, D. & Larocco, S. (1980), Social and psychological correlates of menopausal symptoms. *Psychosom. Med.*, 42, 335–45.

Raymond, C. (1988), Studies question how much role menopause plays in some women's emotional distress. *J. Amer. Med. Ass.*, 259:3522–3523.

Rohrbaugh, J. (1979), *Women: Psychology's puzzle*. New York: Basic Books.

Severne, L. (1979), Psycho-social aspects of the menopause. In: *Psychosomatics in Perimenopause*, ed. A. Haspels & J. Musaph. Baltimore, MD. University Park Press, pp. 101–120.

Sharma, V.K. & Saxena, M.S.L. (1981), Climacteric symptoms: a study in the Indian context. *Maturitas*, 3:11–20.

Sommer, B. (1981), Menstrual cycle research: Yesterday, today and tommorrow. In: *The Menstrual Cycle, Vol. II*, ed. P. Komnenich, M. McSweeney, J. Noack & N. Elder. New York: Springer, pp. 193–199.

Tataryn, I., Lomax, P., Meldrum, D., Bajorek, J., Chesarek, W. & Judd, H. (1981), Objective techniques for the assessment of postmenopausal hot flashes. *Obs. Gyn.*, 57:340–344.

Tulandi, T., Kinch, R., Guyda, H., Maiolo, L. & Lal, S. (1985a), Effect of naloxone infusion on menopausal flushes, skin temperature and luteinizing hormone secretion. *Amer. J. Obs. Gyn.*, 151:277–279.

———— Lal, S. (1985b), Menopausal hot flush. *Obs. Gyn. Survey*, 40:553–563.

Utian, W. (1987), Overview on menopause. *Amer. J. Obs. Gyn.*, 156:1280–1283.

Vara, P. (1970), The climacterium from the gynaecologist's point of view. *Acta Obs. Gyn. Scandinavica*, 49:Supp. 1, 47–55.

Voda, A. (1981a), Alterations of the menstrual cycle: Hormonal and mechanical. In: *The Menstrual Cycle, Vol. II*, ed. P. Komnenich, M. McSweeney, J. A. Noack & N. Elder. New York: Springer, pp. 145–163.

———— (1981b), Climacteric hot flash. *Maturitas*, 3:73–90.

———— & Eliasson, M. (1985), Menopause: The closure of menstrual life. In: *Lifting the Curse of Menstruation*, ed. S. Golub. New York: Harrington Park Press, pp. 137–156.

Voda, A. & George, T. (1986), Menopause. In: *Annual Review of Nursing Research, Vol. 4*, ed. H. Werley, J. Fitzpatrick & R. Taunton. New York: Springer, pp. 55–75.

Walfish, S., Antonovsky, A. & Maoz, B. (1984), Relationship between biological changes and symptoms and health behavior during the climacteric. *Maturitas* 6:9–17.

Weg, R. (1987), Sexuality in the menopause. In: *Menopause: Physiology and Pharmacology*, ed. D. Mishell. Chicago: Year Book Med., pp. 127–138.

Wilbush, J. (1981), What's in a name? Some linquistic aspects of the climacteric. *Maturitas*, 3:1–9.

Wright, A.L. (1983), A cross-cultural comparison of menopausal symptoms. *Med. Anthropol.*, 7:20–35.

III

Endocrinology,
Clinical and Experiential
Studies, and Literary Aspects

8

Endocrinology
of Menopause

LINDA GANNON

An overview of the typical menstrual cycle in women between ages 18 and 40 provides a background against which to appreciate the magnitude of the changes that surround menopause. The events that characterize normal menstrual function rely primarily on the activities of the hypothalamus, the anterior pituitary, and the ovaries. Beginning with menstruation, the hypothalamus produces gonado-tropin releasing hormone (GnRH), which, in turn, stimulates the anterior pituitary to release the gonadotropins-follicle stimulating hormone (FSH) and luteinizing hormone (LH). FSH triggers the initial growth of follicles in the ovary. As these follicles develop, they begin to produce estrogen; eventually, one follicle assumes domi-nance and continues to develop while the others regress. The dominant follicle increases its production of estrogen. This hormone (1) causes proliferation of the endometrium, the lining of the uterus, (2) it exerts a feedback effect on the anterior pituitary and (3) it is responsible for the midcycle surge of LH. This surge is followed by ovulation, which is the release of the mature ovum from the follicle. LH also transforms the ruptured follicle into the corpus luteum.

In the postovulatory phase, the corpus luteum, a short-lived secretory organ, produces estrogen and progesterone. Progesterone transforms the endometrium into a secretory organ in preparation for implantation of the embryo should conception occur. Progesterone also exerts a negative feedback effect on the release of gonadotropins from the pituitary, precluding further follicular growth during this phase. If conception does not occur, the corpus luteum degenerates, accompanied by decreasing levels of estrogen and progesterone. Since the secretory endometrium requires these hormones for maintenance, it also regresses and menstruation occurs. With low levels of estrogen and progesterone, inhibition of the hypothalamus and the anterior pituitary is lifted and a new cycle begins.

Menopause, strictly speaking, refers to the cessation of this cycling activity. The cause of menopause is generally believed to be a considerable reduction in the number of remaining follicles and a lessened responsiveness to gonadotropin stimulation in those remaining (Studd, Chakravarti, and Oram, 1977). Thus, during some menstrual cycles, follicular development may not occur, with consequent lowered levels of estrogen, elevated levels of FSH and LH, a lack of ovulation, and an irregular pattern of bleeding. As this transitional period progresses over five to ten years, more and more cycles become anovulatory until menstruation stops completely.

A problem with this view of menopause is that, extrapolating from follicle counts in menstruating women, one would predict that women at menopausal age would have several thousand follicles remaining. This premise was examined directly by Richardson, Senikas, and Nelson (1987), who assessed the number of follicles remaining in women categorized as menstruating, perimenopausal, or menopausal. Menstruating women were found to have ten times as many follicles as perimenopausal women; follicles were absent in the ovaries of postmenopausal women. Thus, while menopause may be a direct consequence of a considerably diminished follicle reserve, the rate of follicle loss appears to accelerate dramatically in the last decade before menopause; and the cause of this acceleration is yet to be clarified. Indeed, given the fine tuning of the hypothalamic-pituitary-ovarian system required to maintain regular ovulatory cycles, an alteration in any part of the system could initiate the changes that culminate in menopause.

ENDOCRINOLOGICAL CHANGES
ACCOMPANYING THE MENOPAUSE

The natural menopausal process is not a sudden one, but a gradual decrease in ovulatory cycles, with steadily increasing levels of LH and FSH and decreasing levels of estrogen until menstruation ceases completely, usually between the ages of 45 and 55. Adamopoulos, Loraine, and Dove (1971) studied a group of premenopausal women, aged 37 to 42. These women had LH levels approximately seven times greater and FSH levels approximately three times greater than those found in younger women, along with reduced levels of estrogen and progesterone. The authors expressed surprise at the existence of such high levels of gonadotropins in women who were ovulating. In a similar study, Sherman, West, and Korenman (1976) found lowered estradiol concentrations, increased FSH concentrations, but LH concentrations in the normal range in a group of women approaching menopause. Such data argue against the theory that gonadotropins increase as a result of ovarian failure. However, Hammond and Ory (1982) speculate that, given the reduced number of follicles, an increased level of FSH may be required to promote follicular development.

In contrast to this typically gradual process, surgical removal of the ovaries in premenopausal women produces an abrupt menopause. Shortly after surgery, estrogen levels fall dramatically and gonadotropin levels gradually increase (Ostergard, Parlow, and Townsend, 1970; Hunter, Julier, Franklin, and Green, 1977; Utian, Katz, Davey, and Carr, 1978). Monroe, Jaffe, and Midgley (1972) reported that in their sample FSH levels initially rose more rapidly than LH levels and that at one month following surgery the elevated gonadotropin levels had not yet reached postmenopausal levels in all subjects.

Estrogen Production during the Menopause

The postmenopausal ovary is not totally inactive in terms of hormone production. The ovary is divided into two areas: the outer cortex contains granulosa cells, which are the primary source of ovarian estrogen (Longcope, Hunter, and Franz, 1980); these cells are reduced in number and productive capacity after menopause. However, the ovarian stroma, which is capable of synthesizing the androgens—androstendione, dehydroepiandrosterone, and testosterone—continue hormone production after menopause, and these compounds may undergo peripheral conversion to estrogen (Hunter, 1976). Several lines of evidence suggest that the postmenopausal ovary secretes little if any estrogen. Mattingly and Huang (1969) assessed the steroidogenesis of ovarian tissue slices taken from menopausal and postmenopausal women. This tissue was clearly capable of producing dehydroepiandrosterone and testosterone but yielded minimal amounts of estrogen. Furthermore, the similarity between estrogen levels of women with natural versus surgical menopause implies that estrogen is not being secreted by the ovaries (Rader et al. 1973).

More direct data regarding the hormone production of the postmenopausal ovary come from a study by Judd, Judd, Lucas, and Yen (1974). They compared the concentrations of testosterone, androstenedione, estradiol, and estrone in peripheral and ovarian vein blood from ten postmenopausal women. (Estrone, a less biologically active compound than estradiol, is the major estrogen in postmenopausal women.) A higher concentration of all these hormones was found in the ovarian vein than in the peripheral vein; the magnitudes of the differences were 15-fold for testosterone, 4-fold for androstenedione, and 2-fold for both estradiol and estrone. The authors concluded that the postmenopausal ovary secretes primarily androgens while retaining a minimal amount of estrogen secretion. Mattingly and Huang (1969) have suggested that this continued androgen production may contribute to the minor androgenic state of the postmenopausal women, including balding on the scalp, hair growth on the face and chest, and changes in fat distribution.

In spite of the evidence that the ovaries cease to secrete other than minimal amounts of estrogen after menopause, estrogen can be detected in the plasma of postmenopausal women. The mechanism of estrogen production in postmenopausal women is believed to be the conversion of androstenedione to estrogen in peripheral tissue, particularly adipose tissue. Data consistent with this hypothesis have been reported in several studies (Rader et al., 1973; Judd, Lucas, and Yen, 1976; Vermeulen, 1976) that have found estradiol and estrone levels not to be significantly different in oophorectomized women and postmenopausal women with intact ovaries. Hunter (1976) suggested that although the ovarian stroma is capable of synthesizing androstenedione, these cells do not secrete estrogen; and although removal of the ovaries results in a 50% reduction in circulating androstenedione, there is not a corresponding change in estrone because the rate of peripheral conversion is increased to make up for the difference.

Research investigating the percentage of total estrogen that is the product of peripheral conversion has not yielded consistent results. In one study (Grodin, Siiteri, and MacDonald, 1973), the quantity of estrone derived from aromatization of androgens was essentially the same as the absolute levels of estrone, suggesting that all estrone was derived in this manner. In contrast, Judd et al. (1982) assessed the metabolic clearance rate, conversion ratios, and production rates of androgens, estrone, and estradiol. The peripheral conversion of androgens accounted for 24.6% of circulating estrone but accounted for only minimal quantities of estradiol, while the peripheral conversion of estrone accounted for 21.5% of estradiol. The subjects in this study had intact ovaries, but the research cited earlier (Judd et al., 1974) suggests that it is unlikely that the ovaries were the source of the estrogens unaccounted for by peripheral conversion. Age may be a factor of relevance to this issue. Hemsell et al. (1974) found a significant relationship between the efficiency of conversion and age, indicating that as one ages the body becomes more efficient at converting androgens to estrogens. It is interesting that, although the correlations for women were higher, significant correlations between conversion rate and age were reported for both men and women.

Research, then, indicates that the postmenopausal woman has detectable levels of estrogen in her plasma, that the presence or absence of ovaries does not seem to influence significantly the levels of circulating estrogens, and that the peripheral conversion of androgens to estrogen, although a major source of estrogen, may not account for all estrogen. Since the adrenal cortex is capable of synthesizing and secreting androgens, this gland may also be capable of synthesizing estrogen or may contribute significantly to the pool of precursors available for peripheral conversion. Several studies have reported a minimal change in circulating levels of estrone after oophorectomy although androgens were found to decrease (Vermeulen, 1976; Chang and Judd, 1981). These data suggest that the adrenal cortex may secrete estrogens. Some researchers have stimulated the adrenal cortex with adrenocorticotrophic hormone (ACTH) and found significant increases in estrone, progesterone, and androsterodione (Poliak, Smith, Friedlander, and Romney, 1971; Murakami, Yamaji, and Ohsawa, 1976; Vermeulen, 1976). Both Murakami et al. (1976) and Maroulis and Abraham (1976) interpreted these data to mean that the adrenal cortex directly secretes estrone, although this is difficult to determine conclusively since increases in estrone may be due to increased peripheral conversion of androgens to estrone. Thus, the adrenal cortex seems to be a major source of estrone in postmenopausal women, but it is not clear if estrone is secreted directly or if the adrenals secrete androgens, which are then converted to estrogen.

Adipose tissue is a primary site of the peripheral conversion of testosterone and androstenedione to estradiol and estrone in postmenopausal women (Archer, 1982). This process is believed to be the underlying cause of the consistent finding that circulating levels of estrone and estradiol are significantly correlated with body weight and excess fat in postmenopausal women (Badawy, Elliott, Elbadawi, and Marshall, 1979; Judd et al., 1976). Although levels of estrogen would be, in theory, due to the availability of precursors and the rate of conversion, weight has not been found to correlate with circulating androstenedione and testosterone levels. Therefore, the association between weight and estrogen levels is assumed to be due to the increased rate of conversion, which, in turn, is possible because of the greater amount of fat.

Weight has also been found to be negatively correlated with the circulating concentration of sex hormone binding globulin (SHBG), a plasma protein that binds with estradiol and renders it biologically inactive (Erlik, Meldrum, and Judd, 1982). Thus, body fat appears to have a dual effect on estrogen levels: excess body fat is associated with an increased conversion of androgens to estrogens and the lower levels of SHBG exhibited by obese persons suggest that less estrogen is bound, and more is active, than in thin persons. These processes are presumed to account for the greater incidence of hot flashes and osteoporosis among thin postmenopausal women than among the obese.

Gonadotropin Production during the Menopause

There is confusion in the literature as to the cause of the elevated levels of gonadotropins after menopause. Given the feedback mechanisms necessary for normal menstrual cycling during the premenopausal years, it is possible that: (a) the decreasing levels of estrogen cause diminished negative feedback to the hypothalamus, resulting in greater production of gonadotropin releasing hormone (GnRH); (b) the levels of GnRH remain the same but the sensitivity of the pituitary to GnRH increases, resulting in greater production of LH and FSH; or (c) both hypothalamic and pituitary activity is similar to that of premenopausal years but the metabolic clearance rates of LH and FSH are reduced. Rosenblum and Schlaff (1976) reported levels of GnRH in postmenopausal women to be undetectable and concluded that the elevated levels of gonadotropins in postmenopausal women were the result of an increase in pituitary sensitivity owing to low levels of estrogen. However, Archer (1982) has suggested that hypothalamic GnRH is released in a pulsatile manner, and high levels could easily be overlooked unless blood was sampled frequently.

In support of Archer's view, Seyler and Reichlin (1973) sampled blood every ten minutes for several hours and found GnRH in postmenopausal women frequently to be in the range of premeno-pausal values, but seven of the 25 women exhibited values greater than three standard deviations higher. Similarly, Henrik (1982) cited evidence to indicate an increase in levels of GnRH in the menopausal and postmenopausal years. The variability of values found for GnRH in postmenopausal women may well be due to the episodic nature of the release, which is also apparent in the cyclic, pulsatile discharge of FSH and LH from the pituitary at intervals of 60 to 70 minutes. Similar pulses of FSH and LH are present during menstruating years, but the amplitude of the pulses is smaller and the periodicity is asynchronous compared to that of menopausal women (Archer, 1982).

Of recent interest has been the role of endogenous opiates in the regulation of gonadotropins. Reid, Hoff, and Yen (1981) noted a significant decrease in LH concentrations in both men and women after administering synthetic endorphin. Quigley and Yen (1980) administered the opiate antagonist naloxone to menstruating women at various points in their cycle. They observed a significant increase in

LH release in both the late follicular and mid-luteal phases of the cycle; there was no obvious effect on LH concentrations during the early follicular phase. Because the impact of naloxone appeared to be dependent on phase of the menstrual cycle, it was suspected that ovarian steroids were involved. Yen et al. (1985) concluded, "Modulations of frequency and amplitude of GnRH secretory activity appear to be mediated through an inhibitory action of endogenous opioids, and the functional coupling of the opioidergic and GnRH systems is an event dependent on ovarian steroids" (p. 93).

If in menstruating women ovarian steroids are necessary for the release of hypothalamic beta-endorphin, which, in turn, inhibits the release of pituitary gonadotropins, then endogenous opioids may play a role in the high gonadotropin production found with menopause. Aleem and McIntosh (1984) found beta-endorphin levels in 13 postmenopausal women (7 surgical, 6 natural) to be significantly lower than those in 10 normally menstruating controls. Similarly, Yen et al. (1985) reported that infusion of naloxone failed to modify the release of gonadotropins in postmenopausal women, suggesting the absence of endogenous opioid regulation. Further evidence for this link was provided by Dawood, Khan-Dawood, and Ramos (1986), who evaluated responses to naloxone in postmenopausal women and compared those who were medication free with women who had been receiving hormone treatment. The untreated group showed no response to naloxone, whereas LH increased significantly in response to naloxone in women receiving ovarian hormones. The emerging role of endogenous opioids as a link between ovarian steroids and gonadotropin release not only increases our understanding of endocrinological changes associated with the menopause, but also may aid in the development of effective treatment for menopausal symptoms.

Menopause versus Aging

Since menopause typically occurs in women between the ages of 45 and 55, some of the physiological changes that have been attributed to the menopause may, in fact, be due the aging process. If endocrinological changes are primarily due to aging, then one would expect to find a significant relationship between the levels of various hormones and age; alternatively, if such endocrinological changes are due to menopause, the relationship between hormone levels and age would be absent and one would expect to find relatively constant levels prior to menopause, an abrupt shift coincident with menopause, and relatively constant levels subsequent to menopause. The patterns noted for estrogen are consistent with a menopausal hypothesis; that is, estrogen levels decrease at the time of menopause but are not significantly correlated with age or years since menopause (Judd et al., 1976; Reyes, Winter, and Faiman, 1977; Judd et al., 1980; Meldrum, Davidson, Tataryn, and Judd, 1981).

In contrast, Meldrum et al. (1981) assessed hormonal levels in women aged 34 to 83, all of whom had experienced menopause but had intact ovaries. They found a strong negative relationship between age and levels of the androgens dehydroepiandrosterone (DHEA) and dehydroepiandrosterone sulfate (DHEAS); androstendedione and testosterone were significantly lower than levels found in premenopausal women, but levels of these androgens were uncorrelated with age. These authors concluded that adrenal androgen secretion decreases as a function of age. Cumming, Rebar, Hopper, and Yen (1982) measured circulating DHEAS in women with premature ovarian failure, after ovariectomy, and subsequent to menopause. They found that premature ovarian failure and ovariectomy in young, as well as postmenopausal, subjects precipitated an earlier decline in DHEAS levels. The authors concluded that the decline in DHEAS was a function of both age and the cessation of ovarian activity whether it was the result of natural or surgical menopause.

Finally, the effects of age versus menopause on levels of FSH and LH have been investigated. Reyes et al. (1977) reported that although FSH exhibited a significant correlation with age, LH did not but was considerably higher in postmenopause than in premenopause. The obvious explanation for elevated levels of LH and FSH in postmenopausal women is the absence of negative feedback due to lowered levels of estrogen. Henrik (1982) suggests, however, that there may also be age-related, physiological changes that would tend to enhance the increased gonadotropin levels even further. One such change is a decreasing ability of the aging organism to inactivate or excrete LH from the circulation, which would result in the accumulation of gonadotropins; another mechanism may be a reduction in the hormone-binding capacity of the brain due to aging, decreasing the negative feedback effects of the estrogen that is present in the circulation. Thus, the elevated levels of gonadotropins evident in postmenopausal women may be due primarily to the diminished production of estrogen but may be enhanced by other, age-related physiological processes.

In summary, natural menopause is a gradual process with a progressive increase in anovulatory cycles and eventual cessation of menses. The hormonal changes accompanying this process probably originate with a decrease in estrogen production by the ovaries, and the lowered levels of estrogen act to increase levels of the gonadotropins. Although estrogen is usually detectable in postmenopausal women, the primary source of these estrogens is probably the peripheral conversion of androgen with minimal amounts of estrogen directly secreted by the ovaries or the adrenal cortex. Although the inactive ovaries of menopausal women are probably the major determinant of the shift in hormonal profiles of elderly women, other factors, such as physiological changes due to aging and percentage of body fat, are contributory.

MENOPAUSAL SYMPTOMS

The popularized version of the "menopausal syndrome" consists of a variety of unpleasant symptoms and changes—hot flashes, profuse sweating, headaches, increased weight, dryness and thinning of the vaginal walls, increased incidence of vaginal infections, loss of breast firmness, dizziness, sensations of cold in the hands and feet, irritability, depression, insomnia, pruritus of the sexual organs, constipation, atherosclerosis, and osteoporosis (Weideger, 1977). There is a widespread belief, evident in the popular media and, to a lesser extent, in scholarly works, that all women experience the menopausal syndrome and require medical treatment. The research on menopausal symptoms presents a different picture.

Several studies report the results of surveys of large numbers of women of menopausal age. McKinlay and Jeffreys (1974) sent a questionnaire to 638 women between the ages of 45 and 54. Hot flashes and night sweats were consistently associated with menopause and occurred in the majority of women; headaches, dizzy spells, palpitations, sleeplessness, depression, and weight increase showed no direct relationship to the menopause and were reported by 30% to 50% of the sample. In a later postal survey by Ballinger (1975, 1976), 539 women between the ages of 40 and 55 were sent a questionnaire intended to assess depressive and neurotic illness. Subjects were categorized according to premenopausal, menopausal, early postmenopausal and late postmenopausal; the data were also analyzed according to age categories regardless of menopausal status. The only significant difference was that women between the ages of 45 and 49 who were premenopausal had more psychiatric problems than premenopausal women between the ages of 40 to 44. The author interpreted his data to imply that before the menopause there is a rise in psychiatric morbidity that does not persist beyond one year past menopause, but that vasomotor symptoms such as hot flashes and night sweats seem clearly related to the menopausal years. Finally, Chakravarti et al. (1977) surveyed women who had had a bilateral oophorectomy. Vasomotor symptoms were the most common problem reported, followed by depression and sexual dysfunction in the form of loss of libido or dyspareunia. Thus, surveys of symptoms in menopausal women have not consistently supported the universality of the traditional menopausal syndrome.

Similar conclusions were reached in a factor analytic study of climacteric symptoms by Greene (1976). He sampled fifty women between the ages of 40 to 55 who had complained of vasomotor and other symptoms. All completed a 30-item symptom scale on which they indicated the extent of each symptom. Three factors accounting for 38% of the variance emerged from the factor analysis: a psychological factor, which included fatigue, worrying, tension, depression, panic attacks, disturbed sleep, excitability, crying; a somatic factor, which included dizziness, numbness or tingling, weight gain, headaches, blind spots in vision, feelings of suffocation; and a vasomotor factor, which included hot flashes, sweating, cold hands and feet. The labeling of the first two factors seems arbitrary; fatigue, for example, could be viewed as a somatic symptom, and feelings of suffocation might better be considered a psychological symptom. Of primary interest, however, was that the factors were not significantly correlated; that is, suffering from symptoms in one category was unrelated to the probability that the woman would suffer symptoms from another category — again suggesting that the "menopausal syndrome" may not be a valid concept since "syndrome" is typically used to refer to a group of symptoms that tend to occur together.

One difficulty in the interpretation of such research is the lack of a reliable and valid measure of menopausal symptoms. One measure, the Menopausal Index, was developed by Kupperman, Blatt, Wiesbader, and Filler (1953). The Index consists of 11 symptoms: vasomotor complaints, paresthesia, insomnia, nervousness, melancholia, vertigo, weakness or fatigue, arthralgia and myalgia, headaches, palpitations, and formication, the latter being a form of paresthesia in which there is a sensation as of ants running over the skin. In determining a person's score on the Index, symptoms are weighted differently, with vasomotor symptoms being given a "4"; paresthesia, insomnia, and nervousness a weight of "2"; and all others a weight of "1," although the authors do not offer a justification for the differential weighting system. There are no reliability data available for the scale, and there has been no assessment of the validity of the scale as a measure of menopausal symptoms.

The primary theoretical model for conceptualizing menopausal symptoms has been a biomedical one, which states that both physical and psychological symptoms are the direct result of estrogen withdrawal or the result of biochemical changes concomitant with estrogen withdrawal, such as the elevated gonadotropin levels found in menopausal women. Relevant to the evaluation of this model are studies assessing the covariation between symptoms and hormonal levels. Abe et al. (1977) assessed serum levels of estradiol, progesterone, FSH, and LH in 191 premenopausal and postmenopausal women and correlated hormonal levels with symptom severity as measured by Kupperman's Menopausal Index; none of the correlations were significant for the women who were experiencing menopause. Similar results were found in a group of women tested after bilateral ovariectomy; those who experienced vasomotor symptoms did not differ in blood levels of estrogen, LH, or FSH from those who did not experience symptoms (Aksel, Schomberg, Tyrey, and Hammond, 1976). On the other hand, Hutton, Jacobs, Murray, and James (1978) measured plasma levels of estrone and estradiol at 20- to 30-minute intervals for up to 24 hours in postmenopausal or ovariectomized women and compared hormonal levels of groups of women categorized according to symptoms; women with superficial dyspareunia and women with both dyspareunia and vasomotor symptoms had significantly lower levels of estradiol, but not of estrone, than did women with only hot flashes and than did women who were symptom free.

Indirect evidence related to the etiology of menopausal symptoms comes from studies that tested the effects of exogenous estrogen on menopausal symptoms. As early as 1950, Fessler noted that hormonal treatment was effective in relieving hot flashes but not irritability and depression. Kaufman (1967) found that hot flashes and atrophic vaginitis were successfully treated with hormones in close to 100% of the women, while only about 50% experienced relief from common emotional symptoms. In the evaluation of this type of research, improvement due to expectation must be considered. Therefore, the effects of exogenous estrogen should be compared with the effects of placebos in a design in which neither the subjects nor the evaluators are aware of which compound the woman has been given. Only in this way can one evaluate the pharmacological effects of the active treatment.

A treatment study satisfying these criteria was reported by Utian (1972), who evaluated the effectiveness of exogenous estrogen treatment on various menopausal symptoms by comparing estrogen with placebo treatment in women with natural and surgical menopause. Only hot flashes and atrophic vaginitis were relieved by estrogen, but not by placebos, while symptoms of depression, irritability, insomnia, and palpitations responded significantly to both estrogen and placebo therapy. The author concluded that the latter symptoms were, therefore, likely to be of psychological origin. Similar results have been found in several other studies employing a placebo control (George, Utian, Beumont, and Beardwood, 1973; Poller, Thomson, and Coope, 1980; Gerdes, EtPhil, Sonnendecker, and Polakow, 1982).

The relevance of treatment studies to issues of etiology is questionable since one cannot infer the cause of a disease from information on methods of effective treatment. Thus, these studies can not be viewed as strong support for the theory that menopausal symptoms are due to hormonal changes. However, methodological problems, such as the lack of a reliable and valid measure of menopausal symptoms, and the relatively small number of studies preclude any definitive conclusions at this time.

Osteoporosis, although frequently viewed as a menopausal symptom, typically is not studied in conjunction with other menopausal symptoms, since its time course is insidious and diagnosis requires complex medical assessment rather than self-report. It is generally believed that menopause is, at least, a contributory factor in the development of osteoporosis in elderly women. However, it has been difficult to differentiate the effects of menopause from those of aging since menopause occurs at a similar age in most women. Nonetheless, there is no question as to the beneficial effect of estrogen therapy on bone metabolism (see, for example, Abdalla et al., 1985; Ettinger, Genant, and Cann, 1985).

Other models explicating the etiology of menopausal symptoms include: (a) the "domino" theory, which postulates that hormonal factors cause hot flashes, other symptoms, such as insomnia, depression, and irritability, being secondary to the hot flashes; (b) the premorbid personality model, which hypothesizes that psychological symptoms are an exacerbation of or a simple continuation of symptoms that existed prior to menopause; (c) the coincidental stress model, which suggests that the particular stresses that occur during the time of menopause, such as children leaving home or illness or death of parents, predispose women to psychological problems; and (d) the cultural relativist model, which examines the effects of crosscultural, societal, or historical factors, such the influence of attitudes and stereotypes, on menopausal symptoms (Koeske, 1982).

Results of investigations across models and disciplines (for a review of this research, see Gannon, 1985) have been surprisingly consistent in supporting the distinction alluded to within the biomedical model. Thus, theorists in this area have concluded that hot flashes, and perhaps atrophic vaginitis and osteoporosis, are caused by the changing hormonal environment of menopause whereas other somatic and psychological symptoms are the result of aging, historical, cultural, and stress factors (Rakoff, 1975; Christie Brown and Christie Brown, 1976; Dewhurst, 1976; Perlmutter, 1978; Bart and Perlmutter, 1981). Consequently, this chapter will focus on those symptoms most clearly associated with the menopause.

ENDOCRINOLOGICAL AND PHYSIOLOGICAL
ASPECTS OF THE MENOPAUSAL HOT FLASH

The most common complaints of menopausal women are those associated with vasomotor instability. Hot flashes, characterized by sensations of heat usually in the face, neck, and chest and sometimes followed by perspiration, shivering, or both, are frequently noticed prior to the complete cessation of menses and continue through the early years after menopause. They seem to be most frequent and most intense shortly after cessation of menses and shortly after surgery in women having bilateral oophorectomy. There is surprisingly little reliable information on the percentage of women who experience hot flashes during menopause or on the length of time the symptom persists, although it has been assumed that this symptom occurs in the majority of women and that even without treatment hot flashes abate over time and eventually cease completely. Women seeking medical help for hot flashes are typically placed on hormone replacement therapy (HRT) consisting of estrogen or a combination of estrogen and progesterone, both of which tend to alleviate the symptoms.

In the only published descriptive study of the menopausal hot flash, Voda (1982) had 20 menopausal women keep records of their hot flashes for two weeks. She presented the following summary information based on 912 hot flash records: the mean duration was 3.31 minutes; of the 912, 534 started in the neck, head, scalp, and ears, 68 in the neck and/or breasts, 59 below the breasts, 19 in the neck and above the breasts, 118 in the breasts and/or below the breasts, and 114 all over; the direction of spread varied, some up, some down, some both; the time of day or night varied, with no particular time for the majority; and there did not seem to be a common trigger such as eating or stress.

Until recently, the only information on hot flashes came from self-report data. However, in the past several years, attempts have been made to develop objective indices of hot flashes. The most obvious measure of the symptom is body temperature, although researchers have also found changes in other physiological variables to be associated with the occurrence of hot flashes. One of the first studies was reported by Meldrum et al. (1979). They recorded finger temperature for eight hours in seven women who were within two years of surgical or natural menopause and who were experiencing frequent hot flashes; the women were asked to report all subjective feelings of flushing during the recording session. There were 41 significant (one degree centigrade) elevations in finger temperature, 28 of which coincided with subjectively reported hot flashes; for these 28, the mean duration of the skin temperature elevation was 31 minutes and the duration of the subjective sensation was 2.3 minutes. The subjective sensation began an average of 1.2 minutes before and ended 1.1 minutes after the onset of the temperature increase. Five of these subjects received HRT for one to three months and were reassessed; there was a significant reduction in the number of temperature elevations.

Tataryn et al. (1981) studied eight postmenopausal women with frequent and severe hot flashes for 8 or 16 hours, during which time continuous recordings of finger temperature, skin conductance, and core temperature—measured in the external auditory meatus—were taken. They consistently found the first change to be an increase in skin conductance, followed by a rise in finger temperature, followed by a decrease in core temperature. Eighty-two percent, 98%, and 81% of the subjectively reported flashes were associated with changes in finger temperature, skin conductance, and core temperature respectively, and 76% were associated with changes in all three. Four women were reassessed after one month of HRT, and there was a significant reduction in both the subjective sensations and the frequency and magnitude of the finger temperature changes.

Cardiovascular responses associated with hot flashes in six women were measured by Ginsburg, Swinhoe, and O'Reilly (1981). The first circulatory change was a rapid rise in hand blood flow, which in some patients occurred before the subjective sensation. Hand flow increased in each instance of a subjectively reported flash and remained elevated for an average of 2.5 minutes; there was a lesser increase in forearm blood flow. Subjective sensations lasted from one to five minutes, and hand blood flow usually remained elevated for a least a minute after the woman reported that the flush was over. There was a significant increase in heart rate, which occurred after the subjective sensation and returned to control values prior to the end of the flash; there were no significant changes in blood pressure. Although these data indicate consistent cardiovascular changes to be associated with hot flashes, finger temperature and skin conductance seem to be the more popular measures for objectively documenting hot flashes (Erlik et al., 1982; Laufer, Erlik, Meldrum, and Judd, 1982).

These physiological changes accompanying hot flashes are suggestive of alterations in sympathetic nervous system activity—perhaps initiated by transitory changes in central neurotransmitters. These data have been cited as support for the hypothesis that stress may cause or exacerbate hot flashes. Rogers (1956) and Friederich (1982), in their reviews of menopausal symptoms, state that hot flashes occur more often at times of emotional stress but cite no supporting research. Ginsburg, Swinhoe, and O'Reilly (1981) wished to measure physiological changes accompanying hot flashes; the women in their study who did not have spontaneous hot flashes during the recording session were asked to solve mental arithmetic problems intended to induce hot flashes. Unfortunately, the authors did not report if this procedure was effective in inducing hot flashes. In a longitudinal assessment of environmental stress and hot flash frequency and severity, Gannon, Hansel, and Goodwin (1987) reported significant correlations between frequency of hot flashes and frequency of daily stressors for some women but not for others. While these data suggest certain hypotheses concerned with the etiology of hot flashes, they do not address the question of which specific biochemical changes may be responsible for hot flashes.

Estrogen

Originally, it was thought that declining levels of estrogen due to ovarian failure at the time of menopause were the cause of hot flashes. This belief has been bolstered by the fact that exogenous estrogen alleviates hot flashes in the majority of menopausal women who suffer from them. However, research in the last ten years has not consistently supported this theory. Aksel et al. (1976) assessed plasma estrogen levels and vasomotor symptoms in 22 women undergoing bilateral oophorectomy. Estrogen fell on the second day after surgery, and approximately one-third of the women developed hot flashes prior to leaving the hospital; plasma estrogen levels were similar in women with and women without symptoms. Hutton et al. (1978)

determined plasma levels of estrone and estradiol at 20- to 30-minute intervals for up to 24 hours in 26 postmenopausal or ovariectomized women. Women experiencing hot flashes did not have lower estrogen levels than did those not experiencing hot flashes, and there was no obvious relationship between the timing of a flash and estrogen level or change in estrogen level during the 24 hours.

On the other hand, a more recent study in this area did find estrogen levels to be related to hot flashes. Erlik, Meldrum, and Judd (1982) tested 24 postmenopausal women who reported at least 12 hot flashes per day and 24 who had never experienced the symptom. Blood was sampled four times at 15-minute intervals. Mean age, body weight, percentage of ideal weight, total estrone and estradiol, and percentage of nonbound estradiol were significantly lower in symptomatic women than in symptom-free women. Since symptom-free women were heavier, the higher estrogen levels in these women may have been due to the ability of adipose tissue to aromatize androgens to estrogens (Frisch, Canick, and Tulchinsky, 1980). Estrogens produced in this way may reduce vasomotor symptoms in the same way that exogenous estrogen does. Although these data may be interpreted as support for the theory that hot flashes are caused by lowered estrogen levels, other interpretations are possible. The possibility exists that estrogen may alleviate vasomotor symptoms but that the lack of estrogen does not cause such symptoms. Indeed, several researchers in this area (Maddock, 1978; Casper, Yen, and Wilkes, 1979) have argued against lowered estrogen levels as the cause of menopausal hot flashes since other conditions that are characterized by low levels of estrogen, such as primary gonadal failure and gonadal dysgenesis, or by rapidly falling levels of estrogen, such as during the premenstrual phase or prior to labor, are not typically associated with hot flashes.

Luteinizing Hormone

Another theory having to do with the etiology of menopausal hot flashes hypothesizes that the cause lies in the elevated levels or the increased pulsatile amplitude of LH that occurs during menopause. However, in the study by Aksel et al. (1976), plasma levels of LH in women experiencing hot flashes following oophorectomy were similar to those of women who were symptom free. More damaging to the LH theory are two studies reporting hot flashes in women with low levels of LH. Mulley, Mitchell, and Tattersall (1977) described two patients who experienced hot flashes after surgical removal of the pituitary. Similarly, Meldrum, Erlik, Lu, and Judd (1981) studied two women with pituitary insufficiency. In both studies, LH levels were low compared with those of premenopausal women, and the relationships of finger temperature and skin conductance to subjectively reported flashes were identical to that of the typical postmenopausal flush. These women did, however, exhibit LH pulses of low amplitude that had a close temporal association with the finger temperature rise.

Although hot flashes seem unrelated to LH levels, Tataryn et al. (1979) offered support for LH pulse amplitude or frequency as relevant to the symptom. Six postmenopausal women who suffered from frequent hot flashes were studied for eight continous hours. Finger temperature was recorded and blood samples were taken every 15 minutes and every 5 minutes during subjectively reported flashes. Thirty-four temperature changes of at least one degree centigrade were identified. Thirty-two of these were subjectively reported. There were 31 LH pulses, 26 of which occurred simultaneously with a temperature rise. Although these data suggest an association between LH pulses and hot flashes, the temporal parameters of the relationship preclude the assumption of causality. In Tataryn et al. (1979) the peak of the LH pulse occurred, on the average, 13.7 minutes after the onset of the temperature increase and 7.4 minutes after the peak of skin temperature. Similarly, Meldrum et al. (1980) recorded finger temperature continuously for eight hours and drew blood samples in six postmenopausal women. LH changes were significantly correlated with finger temperature, and LH peaked five to ten minutes after the onset of the finger temperature increase. Lightman et al. (1981) found significant increases in LH that occurred after the flush. Finally, clonidine, an alpha-adrenergic agonist, was found to abolish hot flashes in postmenopausal women but did not affect LH pulses (Nagamani, Keever, and Smith, 1987).

Gonadotropin Releasing Hormone

Since hot flashes and LH pulses appear to be temporally but not causally related, it has been hypothesized that the LH pulse and the hot flash are both caused by a third event or process. A logical candidate is hypothalamic GnRH, which stimulates the pituitary to release LH. Evidence to support such a theory would be elevated GnRH levels in postmenopause. Data on GnRH levels in postmenopausal women, presented in a previous section, are contradictory, and GnRH has been found to range from virtually undetectable to levels that were significantly higher than those found in premenopausal women. No conclusions can be drawn from these studies since the typical methodology of sampling blood at regular intervals is not appropriate for evaluating levels of a substance that is released episodically, as is the case with GnRH.

Another theoretical explanation for the temporal, but not causal, relationship between LH pulses and hot flashes is the coincidental anatomic proximity between GnRH secreting neurons and the thermoregulatory center. Meldrum, Erlik, et al. (1981) have speculated that "some of the hypothalamic neurons which contain GnRH and the preoptic/anterior hypothalamic nuclei that regulate body temperature are in a close anatomic relationship, suggesting that neurotransmitter signals associated with GnRH release may modify thermoregulating neurons and trigger a hot flash" (p. 686). This theory is endorsed by Laufer et al. (1982), who successfully treated hot flashes with clonidine, an alpha-adrenergic receptor agonist that stimulates alpha receptors in the depression site of the vasomotor center of the medulla oblongata. They suggest that clonidine was effective treatment because it inhibited catecholamine-induced stimulation in the thermoregulatory center and in the hypothalamic neurons containing GnRH – the latter being a coincidental effect due to the proximity of the two areas and not related to the treatment effectiveness.

Clayden, Bell, and Pollard (1974) have also found clonidine to be a successful treatment for hot flashes; however, their rationale for clonidine treatment was that this drug, which has been successfully used to treat persons with migraine headaches, diminishes vascular reactivity. That menopause is associated with a reduction in peripheral vasomotor control is suggested by Brincat, Lafferty, DeTrafford, and Studd (1984), who found "thermal entrainment" to be significantly reduced in menopausal women, compared with premenopausal women, and that this index of vasomotor control was improved after three months of estrogen therapy. Voda (1982), in her study of twenty menopausal women with hot flashes, noted that all complained of previously experiencing premenstrual headaches and eight reported a longstanding history of premenopausal migraine headaches occurring during the premenstrum. Voda speculated that women who experience hot flashes during the menopause may be those with a predisposition for either thermoregulatory problems or vascular instability or both. Since premenstrual migraines and menopausal hot flashes are both associated with falling levels of estrogen, it is tempting to speculate that estrogen levels are associated with hot flashes because of their influence on vascular reactivity.

Another possible link between regulation of the major thermoregulatory nucleus and the release of GnRH is the level of endogenous opioids. Casper and Yen (1985) argue convincingly that these peptides play a crucial role in the etiology of hot flashes. Evidence relating endorphin levels to phase of menstrual cycle and research on the effects of exogenous estrogen and progesterone on endorphin levels in ovariectomized monkeys and humans (Blankstein, Reyes, Winter, and Faiman, 1981; Ferin et al., 1982; Wardlaw et al., 1982) suggest that in normally cycling, premenopausal women endorphin levels are maintained by adequate levels of ovarian steroids. However, with menopause and decreasing levels of estrogen and progesterone, endogenous opioids may decrease to undetectable levels and cease to regulate GnRH and maintain thermal homeostasis. Tepper et al. (1987) measured plasma beta-endorphins in five postmenopausal women complaining of frequent hot flashes. Significant decreases in beta-endorphins occurred coincidentally with onset of hot flashes, and levels returned to baseline levels within 15 minutes of the end of the flash.

That endorphin levels are significantly reduced after natural or surgical menopause has been demonstrated in several studies (Ferin et al., 1982; Wehrenberg, Wardlaw, Frantz, and Ferin, 1982; Hamilton, Aloi, Mucciardi, & Murphy, 1983; Petraglia et al., 1985; Watts, Butt, Edwards, and Holder, 1985). Furthermore, there is clear evidence that as endorphins increase, the frequency and amplitude of LH pulses decrease (Kalra and Simpkins, 1981; Reid et al., 1981; Russell, Mitchell, Musey, and Collins, 1984) and that the inhibition of LH by endorphins is due to its action on the release of GnRH from the hypothalamus rather than on the pituitary directly (Pang, Zimmermann, and Sawyer, 1977; Meites, 1980). The causal pathway for menopausal hot flashes proposed earlier is consistent with the dramatic effectiveness of exogenous estrogen treatment since increased levels of estrogen would elevate endorphin levels, which, in turn, would regulate GnRH and LH. Although provocative, the theories proposed here are complex and require elaboration and empirical validation if they are to increase understanding and treatment of hot flashes.

In summary, research on the endocrinological and physiological correlates of menopausal hot flashes have not necessarily uncovered their cause. Lowered estrogen levels, LH pulses, and skin conductance changes are associated with hot flashes but there is no empirical support for a causal relationship. Elevated levels or increased pulse amplitudes of GnRH and lowered levels of endogenous opioids are possible, but as yet unverified, causal agents. Research in the last decade, however, is encouraging in that hot flashes, previously considered of insufficient consequence to merit serious investigation, have been the subject of an increasing number of studies, and improved methodologies for the investigation of hot flashes are being developed.

ENDOCRINOLOGICAL AND PHYSIOLOGICAL ASPECTS OF OSTEOPOROSIS

Osteoporosis is characterized by a decrease in skeletal mass or quantity of bone without a change in the quality of the existing bone. New bone is continually formed and existing bone continually resorbed throughout life, but peak bone mass is reached at about age 30 to 35, after which time bone resorption exceeds bone formation and everyone loses bone with advancing age. This reduction in bone mass is regarded as the major factor in osteoporotic fractures, which typically occur in the vertebrae, distal radius, and the hips. The rate of bone loss varies among individuals, and those with high rates of bone loss and demonstrated susceptibility to fractures are viewed as suffering from osteoporosis. It is generally believed that menopause is at least a contributory factor in the development of osteoporosis. Although there are no reliable statistics regarding the percentage of menopausal women who suffer from this disorder, the incidence is believed to be considerably less than the incidence for other symptoms such as hot flashes.

Bone metabolism is a complex process and dependent on a variety of interacting systems for normal activity. Calcium is a crucial ingredient in the making of bone and a byproduct of bone absorption; intestinal absorption of calcium from the diet is the primary source of calcium, and vitamin D is essential for adequate calcium absorption. Vitamin D is converted to its active form, 1,25-dihydroxyvitamin D, in the kidneys, a conversion that requires adequate levels of parathyroid hormone (PTH). Thus, PTH is a primary factor in the regulation of serum calcium levels. Increases in PTH, which can be triggered by falling levels of calcium, cause an accelerated rate of bone resorption and an increase in serum and urinary calcium. Calcitonin, a hormone secreted by the thyroid, has effects opposite those of PTH and decreases the rate of bone remodeling.

Since osteoporosis is characterized by a decrease in skeletal mass, a variety of biochemical measures have been viewed as positive indications of this disorder. These include high serum and urinary concentrations of calcium, low levels of 1,25-dihydroxyvitamin D, high levels of PTH, low levels of calcitonin, as well as direct measures of intestinal absorption of calcium using radioactive isotopes. Similarly, a variety of measures are assumed to reflect bone health, such as bone density, bone size, bone mineral content, and fractures. Given such a wide array of potential variables to study, methodological variation in research on osteoporosis is considerable, and, as might be expected, the results are contradictory.

Those who consider osteoporosis to be a menopausal symptom assume that the decreasing levels of estrogen associated with menopause are responsible for osteoporosis in women (Gallagher and Nordin, 1974). Young and Nordin (1967) assessed plasma and urinary levels of calcium and phosphorus, which they assumed would be elevated in women with an increased rate of bone resorption, in premenopausal and postmenopausal women, and found postmenopausal women to have elevated levels of calcium and phosphorus. These data are suggestive of the etiological nature of menopause in osteoporosis and are consistent with the results of a later study

(Frumar et al., 1980) that found the urinary calcium to creatinine ratio (Ca:Cr), an index of bone resorption, to be significantly and negatively correlated with plasma estrogen in postmenopausal women.

On the other hand, since bone loss is a natural process of aging and since menopause occurs in aging women, it has been difficult to differentiate the effects of menopause from those of aging on the osteoporotic process. Bullamore et al. (1970) measured calcium absorption by plasma radioactivity after ingestion of oral calcium isotopes in men and women between the ages of 20 and 95. Absorption of calcium fell after sixty years of age, and everyone over eighty had significant malabsorption. Since deficits in the intestinal absorption of calcium have been assumed to be a possible factor in osteoporosis, the authors concluded that this malabsorption of calcium associated with the aging process may be etiological in osteoporosis.

To differentiate those effects on bone loss due to aging from those due to menopause, several studies have evaluated bone loss in women who had had bilateral oophorectomy prior to menopause. Aitken et. al. (1973) compared whole bone density in women who had had an hysterectomy with that of women who had had a hysterectomy and bilateral oophorectomy. Neither type of surgery influenced bone density if the woman was over 45 at the time of the surgery. In women who had surgery before age 45, the oophorectomized group had significantly lower values of bone density measured six years post-surgery than did women who had had only hysterectomy. Other researchers (Richelson et al. 1984; Nilas and Christiansen, 1987) have compared women of the same age but different menopausal status and women of similar menopausal status but different age. Data from both studies clearly indicate that menopause has a greater impact on bone loss than does aging. However, the mechanism of action has not been elucidated (Riggs, 1987).

Since the subjects in these studies were not selected on the basis of the presence or absence of osteoporosis, we do not know how many of the subjects actually suffered from this disorder. Positive indications of osteoporosis are more likely at advanced age; menopausal status is correlated with age; the probability of a woman having had a bilateral oophorectomy is correlated with age; and not all postmenopausal women exhibit signs of osteoporosis. The independent contribution of menopause, natural or surgical, to the etiology of osteoporosis has been difficult to establish.

In an effort to address this issue and to evaluate the assumption that if bone loss does increase after menopause or the surgical loss of the ovaries, this loss is due to the decreased levels of estrogen, researchers have compared osteoporotic women with normal postmenopausal women on levels of sex steroids. Davidson et al. (1982) found postmenopausal fracture patients to have a lower percentage of ideal weight and significantly higher concentrations of sex-hormone-binding-globulin (SHBG), resulting in lower concentrations of biologically active estradiol and testosterone than did postmenopausal women without fractures. In contrast are the results from two studies that compared hormone levels in postmenopausal women with vertebral crush fractures to age-matched controls. Riggs et al. (1973) found no group differences in plasma testosterone, serum estrogen, or serum gonadotropins; Davidson, Riggs, Wahner, and Judd (1983) reported no group differences in cortisol, cortisol-binding-globulin, testosterone, androstenedione, dehydroepiandrosterone, estrone, estradiol, or SHBG, but the fracture patients did have significantly lower spinal bone mineral density than the controls. Riggs et al. (1973) concluded that some factor in addition to menopause causes the accelerated bone loss in osteoporotic patients.

In a recent study (Falch, Oftebro, and Haug, 1987), 19 women were followed for eight years, during which time they became menopausal. Appendicular bone mass and serum estrogen were evaluated once a year. According to their data, estrogen levels declined steadily during the four years preceding the cessation of menses and then remained fairly stable. Bone loss exhibited minimal declines prior to menopause; after the final menses, however, the rate of bone loss more than doubled. These data clearly implicate menopause as a contributory factor in bone loss among elderly women but do not necessarily support declining estrogen levels as the responsible agent.

Several recent studies have reported interesting findings: (1) the rate of bone loss after surgical menopause has been found to be about double that which follows natural menopause (Riggs, 1987); (2) smokers have been found to have a higher bone loss and increased hepatic metabolism of exogenously administered estrogens than do nonsmokers (Jensen, Christiansen, and Rodbro, 1985); and (3) bone loss was reported to be significantly and negatively correlated with parity—nulliparous patients lost virtually no bone over a 10-year study period (Abdalla, Hart, Lindsay, and Aitken, 1984). Such data point up that researchers in this area are just beginning to appreciate the truly complex processes underlying osteoporosis.

TREATMENT OF MENOPAUSAL SYMPTOMS

Because of the widespread belief that the symptoms associated with menopause are due to lowered levels of estrogen, the most popular treatment for these symptoms has been exogenous estrogen or Hormone Replacement Therapy. By the 1940s, almost every major drug company offered some form of estrogen for the treatment of menopause. Although this treatment continues to be popular today, research over the past 20 years indicates that the benefits associated with HRT are less and the risks greater than was previously assumed, and, consequently, alternative forms of treatment are currently being investigated.

Hormone Replacement Therapy (HRT)

HRT and Vasomotor Symptoms. Vasomotor symptoms in the form of hot flashes and night sweats are undoubtedly the primary reason for menopausal women to seek medical help. The majority of menopausal women experience such symptoms to some degree, and, for some women, the symptoms are intense and disabling. Although there is little empirical evidence to support the theory that hot flashes are a manifestation of falling levels of estrogen, hormone replacement therapy (HRT) is the most common form of medical treatment for this symptom. Clinical trials of exogenous estrogen administration indicate that estrogen is, indeed, effective in relieving vasomotor symptoms in most women (Reynolds, Kaminester, Foster, and Schloss, 1941; Kaufman, 1967; Martin, Burnier, and Greaney, 1972; Hunter et al., 1977; Larsson-Cohn, Johansson, Kagedal, and Wallentin, 1978;

Lind et al., 1979; Burnier, Martin, Yen, and Brooks, 1981). Furthermore, empirical studies in which estrogen therapy has been compared with placebos have consistently demonstrated estrogen to be superior to placebos in relieving vasomotor symptoms (Utian, 1972; George et al., 1973; Lin, SoBosita, Brar, and Roblete, 1973; Coope, Thomson, and Poller, 1975; Baumgardner et al., 1978; Dennerstein et al., 1978; Poller et al., 1980).

The mechanism by which HRT is an effective treatment for hot flashes is a matter of speculation. Exogenous estrogen does lower levels of LH (Veldhuis et al., 1986) but the temporal relationship between subjective hot flashes and LH pulses argues against LH release as an etiological factor in hot flashes. Some research implicates endogenous opiates as crucial in the pathway of action. Wardlow et al. (1982) assessed effects of HRT on beta-endorphins in ovariectomized monkeys. No change was noted with acute infusion, but beta-endorphins did increase after three weeks of chronic estrogen replacement. At the human level, Dawood et al. (1986) administered the opiate antagonist, naloxone, to postmenopausal women. Those who had not been receiving medication showed no change in LH to naloxone, whereas those who had been receiving HRT exhibited a significant increase in LH in response to naloxone. Although this preliminary research ties endogenous opiates to the impact of HRT on hot flashes, the precise role of these opiates—causal versus correlated—remains to be clarified.

In spite of the success of this treatment, several unresolved issues concerning the treatment of vasomotor symptoms with HRT deserve further research consideration. Given the potentially negative side effects of HRT (discussed later), it would be beneficial for patients to receive the minimal effective dose, and the dosage of estrogen necessary to relieve hot flashes completely or to an acceptable level has not been determined. Meldrum (1987) has suggested (but without substantiation) that prescribing a progestin for at least ten days, in addition to the estrogen, may reduce the negative side effects and may allow for the alleviation of hot flashes with lower doses of estrogen. Second, several authors (Voda, 1981; Archer, 1982) have expressed the belief that when HRT is stopped, vasomotor symptoms return, suggesting that estrogen only postpones the discomfort associated with these symptoms. Jeffcoate (1960) has suggested gradually reducing the dose of estrogen over a period of a few months in order to prevent the reccurrence of vasomotor symptoms, but there is no empirical research to support this as a method of prevention.

HRT and Vaginal Symptoms. The only other menopausal symptom that appears to be treatable with estrogen is atrophic vaginitis. In postmenopause, the walls of the vagina become smooth and dry and produce less lubrication, a condition that has been assumed to be due to a lack of estrogen. The karyopyknotic index (KPI), the percentage of superficial squamous cells with pyknotic nuclei (Morse, Hutton, Murray, & James, 1979), has become a popular method for determining, cytologically, the degree of estrogenicity of the vaginal smear, and the KPI has been found to be significantly correlated with plasma estradiol concentrations (Badawy et al., 1979; Morse et al., 1979). However, contradictory data have been reported by Lind et al. (1979), who noted that vaginal cytology is a poor indicator of estrogen status, and by Kaufman (1967), who found little relationship between vaginal cytology, change in cytology, and severity of other symptoms. Two studies (Kupperman et al., 1953; Lin et al., 1973) found little or no relationship between improvement in vaginal cytology and improvement in other symptoms such as hot flashes.

Notwithstanding doubts concerning the relationship between circulating estrogen and objective measures of vaginal atrophy, estrogen is frequently prescribed to treat vaginal problems during menopause and postmenopause and is generally effective (Utian, 1972; Burnier et al., 1981). Although oral administration of estrogen has been found to produce a significant improvement in vaginal cytology when statistical analyses are applied to group data, Larsson-Cohn et al. (1978) noted that 40% of their subjects exhibited no improvement, and Geola et al. (1980) found that only a relatively high dose of oral estrogen improved the KPI to premenopausal values. Nevertheless, vaginal administration of estrogen has been found more consistently to be effective in relieving the symptoms of atrophic vaginitis (Bercovici, Uretzki, and Patti, 1972; Deutsch, Ossowski, and Benjamin, 1981). Mandel et al. (1983) have reported that quite small doses of conjugated equine estrogens (0.3 mg/day) administered vaginally returned vaginal cytology to premenopausal values. A dose-response relationship was demonstrated in a study by Henzl et al. (1973); postmenopausal women were treated with 5, 20, or 80 mcg of Mestranol per day, and the KPI increased progressively with the dosage.

HRT and Osteoporosis. Although the empirical evidence for low levels of estrogen being etiological in osteoporosis is weak, hormone replacement therapy (HRT) is frequently advocated both as a treatment for osteoporosis and as a prophylactic. Research results have been relatively consistent in demonstrating improvement in parameters associated with osteoporosis in response to the administration of exogenous estrogen. Following estrogen treatment, improvement has been reported in serum calcium and phosphate (Moore, Paterson, Sturdee, and Whitehead, 1981), intestinal absorption of calcium (Canniggia et al., 1970), urinary calcium to creatinine ratio (Frumar et al., 1980; Geola et al., 1980; Mandel et al., 1983), and bone mineral content (Riis, Thomsen, Strom, and Christiansen, 1987). Dose-response relationships were noted by Christiansen, Christensen, Larsen, and Transbol (1982); they administered high, medium, or low doses of estrogen to postmenopausal women and compared the results with those of a group receiving placebos. Bone mineral content declined by 2% in the placebo group, was unchanged in the low estrogen group, and increased by 0.8% and 1.5% in the medium and high groups respectively.

Of perhaps greater importance are the effects of estrogen treatment on fractures. Nachtigall, Nachtigall, Nachtigall, and Beckman (1979) compared an untreated postmenopause group with a group of women who had received HRT for ten years and for whom the treatment was begun within three years of menopause; there were seven fractures in the untreated group but none in the treated group. Jensen, Christiansen, and Transbol (1982) assessed the fracture frequency in groups receiving no HRT, short-term HRT, and long-term HRT: the number of women with postmenopausal fractures was 13% lower in the long-term treatment group than in the no-treatment group.

Some researchers have noted that although HRT may produce beneficial effects on osteoporosis in group comparisons, there is considerable individual variability in the response to estrogen (Lindsay et al., 1978). Gallagher, Riggs, and DeLuca (1980) compared the effects of placebo and estrogen treatment for six months on calcium absorption; the advantage of estrogen was demonstrated by a significant group increase in calcium absorption and in serum 1,25-dihydroxyvitamin D, both of which were unchanged with placebo. However, examination of individual data indicated such improvement in only seven of their twelve subjects. Factors related to individual differences in treatment response are suggested by Williams et al. (1982), who found that the benefits of HRT were greatest for thin women who also smoked. In obese nonsmokers, the risk of neither hip nor of forearm fractures was reduced by exogenous estrogen. Others (Chestnut, 1984; Oyster, Morton, and Linnell, 1984) have questioned the value of HRT by stating that, rather than increasing bone mass or density, it simply slows down the process of bone loss and the benefits of HRT are not sustained if therapy is stopped—indeed, there may even be a rebound effect of accelerated bone loss.

Researchers interested in the relationship between estrogen and osteoporosis have concentrated their efforts on the practical aspects, that is, the effects of HRT on indices of osteoporosis, but have neglected issues concerned with the processes that mediate these effects. Endogenous and exogenous estrogen levels may affect bone metabolism, but the mechanisms that mediate this effect have not been clarified. Hypothesized mechanisms include the following: estrogen may have direct effects on the osteoclasts or may exert effects by increasing calcitonin secretion or by increasing the sensitivity of bones to calcitonin (Aitken, 1976); estrogen may inhibit bone resorption by inhibiting the effects of PTH on the bone (Nordin, 1971); estrogen may increase calcium absorption through effects on vitamin D metabolism (Gallagher et al., 1980); estrogen may reduce the responsiveness of the bone to PTH, reduce calcium loss through excretion, and increase the use of dietary calcium by increasing absorption (Nachtigall et al., 1979); estrogen may improve calcium balance by lowering fecal and urinary calcium (Gallagher and Nordin, 1974); or estrogen may modify endogenous synthesis of 1,25-dihydroxyvitamin D or may enhance calcitonin secretion (Davidson et al., 1982).

Researchers (Young and Nordin, 1967; Davies, Mawer, and Adams, 1977) have pointed out that cause-and-effect relationships in osteoporosis need to be clarified because such treatments as estrogen may be modifying an effect of the disorder rather than a cause of the disorder. For example, increases in bone resorption result in higher levels of calcium in the plasma, and estrogen may reduce plasma levels of calcium without actually decreasing the rate of bone resorption. Clearly, the magnitude of, and the mechanism of, the effect of menopause on bone metabolism, and the magnitude of, and the mechanism of, the effect of exogenous estrogen treatment on osteoporosis have not, thus far, been delineated.

For obvious reasons, calcium supplements have been suggested as a treatment for osteoporosis—both alone and in conjunction with HRT. Not only has it been estimated that the majority of women consume less than 50% of the RDA of calcium, but the body's ability to absorb calcium declines with age; thus, Amschler (1985) has suggested that postmenopausal women may not be consuming adequate amounts of calcium and that the calcium they are getting may not be utilized efficiently. In early studies, calcium supplements were found to reduce bone loss in postmenopausal women (Riggs et al., 1976); and, in a study comparing the effectiveness of calcium supplements and HRT, both were effective in slowing bone loss, but neither was found to increase bone (Gallagher and Nordin, 1974). However, more recent studies have reported that calcium intake was not significantly related to rate of bone loss in postmenopausal women (Riggs et al., 1987) with the possible exception of those with atypically low levels of calcium intake (Dawson-Hughes, Jacques, and Shipp, 1987). Finally, Ettinger et al. (1985) found that the use of calcium supplements in conjunction with HRT provided bone protection at lower doses of estrogen than that required without the calcium.

In conclusion, the foregoing studies suggest that osteoporosis may be a heterogeneous disorder with regard to etiology and that low levels of estrogen may be regarded as one of many possible contributing factors. Consequently, the value of HRT in the treatment of osteoporosis is questionable. The research indicates that to be of value estrogen must be administered on a long-term basis and that treatment must be started soon after menopause and before any signs of osteoporosis appear. However, given that only a small percentage of postmenopausal women experience symptomatic osteoporosis, that estrogen is not beneficial to all women suffering from the disorder, that the mechanisms by which estrogen may be beneficial have not been clarified, and that long-term administration of exogenous estrogen is associated with an increased risk of uterine cancer, the recommendation that all women begin HRT at the time of menopause and continue on it indefinitely (Gallagher and Nordin, 1974; Aitken, 1976) does not reflect an unbiased consideration of the potential risks and benefits. Worley (1981) offers a recommendation more consistent with the empirical evidence—those women in high risk categories for osteoporosis—those who are thin, caucasian, smokers, related to women with postmenopausal osteoporosis, or inactive—should be offered HRT for the prevention of osteoporosis.

HRT and Other Menopausal Symptoms. Studies investigating the benefits of HRT on other menopausal symptoms have already been discussed in previous sections of this chapter. With the exceptions of hot flashes and atrophic vaginitis, the research has not been supportive of HRT as an effective mode of treatment for symptoms commonly attributed to menopause, such as depression, nervousness, insomnia, fatigue, and headaches.

Correlates and Side-Effects of HRT

Hormonal Levels. The assumed mechanism by which HRT improves symptoms of vasomotor instability and atrophic vaginitis is by effecting changes in circulating levels of estrogen or gonadotropins. Regardless of the route of administration, HRT does tend to increase estrone and estradiol concentrations and to reduce FSH and LH in postmenopausal women. In general, studies have found greater increases in estrone than the more biologically active estradiol (see, for example, Lind, 1978) and some reduction in gonadotropins but not to premenopausal levels (see, for example, Stumpf, Maruca, Santen, and Demers, 1982). These effects vary with dose and method of administration of HRT; one study (Thom, Collins, and Studd, 1981) found implants to produce extremely elevated levels of estrogen, decreases in FSH to premenopausal values, and less dramatic decreases in LH.

Similar results have been found with acute administration of estrogen. Within several hours after subjects ingested two milligrams of micronized estradiol, Yen et al., (1975) found significant increases in estradiol and estrone and significant decreases in FSH and LH. Similar results have been reported by Tsai and Yen (1971) and Nillius and Wise (1970). Asch et al. (1983) injected oophorectomized rhesus monkeys with estrogen; during the first 24 hours, FSH and LH levels decreased by 70% to 80% followed by a rebound to 60% to 80% above basal levels at 48 hours. Some animals also received injections of GnRH, which enhanced the negative feedback of estrogen on gonadotropins and diminished the subsequent positive feedback. The authors interpreted their data to mean that exogenous estrogen influences gonadotropin secretion by its action on hypothalamic GnRH.

Because it is thought that oophorectomy results in a more dramatic decrease in estrogen levels than does natural menopause, oophorectomized women are assumed to be particularly susceptible to symptoms. Thus, HRT is frequently begun immediately following surgery in order to prevent changes in estrogen and gonadotropins. Several studies (Ostergard et al., 1970; Simon and diZerega, 1982) have noted that, although HRT begun immediately after surgery resulted in a maintenance of presurgical levels of estrogen, LH and FSH increased to typical postmenopausal levels. In contrast, Hunter et al. (1977) found that estrogen implants prevented both decreases in estrogen and increases in gonadotropins. However, they did not report the actual levels of circulating estrogen resulting from this procedure, which would be relevant information since implants tend to produce levels of estrogen considerably above premenopausal values.

Dose-response relationships between HRT and hormone concentrations have been studied. Mandel et al. (1982, 1983) assessed the effects of various doses of exogenous estrogen on estrogen and gonadotropin levels. Stepwise increases in circulating estrone and estradiol occurred with increasing dosages, but none of the doses tested reduced gonadotropins to premenopausal levels. In a similar study, Utian et al. (1978) found that the highest dose tested (2.5 mg of conjugated estrogen) reduced FSH but not LH levels to premenopausal levels but also resulted in estradiol levels higher than those found in premenopause. Assessing four dosages of HRT on a variety of physical and biochemical markers, Geola et al. (1980) concluded that determining the optimal dosage was difficult since "all doses exerted subphysiological, physiological, and pharmacological responses at different sites of action" (p. 620).

The most popular form of HRT is oral, but this method is relatively ineffective due to poor gastrointestinal absorption. One method of increasing the effectiveness of oral medication is to provide it in micronized form; micronization increases the surface area by reducing the particle size, thereby facilitating dissolution and absorption. Martin et al. (1972) reported that the micronized form was well tolerated and was preferred over the regular form by most subjects. However, Casper and Yen (1981) found that, although absorption was extremely rapid, micronized estrogen, like other forms of oral estrogen, resulted in abnormally high elevations of estrone at the dose required to achieve physiological levels of estradiol.

Estrone increases at a faster rate than does estradiol when HRT is administered orally because the intestines and the liver convert estradiol, the more active form of estrogen, to estrone. Other routes of administration have been studied to discover a method that might bypass the gut and the liver and avoid the rapid conversion of estradiol to estrone. Several studies have compared oral and cutaneous (usually on the abdomen) administration and have reported that both routes increase estradiol and decrease FSH and LH to similar levels, but that oral administration results in considerably higher levels of estrone than does estrogen applied cutaneously (Lyrenas, Karlsrom, Backstrom, and von Schoultz, 1981; Elkik et al. 1982; Fahraeus and Larsson-Cohn, 1982). Fahraeus and co-workers (Fahreus, Larsson-Cohn, and Wallentin, 1982; Fahraeus and Wallentin, 1983) compared these two methods of administration on lipoproteins. They reported a change in lipoproteins with oral but not cutaneous administration; however, the changes noted with the oral route could be viewed as beneficial with respect to atherosclerotic disease.

An alternative method of administering HRT is intravaginally, a method that, like the cutaneous route, bypasses the gut and liver. Deutsch et al. (1981) compared vaginal to oral administration at a variety of dosages and found that, at each dosage level, the vaginal route resulted in significantly lower blood estrogen values than did the oral route. However, relief from vaginal symptoms was achieved in all cases where the hormone was administered vaginally. Rigg et al. (1977) compared vaginal with intranasal administration, and a lower ratio of estrone to estradiol was obtained with the vaginal route. These data are consistent with those comparing oral and cutaneous administrations in that routes of administration that bypass the gut and liver produce a more physiological ratio of estrone to estradiol.

Although a frequently used criterion in determining HRT effectiveness is whether or not the resulting estrogen levels reach premeno-pausal values, this approach is questionable. Since the reason for medicating postmenopausal women is presumably the treatment of symptoms, patient satisfaction with symptom reduction might be a more appropriate criterion. Furthermore, endogenous levels of es-trogen in the postmenopause vary considerably and are influenced by such factors as weight and smoking. Thus, the dose and type of HRT require individualized assessment and follow-up.

Cancer. There is considerable evidence that exogenous estrogen treatment in menopausal women is associated with an increased probability of developing uterine cancer. Studies comparing the rate of uterine cancer among women receiving estrogen therapy with that of women not receiving such therapy have estimated the increased risk associated with estrogen to be four to eight times (Smith et al., 1975; Greenwald, Caputo, and Wolfgang, 1977; Hammond et al., 1979; Gambrell et al., 1980). Stronger evidence for a relationship between exogenous estrogen and uterine cancer comes from studies evaluating the effects of dose and duration of estrogen treatment. Ziel and Finkle (1975, 1976) found duration of estrogen use to be significantly corre-lated with risk of uterine cancer. Ziel and Finkle (1975) reported a risk-ratio estimate of 13.9 for seven years or more of estrogen use. Other researchers (Gray, Christopherson, and Hoover, 1977; Rosen-waks et al., 1979; Stavraky et al., 1981) have found both dose and duration to bear a linear relationship to risk.

Predisposing factors for uterine cancer include obesity, hyperten-sion, diabetes, and nulliparity (Buchman, Kramer, and Feldman, 1978). Investigations of interacting or additive effects of such predis-posing factors and estrogen use on uterine cancer have yielded incon-sistent results. Buchman et al. (1978) found that virtually all their subjects with uterine cancer had either at least one of the predisposing factors or had had estrogen therapy. Data presented by Judd et al. (1982) indicate that the two groups most susceptible to cancer are obese women and slender women on HRT; but these authors noted that such research is difficult to interpret since obese women may be less likely to be on estrogen. Smith et al. (1975) concluded from their research that the increased risk of uterine cancer due to exogenous estrogen is less apparent in patients with characteristics that already predispose them.

The relationships between obesity and uterine cancer, and HRT and uterine cancer suggest, perhaps, that increased blood estrogen levels contribute to the development of uterine cancer, since obese persons exhibit a higher rate of conversion from androgens to estrogen and thus have higher blood concentrations of estrogen. Nisker et al. (1980) found sex-hormone-binding-globulin levels to be significantly lower and free estradiol levels significantly higher in cancer patients than in controls; however, the cancer patients were also more obese. In two studies comparing estrogen levels of women with and without uterine cancer in which subjects were matched for weight, no differences in serum estrogen levels were found (Judd et al., 1976; Lucas and Yen, 1979).

There is some evidence to suggest that exogenous estrogen predisposes one to uterine cancer by its direct effect on the endometrium. Exogenous estrogen administration has been shown to be consistently associated with endometrial hyperplasia (Callantine et al., 1975; Sturdee et al., 1978; Whitehead, McQueen, Minardi, and Campbell, 1978). Aycock and Jollie (1979) compared the cellular response of the postmenopausal endometrium to estrogenic stimulation with the cellular activity in endometrial cancer and found close similarities. Natrajan, Muldoon, Greenblatt, and Mahesh (1981) have suggested that unopposed estrogen stimulation increases the concentration of estrogen receptors, resulting in a state of hyperreceptivity to estrogen, the consequence being hyperplasia and perhaps cancer.

There is considerable controversy over the interpretation of this research and differing conclusions as to the nature of the relationship between exogenous estrogen and uterine cancer, ranging from ". . . I am convinced that estrogens per se are not a cause of endometrial cancer in the human female" (Kistner, 1976, p. 479) to ". . . the U.S. may be observing the close of an unparalleled epidemic of drug-induced cancer" (Walker and Hershel, 1980, p. 733). Consequently, the responses of researchers, practitioners, and patients to the growing evidence of a relationship between HRT and uterine cancer have been mixed. One response of physicians has been to minimize the life-threatening nature of uterine cancer by stating that cancers caused by estrogen therapy are usually diagnosed early and are readily cured (Chu, Schweid, and Weiss, 1982; Kistner, 1976).

A second response has been to develop forms of HRT that are not associated with an increased risk of cancer. Initially, hormone replacement therapy consisted of estrogen administered on a continual basis. Since the increased risk of uterine cancer was thought to be due to the hyperplasic effects of unopposed estrogen on the endometrium, other forms of medication have been advocated. For example, estrogen is sometimes given on a cyclic basis, with 25 days on medication and five days off so as to prevent continuous stimulation of the endometrium. The more common alternative, however, has been to administer estrogen on a cyclic basis and to add progesterone the last five to ten days of the cycle. The rationales for this form of treatment are that it more precisely conforms to premenopausal hormonal levels and, more important, that it prevents hyperplasia. Sturdee et al. (1978) noted that cyclical, unopposed estrogen was associated with a 12% incidence of endometrial hyperplasia, which was reduced to 8% with five days of progesterone, and there was no case of hyperplasia among women with ten or thirteen days of progesterone. Similar results were reported by Whitehead et al. (1978): high dose cyclical estrogen resulted in a 32% incidence of hyperplasia and low dose estrogen a 16% incidence, while estrogen and progesterone administered sequentially resulted in a 6% incidence of hyperplasia with high doses and 3% with low doses. Several researchers (Lind et al., 1979; Flowers et al., 1983) in this area, however, warn that adding progesterone does not produce regular endometrial shedding in all women and it should not be assumed that sequential hormonal therapy entirely eliminates the risk of uterine cancer associated with HRT.

The effect of estrogen on the endometrial lining of the uterus is growth, and continual estrogen causes continual growth with haphazard shedding when the lining outgrows its blood supply. According to Budoff (1980), progesterone protects against hyperplasia by causing differentiation, and, thus, when progesterone and estrogen levels decline, the lining cleanly and precisely sloughs off. King, Whitehead, Campbell, and Minardi (1978) postulate that estrogen increases receptor production in the uterus for both estrogen and progesterone and that progesterone reduces the concentration of estrogen receptors, so that during progesterone therapy, the uterus becomes less responsive to estrogen. Support for these effects has been reported by Natrajan et al. (1981), who assessed the concentrations of estrogen and progesterone receptors in endometrial biopsies of women receiving estrogen alone and those receiving estrogen plus progesterone. Women receiving high doses of estrogen with progesterone or moderate doses of estrogen without progesterone exhibited significantly elevated concentrations of estrogen receptors, while those receiving moderate doses of estrogen with progesterone exhibited estrogen and progesterone receptor concentrations similar to premenopausal women in the proliferative phase of the cycle.

The addition of progesterone to estrogen for the treatment of menopausal symptoms is too new to have been evaluated adequately. However, several studies suggest potential problems with this mode of treatment. First, Hahn, Nachtigall, and Davies (1984) noted compliance difficulties, which they attributed to their patients' objections to the withdrawal bleeding that typically occurs with this regimen. Continuous administration of both estrogen and progesterone has been reported to result in acyclic bleeding in approximately half of the subjects (Luciano, Turksoy, Carleo, and Hendrix, 1988) while producing symptom relief to the same extent as sequential therapy (Weinstein, 1987). Second, Magos et al. (1986) found the addition of progesterone to HRT to result in a syndrome similar to Premenstrual Syndrome. They compared placebos with 5 mg and 2.5 mg of progesterone in a sequential regimen with estrogen. The higher dose was associated with a significantly greater incidence of depression, anxiety, and irritability than was the placebo. The lower dose of progesterone showed a similar trend but was not significantly different from placebo. Thus, while progesterone may offer some protection from uterine cancer, it may result in other problems that women may find unacceptable.

Blood Coagulation. As with estrogen in the form of oral contraceptives, estrogen in the form of HRT has been found to affect blood coagulation adversely by causing a change in the biochemical profile in the direction of increased coagulability (Beller, Nachtigall, and Rosenberg, 1972; Coope et al., 1975; Poller et al., 1980). Some researchers who have reported similar effects of exogenous estrogen on coagulation parameters have interpreted their data as implying a minimal threat for the development of intravascular clots (von Kaulla, Droegemueller, and von Kaulla, 1975; Stangel, Innerfield, Reyniak, and Stone, 1977). At the same time, they suggest that, although a hypercoagulable state does not imply the necessary formation of a clot, the effects of such a state may be additive with the effects of other predisposing factors frequent in the elderly such as vascular endothelial damage or prolonged stasis.

Other research has not supported the increased potential toward coagulation from estrogen. Studd et al. (1978) and Notelovitz, Johnston, Smith, and Kitchens (1987) found no evidence for increased coagulability from exogenous estrogen. Methodological differences, such as choice of dependent measure, type of estrogen, and dose and duration of treatment, are probably the cause of these contradictory results, and there has been no systematic evaluation of the relationship between these procedural variations and coagulation. Hunter, Anderson, and Haddon (1979) found changes in the direction of hypercoagulability in women on HRT but qualified their conclusions by stating that the dose tested was higher than that required to relieve hot flashes and lower doses may have less effect on coagulation. (They do not explain why doses above those required to relieve hot flashes were used.) A final consideration on this issue is suggested by Notelovitz et al. (1981) who found that natural menopause is associated with a shift away from clot formation and toward clot inhibition; thus, exogenous estrogen may change parameters in the direction of clot formation, but this change may simply be a return to the premenopausal level of coagulability and may not reflect an abnormal state. Furthermore, since the liver is assumed to be responsible for these changes in coagulation parameters, the changes may be lessened by administration through vaginal or cutaneous routes.

Cholesterol. Early studies on the impact of HRT on cholesterol levels yielded inconsistent results. HRT containing only estrogen was found either to significantly increase cholesterol and triglyceride levels (Molitch, Oill, and Odell, 1974) or to have no impact (Walter and Jensen, 1977). Lack of significant changes with estrogen therapy was also reported by Paterson, Sturdee, Moore, and Whitehead (1980); however, they also tested the effects of other compounds and found sequential estrogen/progesterone preparations to reduce serum cholesterol to a level similar to that found in premenopausal women; the effect on triglycerides was significant, but the direction of the change was dependent on the exact chemical form of the estrogen and progesterone.

Results of the more recent studies have been relatively consistent in suggesting that HRT has significant and beneficial effects on lipoproteins, which may offer protection against heart disease. HRT consisting of estrogen implants has been found to be associated with decreases in serum cholesterol values (Notelovitz et al., 1987). In two studies by Jensen and colleagues (Jensen, Nilas, and Christiansen, 1986; Jensen, Riis, Strom, and Christiansen, 1987), results indicated that: (1) high density lipoproteins (HDL) increased and low density lipoproteins (LDL) decreased in a dose-related manner with estrogen therapy, and the addition of progesterone in a sequential regimen reduced these beneficial changes but did not eliminate them; and (2) total serum cholesterol and LDL were significantly reduced in postmenopausal women receiving continuous estrogen and progesterone therapy.

All the foregoing studies employed oral forms of HRT. Since the effects of hormones on cholesterol and triglycerides are probably mediated by the liver, nonoral administration may not be associated with these changes. Mandel et al. (1983) assessed the effects of four doses of conjugated estrogen administered vaginally. Although the higher dosages significantly increased hepatic protein synthesis, no dose had a significant effect on circulating levels of triglycerides or cholesterol levels. Similar results were reported by Judd (1987), who found estrogen delivered by way of transdermal patches to have little impact on lipids. On the other hand, Jensen, Riis, Strom, Nilas, and Christiansen (1987) treated postmenopausal women with percutaneous estrogen for one year, then added progesterone to the treatment. Estrogen alone significantly reduced total serum cholesterol and LDL, and these effects were not diminished in the second year when progesterone was added. Thus, it appears that although the most dramatic effects of HRT on lipids occur during oral administration of estrogen, other routes or the addition of progesterone have similar but reduced effects.

Alternative Treatments

Clonidine. Other treatments for vasomotor symptoms associated with menopause have been evaluated, but to a lesser extent than hormonal therapy. Clonidine, an alpha-receptor agonist, is, in high doses, an antihypertensive agent and has been employed as a prophylaxis of migraine headache because of its assumed ability to diminish vascular reactivity. Clayden et al. (1974) and Tulandi and Kinch (1983) evaluated the effectiveness of clonidine in reducing menopausal hot flashes and found it to be significantly more effective than a placebo. Tulandi and Kinch (1983) also reported that clonidine, while reducing the subjective perceptions of flashes, had no discernible effect on episodic elevations of skin temperature or on the number of LH peaks. Laufer et al. (1982) compared various doses of clonidine with a placebo and found clonidine to be significantly more effective; however, the highest dose, 0.4 mg/day, reduced the frequency of hot flashes by only 46%, and four of the ten subjects had to discontinue the medication because of severe side effects. Nagamani et al. (1987) administered clonidine transdermally and reported a reduction in hot flashes but no discernible effect on LH pulses; side-effects appeared to be fewer by this route than those found with oral administration.

The mechanism by which clonidine alleviates hot flashes is unknown. Nagamani et al. (1987) suggest hot flashes may be due to excess catecholamines in the central nervous system since hot flashes are typically accompanied by increases in heart rate and skin conductance. This theory is supported by research by Ginsberg, O'Reilly, and Swinhoe (1985), who administered clonidine to postmenopausal women and evaluated changes in blood-flow responses to various agents. They reported that clonidine reduced the vasomotor response to adrenaline and abolished the typical dilator effects of angiotensin. Simpkins, Katovich, and Chengsong (1983), however, argue that clonidine may act by increasing serum beta-endorphin levels, which, in turn, inhibit LH release.

Other Drug Treatments. Coope, Williams, and Patterson (1978) administered propranolol, an adrenergic, beta-receptor blocking agent effective in treating palpitation and tachycardia, to menopausal women suffering from hot flashes. They reported no significant improvement due to the drug. Similarly, Wheatley (1984) evaluated the treatment effectiveness of Timolol, a beta blocker, and reported the effectiveness did not exceed that of placebo.

Finally, because of the temporal proximity of hot flashes and LH pulses, Lightman, Jacobs, and Maguire (1982) attempted to treat hot flashes with a GnRH analog. Initially LH increased dramatically, but within one week levels fell to pretreatment values and remained within the postmenopausal range. Although levels of neither LH nor FSH were significantly reduced during the five-week treatment period, the treatment was effective in abolishing the pulsatile release of LH in all subjects. Unfortunately, the frequency of subjectively reported hot flashes remained unaltered. The authors concluded that although the pulsatile release of LH is temporally associated with the occurrence of a hot flash, the relationship is not a causal one.

Exercise. Exercise has been proposed as an alternative to medication for the alleviation of menopausal symptoms (Gannon, 1988). Exercise tends to increase endorphin levels and thus may decrease LH levels and perhaps hot flashes. Cumming et al. (1985) found a significant reduction in the frequency of LH pulses after exercise, compared with before exercise, in six premenopausal runners, thus suggesting the potential for a similar effect in postmenopausal women. The one study thus far that evaluated the effect of exercise on hot flashes is encouraging. Wallace et al. (1982) tested pre- and postmenopausal women before and after an aerobic conditioning program. Both groups showed a significant increase in levels of estrogen, and 55% of the postmenopausal women reported a decrease in severity of hot flashes. Although the effectiveness of aerobic exercise on hot flashes requires further empirical evaluation and although such a treatment would be appropriate only for those physically able to engage in exercise, the possibility is promising.

The benefical effect of weight-bearing exercise on bone density and size, as well as the detrimental effects of immobility, have been known for decades. Research comparing exercising and sedentary postmenopausal women has consistently found exercise to be beneficial to bone health as measured by calcium balance (Aloia et al., 1978), bone mineral content (Smith and Reddan, 1976; Smith, Reddan and Smith, 1981; Krolner et al., 1983), bone density (Lutter and Lutter, 1984), and cortical diameter (Oyster et al., 1984). Particularly encouraging is that exercise has been found not only to prevent bone loss, but actually to increase bone mass. In Smith's 1981 study of women aged 69 to 95, sedentary controls lost an average of 3.29% of bone mineral over 36 months, while those in an exercise program increased bone mineral by 2.29%.

Some have argued that exercise in postmenopausal women may reduce adipose tissue, which converts androgens to estrogen, and thus may reduce estrogen and increase the risk of osteoporosis. However, this does not seem to be the case. Brewer et al. (1983) compared 42 women, aged 30 to 49, who had participated in a running program for at least two years, with 39 sedentary controls of similar age. Although the sedentary women were significantly heavier, they experienced a significant bone loss with age whereas the runners had either stable or increased bone mineral content with age. Collectively, research concerned with the treatment and prevention of osteoporosis suggests that regular exercise may be more effective than HRT or calcium supplements although comparative studies are clearly needed. Furthermore, exercise may be associated with additional benefits such as weight reduction and stress reduction.

Summary

Hormone replacement therapy is the most common form of treatment for menopausal symptoms, and the research clearly indicates that this treatment is effective in alleviating vasomotor instability, atrophic vaginitis, and, to some extent, osteoporosis. On the other hand, as discussed in previous sections of this chapter, there is little empirical evidence to endorse treatment with hormones for the alleviation of psychological symptoms. The increased risk of uterine cancer associated with HRT renders this form of treatment less than ideal. Anecdotal evidence from my own research in this area suggests that stress reduction, a regular exercise program, vitamin E therapy, or all of these are potentially useful in reducing the frequency and severity of hot flashes, although none of these has yet been tested systematically for its effectiveness. As the research on HRT becomes more widely available, physicians will be more reluctant to prescribe it and women more reluctant to take it. Consequently, researchers in both medical and nonmedical areas may be encouraged to develop and test alternative forms of treatment.

Apparent in most of the literature on HRT is an underlying conceptual framework within which menopause, and not the symptoms associated with it, is viewed as the problem to be treated. Evidence for the pervasiveness of this perspective is the emphasis on the effects of HRT on blood estrogen levels and the relative lack of interest in the alleviation of symptoms. A considerable amount of research has been done on the effects of dosage, chemical configuration, and mode of administration of HRT on plasma concentrations of estrogen, LH, and FSH; resulting concentrations are typically compared with those found in premenopausal women. The underlying, and often explicitly stated, justification for such research is that the purpose of HRT is to restore premenopausal levels of these hormones, particularly estrogen. Since the severity and frequency of hot flashes are not necessarily related to hormone levels, this rationale implies a belief that menopause itself is the disorder to be treated.

The view that menopause is a disease and that the goal of HRT is to restore the premenopausal physiological state can perhaps be explained within a sociocultural framework. The roles for women in our society have traditionally been the biological ones of having and raising children; thus, the physiological state of their reproductive years is considered normal and ideal, and efforts are made to maintain this state. With the feminist movement have come new theoretical conceptualizations within which menopause is viewed as a natural event, and alternative treatment approaches for menopausal symptoms are promoted to integrate psychological and cultural as well as physiological factors. At the same time, statements like, "I now believe the menopause may be considered an endocrinopathy" (Utian, 1987, p. 1281) and "Currently cessation of ovarian function [menopause] is the only form of end organ failure in endocrinology that is not routinely replaced" (Quigley et al., 1987, p. 1520) suggest that a natural view of menopause is still not accepted by mainstream medicine. In contrast, biology in men is viewed as secondary to their abilities to think, perform, and earn money; although levels of testosterone in men diminish rapidly after age 40, testosterone replacement therapy is not typically recommended.

Nevertheless, attributing the disease concept of menopause to cultural values does not negate the fact that two symptoms clearly related to menopausal status—hot flashes and atrophic vaginitis—can be disabling or particularly distressing for some women. Hormone Replacement Therapy does reliably alleviate these symptoms in most women and, if a woman can avoid the discomfort without exposing herself to an unacceptably high risk of cancer, cyclical estrogen with progesterone added during the last ten days of the cycle is the current treatment of choice. Future research in this area should not only develop and evaluate alternative forms of treatment but also be concerned with determining the lowest dose of HRT that is effective in alleviating hot flashes and atrophic vaginitis and should investigate the possibility of gradually diminishing the dose of HRT without a reccurrence of symptoms.

SUMMARY

Research concerned with the etiology of menopausal symptoms has been characterized by a strong focus on biomedical conceptualizations and methodologies. As a result of such a focus, the physiological event of menopause has been emphasized and the sociological and psychological aspects of the climacteric transition have been virtually ignored. Although most symptoms that occur prior to and subsequent to menopause probably have multiple, interacting etiologies, the research in general indicates that only hot flashes and atrophic vaginitis are best viewed from a biological perspective. Other menopausal symptoms, such as depression, anxiety, fatigue, and weight gain, are perhaps more appropriately termed climacteric symptoms, since the evidence suggests that these symptoms bear a stronger relationship to the stress associated with, and the psychological manifestations of, cultural attitudes toward aging and menopause than to physiology.

Because the literature concerned with the treatment of menopausal symptoms is also almost exclusively grounded in a biomedical conceptualization system, this body of literature is relevant to only a few of the many difficulties women experience during the climacteric transition. Tranquilizers and individual psychotherapy have occasionally been advocated for those symptoms which do not respond to hormonal treatment. However, such treatment must be viewed as symptomatic rather than curative, since the problem is not one of individual psychopathology but one of cultural pathology. Although cultural values and attitudes are neither easily nor readily modified, newly developing areas in sociology, psychology, and medicine are beginning to focus on system-centered rather than person-centered theories, and the eventual application of these theories may provide a context for viewing menopause as a natural, and potentially positive, experience in which freedom and wisdom are emphasized and valued rather than childbearing and youthful beauty.

In conclusion, although menopause strictly refers to a physiological event, the cessation of menses, the psychological manifestations, and the social impact and implications of menopause cannot be ignored in the study of symptoms associated with menopause. Women's roles have traditionally been limited to biological ones, women's femininity has been judged according to their reproductive capacity, and their value has been determined by their youth and beauty. Thus, although aging is psychologically difficult for everyone to accept, it is not surprising that it is particularly difficult for women, and menopause is clearly a sign of aging. There is no question but that stress, beliefs, and attitudes influence central and peripheral nervous system activity, reactivity to stress, susceptibility to disease, psychological and behavioral parameters, and the subjective report of symptoms. Thus, the study of menopause necessitates the consideration of psychological, social, and cultural, as well as physiological, factors.

REFERENCES

Abdalla, H.I., Hart, D.M., Lindsay, R. & Aitken, M. (1984), Determinants of bone mass and bone loss response to oestrogen therapy In oophorectomized women. Presented at the Fourth International Congress on the Menopause, Orlando, FL.
_____ McKay, D., Lindsay, R., Leggate, I. & Hooke, A. (1985), Prevention of bone mineral loss in postmenopausal women by norethisterone. *Obs. Gyn.*, 66:789–792.
Abe, T., Furuhashi, N., Yamaya, Y., Wada, Y., Hoshiai, A. & Suzuki, M. (1977). Correlation between climacteric symptoms and serum levels of estradiol, progesterone, follicle-stimulating hormone, and luteinizing hormone. *Amer. J. Obs. Gyn.*, 129:65–67.
Adamopoulos, D.A., Loraine, J.A. & Dove, G.A. (1971), Endocrinological studies in women approaching the menopause. *J. Obs. Gyn. of the Brit. Commonwealth*, 78:62–79.
Aitken, J.M. (1976), Bone metabolism in post-menopausal women. In: *The Menopause, ed. R.J. Beard.* Baltimore, MD: University Park Press, pp. 95–142
_____ Hart, D.M., Anderson, J.B., Lindsay, R., Smith, D.A. & Speirs, S.F. (1973), Osteoporosis after oophorectomy for non-malignant disease in pre-menopausal women. *Brit. Med. J.*, 2:325–328.
Aksel, S., Schomberg, D.W., Tyrey, L. & Hammond, C.B. (1976), Vasomotor symptoms, serum estrogens and gonadotropin levels in surgical menopause. *Amer. J. Obs. Gyn.*, 126:165–169.

Aleem, Fatma A. & McIntosh, Tracy K. (1984), Plasma b-endorphin in postmenopausal women. Presented at the Fourth International Congress on the Menopause, Orlando, FL.

Aloia, J.F., Cohn, S.H., Zanzi, I., Abesamis, C. & Ellis, K. (1978), Hydroxyproline peptides and bone mass in postmenopausal and osteoporotic women. *J. Clin. Endocrinol. Metab.*, 47:314–318.

Amschler, D.H. (1985), Calcium intake: A lifelong proposition. *J. School Health*, 55:360–362.

Archer, D.F. (1982), Biochemical findings and medical management of menopause. In: *Changing Perspectives on Menopause*, ed. A.M. Voda, M. Dinnerstein & S.R. O'Connell. Austin: University of Texas Press, pp. 29–45.

Asch, E.H., Balmaceda, J.P., Borghi, M.R., Niesvisky, R., Coy, D.H. & Schally, A.V. (1983), Suppression of the positive feedback of estradiol benzoate on gonadotropin secretion by an inhibitory analog of luteinizing hormone-releasing hormone (LRH) in oophorectomized rhesus monkeys: Evidence for a necessary synergism between LRH and estrogens. *J. Clin. Endocrinol. Metab.*, 57:367–372.

Aycock, N.R. & Jollie, W.P. (1979), Ultrastructural effects of estrogen replacement on postmenopausal endometrium. *Amer. J. Obs. Gyn.*, 135:461–466.

Badawy, S.Z.Z., Elliott, L.J., Elbadawi, A. & Marshall, L.D. (1979), Plasma levels of oestrone and oestradiol-17B in postmenopausal women. *Brit. J. Obs. Gyn.*, 86:56–63.

Ballinger, C.B. (1975), Psychiatric morbidity and the menopause: Screening of general population sample. *Brit. Med. J.*, 3:344–346.

_____ (1976), Subjective sleep disturbance at menopause. *J. Psychosom. Res.*, 20:509–513.

Bart, P. & Perlmutter, E. (1981), The menopause in changing times. In: B. Justice *Toward the Second Decade*, Westport, CT.: Greenwood, pp. 93–117.

Baumgardner, S.B., Condrea, H., Daane, T.A., Dorsey, J.H., Jurow, H.N., Shively, J.P., Wachsman, M., Wharton, L.R. & Zibel, M.J. (1978), Replacement estrogen therapy for menopausal vasomotor flushes: Comparison of Quinestrol and conjugated estrogens. *Obs. Gyn.*, 51:445–452.

Beller, F.K., Nachtigall, L. & Rosenberg, M. (1972), Coagulation studies of menopausal women taking estrogen replacement. *Obs. Gyn.*, 39:775–778.

Bercovici, B., Uretzki, G. & Patti, Y. (1972), The effects of estrogens on cytology and vascularization of the vaginal epithelium in climacteric women. *Amer. J. Obs. Gyn.*, 113:98–103.

Blankstein, J., Reyes, F.I., Winter, J.S.D. & Faiman, C. (1981), Endorphins and the regulation of the human menstrual cycle. *Clin. Endocrinol.*, 14:287–294.

Brewer, V., Meyer, B.M., Keele, M.S., Upton, S.J. & Hagan, R.D. (1983), Role of exercise in prevention of involutional bone loss. *Med. & Sci. in Sports & Exercise*, 15:445–449.

Brincat, M., Lafferty, K., De Trafford, J. & Studd, J.W. (1984), Thermal entrainment testing–a new way of looking at menopausal flushing. Presented at the Fourth International Congress on the Menopause, Orlando, FL.

Buchman, M.I., Kramer, E. & Feldman, G.B. (1978), Aspiration curettage for asymptomatic patients receiving estrogen. *Obs. Gyn.*, 51:339–341.

Budoff, P.W. (1980), *No More Menstrual Cramps and Other Good News*. New York: G.P. Putnam's Sons.

Bullamore, J.R., Gallagher, J.C., Wilkinson, R., Nordin, B.E.C. & Marshall, D.H. (1970), Effect of age on calcium absorption. *Lancet*, Sept.:535–537.

Burnier, A.M., Martin, P.L., Yen, S.S.C. & Brooks, P. (1981), Sublingual absorption of micronized 17B-estradiol. *Amer. J. Obs. Gyn.*, 140:146–149.

Callantine, M.R., Martin, P.L., Bolding, O.T., Warner, P.O. & Greaney, M.O. (1975), Micronized 17B-estradiol for oral estrogen therapy in menopausal women. *Obs. Gyn.*, 46, 37–41.

Canniggia, A., Gennari, C., Borrello, G., Bencini, M., Cesari, L., Poggi, C. & Escobar, S. (1970), Intestinal absorption of calcium-47 after treatment with oral oestrogen-gestogens in senile osteoporosis. *Brit. Med. J.*, 4:30–32.

Casper, R.F. & Yen, S.S.C. (1981). Rapid absorption of micronized estradiol-17B following sublingual administration. *Obs. Gyn.*, 57:62–64.

_____ _____ (1985), Neuroendocrinology of menopausal flushes: An hypothesis of flush mechanism. *Clin. Endocrinol.*, 22:293–312.

_____ _____ Wilkes, M.M. (1979), Menopausal flushes: A neuroendocrine link with pulsatile luteinizing hormone secretion. *Science*, 205:823–825.

Chakravarti, S., Collins, W.P., Newton, J.R., Oram, D.H. & Studd, J.W.W. (1977), Endocrine changes and symptomatology after oophorectomy in premenopausal women. *Brit. J. Obs. Gyn.*, 84:769–775.

Chang, R.J. & Judd, H.L. (1981), The ovary after menopause. *Clin. Obs. Gyn.*, 24:181–191.

Chestnut, C. (1984), An appraisal of the role of estrogens in the treatment of postmenopausal osteoporosis. *J. Amer. Geriat. Soc.*, 32:604–608.

Christiansen, C., Christensen, M.S., Larsen, N.E. & Transbol, I. (1982). Pathophysiological mechanism of estrogen effect on bone metabolism. Dose-response relationships in early postmenopausal women. *J. Clin. Endocrinol. Metab.*, 55:1124–1130.

Christie Brown, J.R.S. & Christie Brown, M.E. (1976), Psychiatric disorders associated with the menopause. In: *The Menopause*, ed. R.J. Beard. Baltimore, MD: University Park Press, pp. 57–59.

Chu, J., Schweid, A.I. & Weiss, N.S. (1982), Survival among women with endometrial cancer: A comparison of estrogen users and non-users. *Amer. J. Obs. Gyn.*, 143:569.

Clayden, J.R., Bell, J.W. & Pollard, P. (1974), Menopausal flushing: Double-blind trial of non-hormonal medication. *Brit. Med. J.*, 1:409–412.

Coope, J., Thomson, J.M. & Poller, L. (1975), Effects of "natural oestrogen" replacement therapy on menopausal symptoms and blood clotting. *Brit. Med. J.*, 4:139–143.

_____ Williams, S. & Patterson, J.S. (1978), A study of the effectiveness of propranolol in menopausal hot flushes. *Brit. J. Obs. Gyn.*, 85:474–475.

Cumming, D.C., Rebar, R.W., Hopper, B.R. & Yen, S.S.C. (1982), Evidence for an influence of the ovary on circulating dehydroepianodrosterone sulfate levels. *J. Clin. Endocrinol. Metab.*, 54:1069–1071.

_____ Vickovic, M.M., Wall, S.R., Flukar, M.R. & Belcastro, A.N. (1985), The effect of acute exercise on pulsatile release of luteinizing hormone in women runners. *Amer. J. Obs. Gyn.*, 153:482–485.

Davidson, B.J., Riggs, B.L., Wahner, H.W. & Judd, H.L. (1983), Endogenous cortisol and sex steroids in patients with osteoporotic spinal fractures. *Obs. Gyn.*, 61:275–278.

_____ Ross, R.K., Paganini-Hill, A., Hammond, G., Siiteri, P.K. & Judd, H.L. (1982), Total and free estrogens and androgens in postmenopausal women with hip fractures. *J. Clin. Endocrinol. Metab.*, 54:115–120.

Davies, M., Mawer, E.B. & Adams, P.H. (1977), Vitamin D metabolism and the response to 1,25-Dihydroxycholecalciferol in osteoporosis. *J. Clin. Endocrinol. Metab.*, 45:199–208.

Dawood, M.Y., Khan-Dawood, F.S. & Ramos, J. (1986), The effect of estrogen-progestin treatment on opioid control of gonadotropin and prolactin secretion in postmenopausal women. *Amer. J. Obs. Gyn.*, 155:1246–1251.

Dawson-Hughes, B., Jacques, M.S. & Shipp, C. (1987), Dietary calcium intake and bone loss from the spine in healthy postmenopausal women. *Amer. J. Clin. Nut.*, 46:685–687.

Dennerstein, L., Burrows, G.D., Hyman, G. & Wood, C. (1978), Menopausal hot flushes: A double blind comparison of placebo, ethinyl oestradiol and norgestrel. *Brit. J. Obs. Gyn.*, 85:852–856.

Deutsch, S., Ossowski, R. & Benjamin, I. (1981), Comparison between degree of systemic absorption of vaginally and orally administered estrogens at different dose levels in postmenopausal women. *Amer. J. Obs. Gyn.*, 139:967–968.

Dewhurst, C.J. (1976), The role of estrogen in preventative medicine. In: *The Menopause*, ed. R.J. Beard. Baltimore, MD: University Park Press, pp. 219–245.

Erlik, R., Gompel, A., Mercier-Bodard, C., Kuttenn, F., Guyenne, P.N., Corvol, P. & Mauvais-Jarvis, P. (1982), Effects of percutaneous estradiol and conjugated estrogens on the level of plasma proteins and triglycerides in postmenopausal women. *Amer. J. Obs. Gyn.*, 143:888–892.

Erlik, Y., Meldrum, D.R. & Judd, H.L. (1982). Estrogen levels in postmenopausal women with hot flashes. *Obs. Gyn.*, 59:403–407.

Ettinger, B., Genant, H.K. & Cann, C.E. (1985). Long term estrogen replacement therapy prevents bone loss and fractures. *Annals of Internal Medicine*, 102:319–324.

Fahraeus, L. & Larsson-Cohn, U. (1982), Oestrogens, gonadotrophins and SHBG during oral and cutaneous administration of oestradiol-17B to menopausal women. *Acta Endocrinol.*, 101:592–596.

_____ _____ Wallentin, L. (1982), Lipoproteins during oral and cutaneous administration of oestradiol-17B to menopausal women. *Acta Endocrinol.*, 101:597–602.

_____ Wallentin, L. (1983), High density lipoprotein subfractions during oral and cutaneous administration of 17B-estradiol to menopausal women. *J. Clin. Endocrinol. Metab.*, 56:797–801.

Falch, J., Oftebro, H. & Haug, E. (1987), Early postmenopausal bone loss is not associated with a decrease in circulating levels of 25-hydroxyvitamin D, 1,25-Dihydroxyvitamin D, or Vitamin D-binding protein. *J. Clin. Endocrinol. Metab.*, 64:836–840.

Ferin, M., Wehrenberg, W.B., Lam, N.Y., Alston, E.J. & VandeWiele, R.L. (1982), Effects and site of action of morphine on gonadotropin secretion in the female rhesus monkey. *Endocrinol.*, 111:1652–1656.

Fessler, L. (1950), The psychopathology of climacteric depression. *Psychoanal. Quart.*, 19:27–41.

Flowers, C.E., Wilborn, W.H. & Hyde, B.M. (1983), Mechanisms of uterine bleeding in postmenopausal patients receiving estrogen alone or with a progestin. *Obs. Gyn.*, 61:135–143.

Friederich, M.A. (1982), Middle-aged women's experience and perception of menopause. In: *Changing Perspectives on Menopause*, ed. A.M. Voda, M. Dinnerstein & S.R. O'Connell. Austin: University of Texas Press, pp. 173–210.

Frisch, R.E., Canick, J.A. & Tulchinsky, D. (1980), Human fatty marrow aromatizes androgen to estrogen. *J. Clin. Endocrinol. Metab.*, 51:394–396.

Frumar, A.M., Meldrum, D.R., Geola, F., Shamonki, I.M., Tataryn, I.V., Deftos, L.J. & Judd, H.L. (1980), Relationship of fasting urinary calcium to circulating estrogen and body weight in postmenopausal women. *J. Clin. Endocrinol. Metab.*, 50:70–75.

Gallagher, J.C. & Nordin, B.E.C. (1974), Calcium metabolism and the menopause. In: *Biochemistry of Women*, ed. A.S. Curry & J.V. Hewitt. Cleveland, OH: CRC Press, pp. 145–164.

_____ Riggs, B.L. & De Luca, H.F. (1980), Effect of estrogen on calcium absorption and serum vitamin D metabolites in postmenopausal osteoporosis. *J. Clin. Endocrinol. Metab.*, 51:1359–1364.

Gambrell, R.D., Massey, F.M., Castaneda, T.A., Ugenas, A.J., Ricci, C.A. & Wright, J.M. (1980), Use of progestogen challenge test to reduce the risk of endometrial cancer. *Obs. Gyn.*, 55:732–738.

Gannon, L.R. (1985), *Menstrual Disorders and Menopause*. New York: Praeger.

_____ (1988), The potential role of exercise in the alleviation of menstrual disorders and menopausal symptoms: A theoretical synthesis of recent research. *Women & Health*, 14:105–127.

_____ Hansel, S. & Goodwin, J. (1987), Correlates of menopausal hot flashes. *J. Beh. Med.*, 10:277–285.

Geola, F.L., Frumar, A.M., Tataryn, I.V., Lu, K.H., Hershman, J.M., Eggena, P., Sambhi, M.P. & Judd, H.L. (1980), Biological effects of various doses of conjugated equine estrogens in postmenopausal women. *J. Clin. Endocrinol. Metab.*, 51:620–625.

George, G.C.W., Utian, W.H., Beumont, P.J.V. & Beardwood, C.J. (1973), Effect of exogenous oestrogens on minor psychiatric symptoms in postmenopausal women. *S. African Med. J.*, 47:2387–2388.

Gerdes, L.C., EtPhil, D.L., Sonnendecker, E.W.W. & Polakow, E.S. (1982), Psychological changes effected by estrogen-progesterone and clonidine treatment in climacteric women. *Amer. J. Obs. Gyn.*, 142:98–104.

Ginsburg, J., O'Reilly, B. & Swinhoe, J. (1985), Effect of oral clonidine on human cardiovascular responsiveness: A possible explanation of the therapeutic action of the drug in menopausal flushing and migraine. *Brit. J. Obs. Gyn.*, 92:1169–1175.

_____ Swinhoe, J. & O'Reilly, B. (1981), Cardiovascular responses during the menopausal hot flush. *Brit. J. Obs. Gyn.*, 88:925–930.

Gray, L.A., Christopherson, W.M. & Hoover, R.N. (1977), Estrogens and endometrial carcinoma. *Obs. Gyn.*, 49:385–389.

Greene, J.G. (1976), A factor analytic study of climacteric symptoms. *J. Psychosom. Res.*, 20:425–430.

Greenwald, P., Caputo, T.A. & Wolfgang, P.E. (1977), Endometrial cancer after menopausal use of estrogens. *Obs. Gyn.*, 50:239–243.

Grodin, J.M., Siiteri, P.K. & MacDonald, P.C. (1973), Source of estrogen production in postmenopausal women. *J. Clin. Endocrinol. Metab.*, 36:207–214.

Hahn, R., Nachtigall, R.D. & Davies, T.C. (1984), Compliance difficulties with progestin-supplemented estrogen replacement therapy. *J. Fam. Pract.*, 18:411–414.

Hamilton, J.A., Aloi, J., Mucciardi, B. & Murphy, D.L. (1983), Human plasma beta-endorphin through the menstrual cycle. *Psychopharm. Bull.*, 19:586–587.

Hammond, C.B., Jelovsek, F.R., Lee, K.L., Creasman, W.T. & Parker, R.T. (1979), Effects of long-term estrogen replacement therapy. II. Neoplasia. *Amer. J. Obs. Gyn.*, 133:537–547.

_____ C.B. & Ory, S.J. (1982), Endocrine problems in the menopause. *Clin. Obs. Gyn.*, 25:19–38.

Hemsell, D.L., Grodin, J.M., Brenner, P.F., Siiteri, P.K. & MacDonald, P.C. (1974), Plasma precursors of estrogen. II. Correlation of extent of conversion of plasma and androstenedione to estrone with age. *J. Clin. Endocrinol. Metab.*, 38:476–479.

Henrik, E. (1982), Neuroendocrine mechanisms of reproductive aging in women and female rats. In: *Changing Perspectives on Menopause* ed. A.M. Voda, M. Dinnerstein & S.R. O'Connell. Austin: University of Texas Press, pp. 46–59.

Henzl, M.R., Moyer, D.L., Townsend, D., Valand, R.S. & Segre, E.J. (1973), Quantification of the estrogenic effects of mestranol on human endometrium and vaginal mucosa. *Amer. J. Obs. Gyn.*, 115:401–406.

Hunter, D.J.S. (1976), Oophorectomy and the surgical menopause. In: *The Menopause*, ed. R.J. Beard. Baltimore, MD: University Park Press, pp. 203–217.

_____ Anderson, A.B.M. Haddon, M. (1979), Changes in coagulation factors in postmenopausal women on ethinyl oestradiol. *Brit. J. Obs. Gyn.*, 86:488–490.

_____ Julier, D., Franklin, M. & Green, E. (1977), Plasma levels of estrogen, lutenizing hormone, and follicle stimulating hormone following castration and estradiol implant. *Obs. Gyn.*, 49:180–185.

Hutton, J.D., Jacobs, H.S., Murray, M.A.F. & James, V.H.T. (1978), Relation between plasma oestrone and oestradiol and climacteric symptoms. *Lancet*, April:678–681.

Jeffcoate, T.N.A. (1960), Drugs for menopausal symptoms. *Brit. Med. J.*, 1:340–342.

Jensen, J., Christiansen, C. & Rodbro, P. (1985), Cigarette smoking, serum estrogens, and bone loss during hormone-replacement therapy early after menopause. *New Eng. J. Med.*, 313:973–975.

_____ _____ Transbol, I.B. (1982), Fracture frequency and bone preservation in postmenopausal women treated with estrogen. *Obs. Gyn.*, 60:493–496.

_____ Nilas, L. Christiansen, C. (1986), Cyclic changes in serum cholesterol and lipoproteins following different doses of combined postmenopausal hormone replacement therapy. *Brit. J. Obs. Gyn.*, 93:613–618.

_____ Riis, B.J., Strom, V. & Christiansen, C. (1987), Continuous oestrogen-progestogen treatment and serum liproproteins in postmenopausal women. *Brit. J. Obs. Gyn.*, 94:130–135.

_____ _____ _____ Nilas, L. & Christiansen, C. (1987), Long-term effects of percutaneous estrogens and oral progesterone on serum lipoproteins in postmenopausal women. *Amer. J. Obs. Gyn.*, 156:66–71.

Judd, H.L. (1987), Efficacy of transdermal estradiol. *Amer. J. Obs. Gyn.*, 156:1326–1331.

_____ Davidson, B.J., Frumar, A.M., Shamonki, I.M. & Logasse, L.D. (1982), Origin of serum estradiol in postmenopausal women. *Obs. Gyn.*, 59:680–686.

_____ _____ _____ _____ _____ Ballon, S.C. (1980), Serum androgens and estrogens in postmenopausal women with and without endometrial cancer. *Amer. J. Obs. Gyn.*, 136:859–866.

_____ Judd, G.E., Lucas, W.E. & Yen, S.S.C. (1974), Endocrine function of the postmenopausal ovary: Concentration of androgens and estrogens in ovarian and peripheral vein blood. *J. Clin. Endocrinol. Metab.*, 39:1020–1024.

_____ Lucas, W.E. & Yen, S.S.C. (1976), Serum 17B-estradiol and estrone levels in postmenopausal women with and without endometrial cancer. *J. Clin. Endocrinol. Metab.* 43:272–278.

Kalra, S.P. & Simpkins, J.W. (1981), Evidence for noradrenergic mediation of opioid effects on luteinizing hormone secretion. *Endocrinol.*, 109:776–782.

Kaufman, S.A. (1967), Limited relationship of maturation index to estrogen therapy for menopausal symptoms. *Obs. Gyn.*, 54:399–407.

King, R.J.B., Whitehead, M.I., Campbell, S. & Minardi, J. (1978), Effects of estrogens and progestogens on the biochemistry of the postmenopausal endometrium. In: *The Role of Estrogen/Progesterone in the management of the menopause.*, ed. I.D. Cooke. Baltimore, MD: University Park Press, pp. 111–119.

Kistner, R.W. (1976), Estrogens and endometrial cancer: An editorial. *Obs. Gyn.*, 48:479–482.

Koeske, R. (1982). Toward a biosocial paradigm for menopausal research: Lessons and contributions from behavioral sciences. In: *Changing Perspectives on Menopause*, ed. A. Voda, M. Dinnerstein & S.R. O'Connell. Austin: University of Texas Press, pp. 159–172.

Krolner, B., Toft, B., Nielsen, S.P. & Tondevold, E. (1983), Physical exercise as prophylaxis against involutional vertebral bone loss: A controlled trial. *Clin. Sci.*, 64:541–546.

Kupperman, H.S., Blatt, M.H.G., Wiesbader, H. & Filler, W. (1953), Comparative clinical evaluation of estrogenic preparations by the menopausal and amenorrheal indices. *J. Clin. Endocrinol. Metab.*, 13:688–701.

Larsson-Cohn, U., Johansson, E.D.B., Kagedal, B. & Wallentin, L. (1978), Serum FSH, LH, and oestrone levels in postmenopausal patients on oestrogen therapy. *Brit. J. Obs. Gyn.*, 85:367–372.

Laufer, L.R., Erlik, Y., Meldrum, D.R. & Judd, H.L. (1982), Effect of clonidine on hot flashes in postmenopausal women. *Obs. Gyn.*, 60:583–586.

Lightman, S.L., Jacobs, H.S. & Maguire, A.K. (1982), Down-regulation of gonado-tropin secretion in postmenopausal women by a superactive LHRH analogue: Lack of effect of menopausal flushing. *Brit. J. Obs. Gyn.*, 89:977–980.

―――― ―――― ―――― McGarrick, G. & Jeffcoate, S.L. (1981). Climacteric flushing: Clinical and endocrine response to infusion of naloxone. *Brit. J. Obs. Gyn.*, 88:919–924.

Lin, T., SoBosita, J.L., Brar, H.K. & Roblete, B.V. (1973), Clinical and cytologic responses of postmenopausal women to estrogen. *Obs. Gyn.*, 41:97–107.

Lind, T. (1978), A prospective controlled trial of six forms of hormone replacement therapy after the menopause. In: *The Role of Estrogen/Progesterone in the Management of the Menopause*, ed. I.D. Cooke. Baltimore, MD: University Park Press, pp. 89–99.

―――― Cameron, E.C., Hunter, W.M., Leon, C., Moran, P.F., Oxley, A., Gerrard, J. & Lind, U.C.G. (1979), A prospective, controlled trial of six forms of hormone replacement therapy given to postmenopausal women. *Brit. J. Obs. Gyn.*, 86, Suppl. 3:1–29.

Lindsay, R., Hart, D.M., Maclean, H.A., Garwood, J., Aitken, J.M., Clark, A.C. & Coutts, J.R.T. (1978), Pathogenesis and prevention of post-menopausal osteoporosis. In: *The Role of Estrogen/Progesterone in the Management of the Menopause*, ed. I.D. Cooke. Baltimore, MD: University Park Press, pp. 9–27.

Longcope, C., Hunter, R. & Franz, C. (1980), Steroid secretion by the postmenopausal ovary. *Amer. J. Obs. Gyn.*, 138:564–568.

Lucas, W.E. & Yen, S.S.C. (1979), A study of endocrine and metabolic variables in postmenopausal women with endometrial carcinoma. *Amer. J. Obs. Gyn.*, 134:180–186.

Luciano, A.A., Turksoy, R.N., Carleo, J. & Hendrix, J.W. (1988), Clinical and metabolic responses of menopausal women to sequential versus continuous estrogen and progestin replacement therapy. *Obs. Gyn.*, 71:39–50.

Lutter, L.D. & Lutter, J.M. (1984), Osteoporosis in menopausal women related to level of physical activity. Presented at the Fourth International Congress on the Menopause, Orlando, FL.

Lyrenas, S., Karlstrom, K., Backstrom, T. & von Schoultz, B. (1981), A comparison of serum oestrogen levels after percutaneous and oral administration of oestradiol-17B. *Brit. J. Obs. Gyn.*, 88:181–187.

Maddock, J. (1978), Gonadal and pituitary hormone profiles in perimenopausal patients. In: *The Role of Estrogen/Progesterone in the Management of the Menopause*, ed. I.D. Cooke. Baltimore, MD: University Park Press, pp. 77–88.

Magos, A.L., Brewster, E., Singh, R., O'Dowd, T., Brincat, M. & Studd, J.W. (1986). The effects of norethesterone in postmenopausal women on oestrogen replacement therapy: A model for the pre-menstrual syndrome. *Brit. J. Obs. Gyn.*, 93:1290–1296.

Mandel, F.P., Geola, F.L., Lu, J.H.K., Eggena, P., Sambhi, M.P., Hershman, J.M. & Judd, H.L. (1982), Biologic effects of various doses of ethinyl estradiol in postmenopausal women. *Obs. Gyn.*, 59:673–679.

―――― ―――― Meldrum, D.R., Lu, J.H.K., Eggena, P., Sambhi, M.P., Hershman, J.M. & Judd, H.L. (1983), Biological effects of various doses of vaginally administered conjugated equine estrogens in postmenopausal women. *J. Clin. Endocrinol. Metab.* 57:133–139.

Maroulis, G.B. & Abraham, G.E. (1976), Ovarian and adrenal contributions to peripheral steroid levels in postmenopausal women. *Obs. Gyn.*, 48:150–154.

Martin, P.L., Burnier, A.M. & Greaney, M.O. (1972), Oral menopausal therapy using 17-B micronized estradiol. *Obs. Gyn.*, 39:771–774.

Mattingly, R.F. Huang, W.Y. (1969), Steroidogenesis of the menopausal and postmenopausal ovary. *Amer. J. Obs. Gyn.*, 103:679–690.

McKinlay, S.M. & Jeffreys, M. (1974), The menopausal syndrome. *Brit. J. Prevent. Soc. Med.*, 28:108–115.

Meites, J. (1980), Relation of endogenous opioid peptides to secretion of hormones. *Fed. Proc.*, 39:2531–2532.

Meldrum, D.R. (1987), Treatment of hot flushes. In: *Menopause*, ed. D.R. Mishell. Chicago: Yearbook Medical, pp. 141–150.

——— Davidson, B.J. Tataryn, I.V. & Judd, H.L. (1981), Changes in circulating steroids with aging in postmenopausal women. *Obs. Gyn.*, 57:624–628.

——— Erlik, Y., Lu, J.K.H. & Judd, H.L. (1981), Objectively recorded hot flashes in patients with pituitary insufficiency. *J. Clin. Endocrinol. Metab.*, 52:684–687.

——— Shamonki, I.M., Frumar, A.M., Tataryn, I.V., Chang, R.J. & Judd, H.L. (1979), Elevations in skin temperature of the finger as an objective index of postmenopausal hot flashes: Standardization of the technique. *Amer. J. Obs. Gyn.*, 135:713–717.

——— Tataryn, I.V., Frumar, A.M., Erlik, Y., Lu, K.H. & Judd, H.L. (1980), Gonadotropins, estrogens and adrenal steroids during the menopausal hot flash. *J. Clin. Endocrino. Metab.*, 50:685–689.

Molitch, M.E., Oill, P. & Odell, W.D. (1974), Massive hyperlipemia during estrogen therapy. *J. Amer. Med. Ass.*, 227:522–525.

Monroe, S.E., Jaffe, R.B. Midgley, A.T. (1972). Regulation of human gonadotropins. XII. Increase in serum gonadotropins in response to estradiol. *J. Clin. Endocrinol. Metab.*, 34:342–347.

Moore, B., Paterson, M.E.L., Sturdee, D.W. & Whitehead, T.P. (1981), The effect of menopausal status and sequential mestranol and norethisterone on serum biochemical profiles. *Brit. J. Obs. Gyn.*, 88:853–858.

Morse, A.R., Hutton, J.D., Murray, M.A.F. & James, V.H.T. (1979), Relation between the karyopyknotic index and plasma oestrogen concentrations after the menopause. *Brit. J. Obs. Gyn.*, 86:981–983.

Mulley, G., Mitchell, J.R.A. & Tattersall, R.B. (1977), Hot flushes after hypophysectomy. *Brit. Med. J.*, 2:1062.

Murakami, T., Yamaji, T. & Ohsawa, K. (1976), The effect of ACTH administration on serum estrogens, LH and FSH in the aged. *J. Clin. Endocrinol. Metab.*, 42:88–90.

Nachtigall, L.E., Nachtigall, R.H., Nachtigall, R.D. & Beckman, E.M. (1979), Estrogen replacement therapy: A 10-year prospective study in the relationship to osteoporosis. *Obs. Gyn.*, 53:277–281

Nagamani, M., Keever, M.E. Smith, E.R. (1987), Treatment of menopausal hot flashes with transdermal administration of clonindone. *Amer. J. Obs. Gyn.*, 156:561–565.

Natrajan, P.K., Muldoon, T.G., Greenblatt, R.B. & Mahesh, V.B. (1981). Estradiol and progesterone receptors in estrogen-primed endometrium. *Amer. J. Obs. Gyn.*, 140:387–392.

Nilas, L. & Christiansen, C. (1987), Bone mass and its relationship to age and the menopause. *J. Clin. Endocrinol. Metab.*, 65:697.

Nillius, S.J. & Wise, L. (1970), Effects of oestrogen on serum levels of LH and FSH. *Acta Endocrinol.*, 65:583–594.

Nisker, J.A., Hammond, G.L., Davidson, B.J., Frumar, A.M., Takaki, N.K., Judd, H.L. & Siiteri, P.K. (1980), Serum sex-hormone-binding-globulin capacity and the percentage of free estradiol in postmenopausal women with and without endometrial carcinoma. *Amer. J. Obs. Gyn.*, 138:637–642.

Nordin, B.E.C. (1971), Clinical significance and pathogenesis of osteoporosis. *Brit. Med. J.*, 1:571–576.

Notelovitz, M., Johnston, M., Smith, S. & Kitchens, C. (1987), Metabolic and hormonal effects of 25-mg and 50-mg 17B-estradiol implants in surgically menopausal women. *Obs. Gyn.*, 70:749.

—————— Kitchens, C.S., Rappaport, V., Coone, L. & Dougherty, M. (1981), Menopausal status associated with increased inhibition of blood coagulation. *Amer. J. Obs. Gyn.*, 141:149–152.

Ostergard, D.R., Parlow, A.F. Townsend, D.E. (1970), Acute effect of castration on serum FSH and LH in the adult woman. *J. Clin. Endocrinol. Metab.*, 31:43–47.

Oyster, N., Morton, M. & Linnell, S. (1984), Physical activity and osteoporosis in post-menopausal women. *Med. Sci. in Sports & Exercise*, 16:44–50.

Pang, C.N., Zimmermann, E. & Sawyer, C.H. (1977), Morphine inhibition of the preovulatory surges of plasma luteinizing hormone and follicle stimulating hormone in the rat. *Endocrinol.*, 101:1726–1732.

Paterson, M.E.L., Sturdee, D.W., Moore, B. & Whitehead, T.P. (1980), The effect of various regimens of hormone therapy on serum cholesterol and triglyceride concentrations in postmenopausal women. *Brit. J. Obs. Gyn.*, 87:552–560.

Perlmutter, J.F. (1978), A gynecological approach to menopause. In: *Sexual and Reproductive Aspects of Women's Health Care*, ed. M.T. Notman & C.C. Nadelson New York: Plenum Press, pp. 323–336.

Petraglia, F., Segre, A., Facchinetti, F., Campanini, D., Ruspa, M. & Genazzani, A.R. (1985), B-endorphin and met-enkephalin in peritoneal and ovarian follicular fluids of fertile and postmenopausal women. *Fertil. Steril.*, 44:615–621.

Poliak, A., Smith, J.J., Friedlander, D. & Romney, S.L. (1971), Estrogen synthesis in castrated women: The action of human chorionic gonadotropin and corticotropin. *Amer. J. Obs. Gyn.*, 110:376–379.

Poller, L., Thomson, J.M. & Coope, J. (1980), A double-blind cross-over study of piperazine oestrone sulphate and placebo with coagulation studies. *Brit. J. Obs. Gyn.*, 87:718–725.

Quigley, M.E.T., Martin, P.L., Burnier, A.M. & Brooks, P. (1987), Estrogen therapy arrests bone loss in elderly women. *Amer. J. Obs. Gyn.*, 156:1516–1523.

—————— Yen, S.S.C. (1980), The role of endogenous opiates on LH secretion during the menstrual cycle. *J. Clin. Endocrinol. Metab.*, 51:179–181.

Rader, M.D., Flickinger, G.L., de Villa, G.O., Mikuta, J.J. & Mikhail, G. (1973),

Plasma estrogens in postmenopausal women. *Amer. J. Obs. Gyn.*, 116:1069–1073.

Rakoff, A.E. (1975), Female climacteric: Premenopause, menopause, postmenopause. In: *Gynecologic Endocrinology*, ed. J.J. Gold. New York: Harper & Row, pp. 356–376.

Reid, R.L., Hoff, J.D. & Yen, S.S.C. (1981), Effects of exogenous B-endorphin on pituitary hormone secretion and its disappearance rate in normal human subjects. *J. Clin. Endocrinol. Metab.*, 52:1179–1184.

Reyes, F.I., Winter, J.S.D. Faiman, C. (1977), Pituitary-ovarian relationships preceding the menopause. I. A cross-sectional study of serum follicle-stimulating hormone, luteinizing hormone, prolactin, estradiol, and progesterone levels. *Amer. J. Obs. Gyn.*, 129:557–564.

Reynolds, S.R., Kaminester, S., Foster, F.L. & Schloss, S. (1941), Psychogenic and somatogenic factors in the flushes of the surgical menopause. *Amer. J. Obs. Gyn.*, 41:1022–1029.

Richardson, S.J., Senikas, V. & Nelson, J.F. (1987), Follicular depletion during the menopausal transition: Evidence for accelerated loss and ultimate exhaustion. *J. Clin. Endocrinol. Metab.*, 65:1231–1237.

Richelson, L.S., Heinz, W., Wahner, H.W., Melton, L.J. & Riggs, B.L. (1984), Relative contributions of aging and estrogen deficiency to postmenopausal bone loss. *New Eng. J. Med.*, 311:1273–1275.

Rigg, L.A., Milanes, B., Villaneuva, B. & Yen, S.S.C. (1977), Efficacy of intravaginal and intranasal administration of micronized estradiol-17B. *J. Clin. Endocrinol. Metab.* 45:1261–1264.

Riggs, B.L. (1987), Pathogenesis of osteoporosis. *Amer. J. Obs. Gyn.*, 156:1342–1346.

_____ Jowsey, J., Kelly, P.J., Hoffman, D.L. & Arnaud, C.D. (1976), Effects of oral therapy with calcium and vitamin D in primary osteoporosis. *J. Clin. Endocrinol. Metab.*, 42:1139–1144.

_____ Ryan, R.J., Wahner, H.W., Jiang, K. & Mattox, V.R. (1973), Serum concentrations of estrogen, testosterone and gonadotropins in osteoporotic and nonosteoporotic postmenopausal women. *J. Clin. Endocrinol. Metab.*, 36:1097–1099.

_____ Wahner, H.W., Melton, L.R., Richelson, L.S., Judd, H.L. & O'Fallon, W.M. (1987), Dietary calcium intake and rates of bone loss in women. *J. Clin. Invest.*, 80:979–982.

Riis, B.J., Thomsen, K., Strom, V. & Christiansen, C. (1987), The effect of percutaneous estradiol and natural progesterone on postmenopausal bone loss. *Amer. J. Obs. Gyn.*, 156:61–65.

Rogers, J. (1956), The menopause. *New Eng. J. Med.*, 254:697–704.

Rosenblum, H.G. & Schlaff, S. (1976), Gonadotropin-releasing hormone radioimmunoassay and its measurement in normal human plasma, secondary amenorrhea, and postmenopausal syndrome. *Amer. J. Obs. Gyn.*, 124:340–347.

Rosenwaks, Z., Wentz, A.C., Jones, G.S., Urban, M.D., Lee, P.A., Migeon, C.J., Parmley, T.H. & Woodruff, J.D. (1979), Endometrial pathology and estrogens. *Obs. Gyn.*, 53:403–410.

Russell, J.B., Mitchell, D., Musey, P.I. & Collins, D.C. (1984), The role of B-endorphins and catechol estrogens on the hypothalamic-pituitary axis in female athletes. *Fertil. Steril.*, 42:690–695.

Seyler, L.E. & Reichlin, S. (1973), Luteinizing hormone-releasing factor (LRF) in plasma of postmenopausal women. *J. Clin. Endocrinol. Metab.*, 37:197–203.

Sherman, L.M., West, J.H. & Korenman, S.G. (1976), The menopausal transition: Analysis of LH, FSH, estradiol, and progesterone concentrations during menstrual cycles of older women. *J. Clin. Endocrinol. Metab.* 42:629–636.

Simon, J.A. & diZerega, G.S. (1982), Physiologic estradiol replacement following oophorectomy: Failure to maintain precastration gonadotropin levels. *Obs. Gyn.*, 59:511–513.

Simpkins, J.W., Katovich, M.J. & Chengsong, I. (1983), Similarities between morphine withdrawal in the rat and the menopausal hot flush. *Life Sci.*, 32:1957–1966.

Smith, D.C., Prentice, R., Thompson, D.J., and Herrmann, W.L. (1975). Association of exogenous estrogen and endometrial carcinoma. *New Eng. J. Med.*, 293:1164–1167.

Smith, E.L. & Reddan, W. (1976), Physical activity: A modality for bone accretion in the aged. *Amer. J. Roentgenol.*, 126:1297.

Smith, E.L., Reddan, W. & Smith, P.E. (1981), Physical activity and calcium modalities for bone mineral increase in aged women. *Med. Sci. in Sports & Exercise*, 13:60–64.

Stangel, J.J., Innerfield, I., Reyniak, J.V. & Stone, M.L. (1977), The effect of conjugated estrogens on coagulability in menopausal women. *Obs. Gyn.*, 49:314–316.

Stavraky, K.M., Collins, J.A., Donner, A. & Wells, G.A. (1981), A comparison of estrogen use by women with endometrial cancer, gynecologic disorders, and other illnesses. *Amer. J. Obs. Gyn.*, 141:547–555.

Studd, J.W.W., Chakravarti, S. & Oram, D. (1977), The climacteric. In: *The Menopause: Clinics in Obstetrics and Gynecology*, Vol. 4 ed. R.B. Greenblatt & J. Studd. London: Saunders, pp. 78–91.

_____ Dubiel, M., Kakkar, V.V., Thom, M., and White, P.J. (1978). The effect of hormone replacement therapy on glucose tolerance clotting factors, fibrinolysis and platelet behavior in postmenopausal women. In: *The Role of Estrogen/Progesterone in the Management of the Menopause*, ed. I.D. Cooke. Baltimore, MD: University Park Press, pp. 41–62.

Stumpf, P.G., Maruca, J., Santen, R.J., and Demers, L.M. (1982). Development of a vaginal ring for achieving physiological levels of 17B-estradiol in hypoestrogenic women. *J. Clin. Endocrinol. Metab.*, 54:208–210.

Sturdee, D.W., Wade-Evans, T., Paterson, M.E.L., Thom, M. & Studd, J.W.W. (1978), Relations between bleeding pattern, endometrial histology, and oestrogen treatment in menopausal women. *Brit. Med. J.*, 1:1575–1577.

Tataryn, I.V., Lomax, P., Meldrum, D.R., Bajorek, J.G., Chesarek, W. & Judd, H.L. (1981), Objective techniques for the assessment of postmenopausal hot flashes. *Obs. Gyn.*, 57:340–344.

_____ Meldrum, D.R., Lu, K.H., Frumar, A.M. & Judd, H.L. (1979). LH, FSH, and skin temperature during the menopausal hot flash. *J. Clin. Endocrinol. Metab.*, 49:152–154.

Tepper, R., Neri, A., Kaufman, H., Schoenfeld, A. & Ovadia, J. (1987), Menopausal hot flushes and plasma B-endorphins. *Obs. Gyn.*, 70:150–152.

Thom, M., Collins, W.P. & Studd, J.W.W. (1981), Hormonal profiles in postmenopausal women after therapy with subcutaneous implants. *Brit. J. Obs. Gyn.*, 88:426–433.

Tsai, C.C. & Yen, S.S.C. (1971), Acute effects of intravenous infusion of 17B-estradiol on gonadotropin release in pre- and post-menopausal women. *J. Clin. Endocrinol. Metab.*, 32:766–771.

Tulandi, T., Lal, S. & Kinch, R.A. (1983), Effect of intravenous clonidine on menopausal flushing and luteinizing hormone secretion. *Brit. J. Obs. Gyn.*, 90:854–857.

Utian, W.H. (1972), The mental tonic effect of oestrogens administered to oophorectomized females. *S. African Med. J.*, 46:1079–1082.

_____ (1987), Overview on menopause. *Amer. J. Obs. Gyn.*, 156:1280–1283.

_____ Katz, M., Davey, D.A., and Carr, P.J. (1978), Effect of premenopausal castration and incremental dosages of conjugated equine estrogens on plasma follicle-stimulating hormone, luteinizing hormone, and estradiol. *Amer. J. Obs. Gyn.*, 132:297–302.

Veldhuis, J.C., Samojlik, E., Evans, W.S., Rogol, A.D., Ridgeway, C., Crowley, W.F., Kolp, L., Checinska, E., Kirschner, M.A., Thorner, M.O. & Stumpf, P. (1986), Endocrine impact of pure estradiol replacement in postmenopausal women: Alterations in anterior pituitary hormone release and circulating sex steroid hormone concentrations. *Amer. J. Obs. Gyn.*, 155:334–339.

Vermeulen, A. (1976), The hormonal activity of the postmenopausal ovary. *J. Clin. Endocrinol. Metab.*, 42:247–253.

Voda, A. (1981), Alterations of the menstrual cycle: Hormonal and mechanical. In: *The Menstrual Cycle, Vol. 2*, ed. P. Komnenich, M. McSweeney, J.A. Noack & N. Elder. New York: Springer, pp. 141–165.

_____ (1982), Menopausal hot flash. In: *Changing Perspectives on Menopause*, ed. A. Voda, M. Dinnerstein, & S. R. O'Connell. Austin: University of Texas Press, pp. 110–136.

von Kaulla, E., Droegemueller, W. & von Kaulla, K.N. (1975), Conjugated estrogens and hypercoagulability. *Amer. J. Obs. Gyn.*, 122:688–692.

Walker, A.M. & Hershel, J. (1980), Declining rates of endometrial cancer. *Obs. Gyn.*, 56:733–736.

Wallace, J.P., Lovell, S., Talano, C., Webb, M.L. & Hodgson, J.L. (1982), Changes in menstrual function, climacteric syndrome, and serum concentrations of sex hormones in pre- and post-menopausal women following a moderate intensity conditioning program. *Med. Sci. in Sports & Exercise*, 14:154.

Walter, S. & Jensen, H.K. (1977), The effect of treatment with estradiol and estriol on fasting serum cholesterol and triglyceride levels in postmenopausal women. *Brit. J. Obs. Gyn.*, 84:869–872.

Wardlaw, S.L., Wehrenberg, W.B., Ferin, M., Antunes, J.L. & Frantz, A.G. (1982), Effect of sex steroids on B-endorphin in hypophyseal portal blood. *J. Clin. Endocrinol. Metab.* 55:877–881.

Watts, J.F.F., Butt, W.R., Edwards, R.L. & Holder, G. (1985), Hormonal studies in women with premenstrual tension. *Brit. J. Obs. Gyn.*, 92:247–255.

Wehrenberg, W.B., Wardlaw, S.L., Frantz, A.G. & Ferin, M. (1982), B-endorphin in hypophyseal portal blood: Variations throughout the menstrual/cycle. *Endocrinol.*, 11:879–881.

Weideger, P. (1977), *Menstruation and Menopause*. New York: Knopf.

Whitehead, M.I., McQueen, J., Minardi, J. & Campbell, S. (1978), Progestogen modification of estrogen-induced endometrial proliferation in climacteric women. In: *The Role of Estrogen/Progesterone in the Management of the Menopause*, ed. I.D. Cooke. Baltimore, MD: University Park Press, pp. 121–137.

Weinstein, L. (1987), Efficacy of a continuous estrogen-progestin regimen in a menopausal patient. *Obs. Gyn.*, 69:929–932.

Wheatley, D. (1984), Trial of an adrenergic beta-blocker in the menopause. *Psychosomat.*, 25:208–220.

Williams, A.R., Weiss, N.S., Ure, C.L., Ballard, J. & Daling J.R. (1982), Effect of weight, smoking, and estrogen use on the risk of hip and forearm fractures in postmenopausal women. *Obs. Gyn.*, 60:695–699.

Worley, R.J. (1981), Age, estrogen, and bone density. *Clin. Obs. Gyn.*, 24:203–218.

Yen, S.S.C., Martin, P.L., Burnier, A.M., Czekala, N.M., Greaney, M.O. & Callantine, M.R. (1975), Circulating estradiol, estrone, and gonadotropin levels following the administration of orally active 17B-estradiol in postmenopausal women. *J. Clin. Endocrinol. Metab.*, 40:518–521.

_____ Quigley, M.E., Reid, R.L., Robert, J.F. & Cetel, N.S. (1985), Neuroendocrinology of opioid peptides and their role in the control of gonadotropin and prolactin secretion. *Amer. J. Obs. Gyn.*, 152:485–493.

Young, M.M. & Nordin, B.E.C. (1967), Effects of natural and artificial menopause on plasma and urinary calcium and phosphorus. *Lancet*, July:118–120.

Ziel, H.K. & Finkle, W.D. (1975), Increased risk of endometrial carcinoma among users of conjugated estrogens. *New Eng. J. Med.*, 293:1167–1170.

_____ _____ (1976), Association of estrone with the development of endometrial carcinoma. *Amer. J. Obs. Gyn.*, 124:735–740.

9

Varieties of Menopausal Experience

Case Histories

MALKAH T. NOTMAN

Sparked by the women's movement and influenced by the increased consumerism and the antimedical sentiment of the late 1980s, two different attitudes toward women's health have emerged. On one hand, attributes that were thought characteristically female or femi-nine have been reconsidered: Are these attributes "truly" female and feminine, or are they socially produced? On the other hand, acknowl-edgment of those characteristics and of the experiences of mind and body that do belong to women has been strongly urged by feminists. Recognition of the enormous role of socialization in creating traits and establishing norms previously considered biological and innate has cast doubt on the existence of innately "feminine" characteristics, and the close connection between the feminine and the biological has been questioned. The inevitability and significance of experiences that are uniquely female has also been deemphasized.

Consequently, the effort to take an egalitarian approach to women and to men has also served to diminish the importance of those experiences which are uniquely women's. It is clear that if women are really to be included fully in the total society, their experiences cannot be represented by male-derived norms. Concepts need to be changed and women's particular ways of feeling, knowing and judging must be acknowledged. More attention must be paid to the actual nature of women's experiences. Events that are unquestionably female, such as those of the menstrual cycle, must be studied and their significance assessed rather than denied or minimized. This does not mean that these experiences signify vulnerability or weakness. In the move to liberate women, some of the distinctive aspects of their lives have been minimized—pregnancy, menses, menopause. Since these are also sexual functions, they share with sexuality highly charged attitudes about sex and reproduction and the values connected with childbearing, and, indirectly, inheritance, and property.

Myths and superstitions surrounding menstruation, pregnancy, and menopause have multiple origins. The hidden location of the female reproductive organs invites fantasy. The central role of sex and reproduction in all aspects of human existence inevitably evokes a sense of mystery, as do the ability to give life and to nurture the young.

The reproductive system has not been as well studied as other functions, and many aspects of reproductive functioning were not well understood until relatively recently. Research is now underway in many areas previously neglected, but the absence of women as researchers and in positions to set research priorities also has been responsible for the relative scarcity of research about women's reproductive experience.

Menopause has been particularly poorly understood and subject to distortions and misconceptions. It has mostly been thought of as synonymous with loss, needing to be mourned. All difficulties of middle-aged women have been blamed on the menopause. This tendency is compounded by the deprecation of the older woman, that is, the woman who is past the peak of her youthful sexual attractiveness and is no longer able to produce children. Adult development, especially "midlife," has also received less attention from theorists and students than has early development—partly because life expectancy was so much shorter in the past. "Midlife" was conceptualized as primarily a time of preparation for death.

Further complicating our understanding is that the effects of menopause have been confounded with the effects of aging. Hormonal changes and their mysterious consequences have been blamed for conditions that actually are due to lack of exercise, poor nutrition, and physiological changes that accompany aging.

The normal course of women's lives also has received scant attention. A now familiar complaint is that developmental models have been derived from males and reflect male lives. Thinking about male development has been a linear process, such as that of Erikson (1963), who described development as progressing through a sequence of life events and experiences moving from one stage to the next. Events related to career and work either precede or accompany the establishment of a family. In contrast to this linear model, the life cycle for women can proceed along a number of different paths at the same time, not necessarily sequentially. Some women follow a course similar to that of men, with work first and family at the same time, but others do not. It is possible for a woman to have a family first and then work outside of the home, or to pursue training and a career and then have a family, or to do both at once. The reproductive limitation, the "biological clock," provides a context within which these pursuits occur. Because the years of childbearing are limited, women are not as free as men are to develop a career and *then* have a family (Notman, 1979). Anxiety about approaching menopause thus can provide an impetus to make childbearing decisions; this sense of finiteness is one of the key experiences defining middle age (Neugarten, 1975). This anxiety can also stimulate fantasies about menopause and give shape to many other concerns. It also provides the potential for displacement for work-related anxieties, so that a woman can worry about childbearing rather than face conflicts about work.

In the last few years there has been converging information that menopause itself is not as major a source of symptoms and difficulties as had been supposed. The actual menopause is not accompanied by depression (Weissman and Klerman, 1977), nor by an increase in visits for medical care (McKinlay, McKinlay, and Brambilla, 1987). Neugarten and her co-workers (1968) began to question prevailing ideas about menopause in a series of studies in the 50s. Their findings have been expanded in recent years but, regrettably, have not yet found their way into the literature; and older ideas prevail in many quarters.

In understanding menopause, it is important to consider its symbolic meaning, as well as to study the actual experiences that accompany menopause. There have been changes in the significance of motherhood (Notman and Nadelson, 1982) as a unique source of self-esteem and identity for women. Although parenthood as a source of fulfillment for men and women has long been recognized—it provides fulfillment of one's ego ideal and identifications with one's own parents, and in many ways is a major representation of adult-hood—not everyone wants to be a parent. Some women have felt hindered by the isolation and constraints of the patterns of child-bearing in the nuclear family; some have felt personally unsuited for motherhood. Not choosing motherhood was a socially deviant posi-tion until the recent shifts in social roles and widening work opportu-nities. Many women who chose career priorities are now regretting that they did not feel a sense of urgency toward forming a family and becoming a mother. Menopause, then, is a more compelling threat for those women who feel pressed by the short period remaining for them to become pregnant. For them the symbolic loss of youth and status may be less important; for those who have delayed childbearing, the actual loss is the larger problem.

Menopause has also been confused with the developmental changes of midlife. At the time a woman is likely to become menopausal, she is in a life phase when major changes may be occurring. If she had children near the beginning of her reproductive life, when she was in her 20s, they are either becoming adolescent or starting their own families or their own lives outside the family. Competitive conflicts with adolescents are likely to become intensified. The older woman may be confronted with her young daughter, now sexually more attractive and potentially threatening. This conflict has been repre-sented in fairy tales, for instance, Snow White, in which the wicked stepmother asks her mirror, "Who is the fairest of them all?" When the mirror tells her it is Snow White, she plans revenge.

The well-known midlife reassessment described for men occurs with women as well, although the ingredients are likely to be different. For both women and men there may be a sense of disappointment with what has been accomplished and a shift of investment, emotional and actual. For the man, this sense can be projected and experienced not as disappointment in himself, but as disappointment in his wife, and he may abandon the marriage. Women historically have not been as ready as men to leave their marriages because women's ability to support themselves well has been more limited and the stigma of divorce has been greater for women. The woman whose marriage is threatened in middle age is likely to become depressed. If this threat coincides with menopause, menopause may be blamed for the depression.

The entry, or reentry, of women into the paid work force at the time that children become more independent or leave home is accompanied by particular stresses for many women. Being a new student or entering a new job situation may evoke old anxieties about aggression, competition, and performance, with a need to establish herself and develop a sense of control. Her control over herself can seem threatened by unpredictable menopausal symptoms, such as irregular, profuse menstrual bleeding or hot flashes that interfere with sleep.

Sexual changes also occur in midlife. Many couples seek help then because of sexual changes that create sexual difficulties. Women's interest in sex is maintained as they get older and often is greater when the distractions, fatigue, and lack of privacy connected with having young children are over. Postmenopausal women also experience relief at not having to worry about pregnancy, and they feel sexually freer and more responsive. However, endocrine changes do affect the vaginal mucosa. Diminished estrogen causes diminished vaginal lubrication, with a longer time necessary for foreplay. The midlife sexual changes characteristic of men result in longer time before ejaculation, sometimes with difficulty in maintaining an erection. Men's performance anxiety often increases or is intensified if the partner takes longer to become aroused and therefore appears less responsive. These changes can reverberate with a man's concerns about his own attractiveness, power, control, and with both satisfactions and disappointments in his life. Similar issues pertain to a woman, but she may be more worried about her attractiveness and her body and less explicitly with her "power." She may express these issues in worry about her remaining "feminine."

The concept of "femininity," however, is vague and confused. It contains elements that are descriptive of predominant ways of behaving and feeling in a particular society. It also has a normative aspect, prescribing what is "normal" and "right" for women. There are some fundamental components of the "femininity" concept that result from (1) women's reproductive and nurturant roles, (2) the female body and its potential, and (3) the body image that derives from it. "Femininity" has always included reproductive potential and has often been primarily limited to it. To the extent that a woman's self-concept, gratifications, and social roles depend on her continuing to bear children, she will feel a loss at menopause.

In the psychoanalytic writings of the 1940s and 1950s, menopause was conceptualized in terms of loss, which was a dominant element in thinking about this event or series of events. Deutsch (1945) described menopause as a "narcissistic mortification that is difficult to overcome" and said that at menopause, a woman "loses all she received at puberty" (p. 457). Reproductive potential is thus considered literally, not as creativity or nurturance, or "generativity" in Erikson's (1963) terms. Another view held that a woman's reactions to menopause resembled her responses to menarche and pregnancy, representing her overall adaptation to "femininity" and to its stresses (Bibring, 1961). Women who had not borne children, or who had had abortions, were thought to have a more difficult time at menopause. To some extent, it is true that reactions to menarche and pregnancy presage responses to menopause in that they are part of a general similarity in a woman's adaptive potential and patterns. Menopause, however, is less an "event" than is pregnancy or than are the complex adolescent changes of which menarche is a part. That childless women have a more difficult time at menopause is not supported by data. Childless women do indeed have to come to terms with their state at some time and may then mourn their unrealized potential. But, for many, the awareness that they are unlikely to have children takes place in the context of other events in their lives, such as the breaking up of a close relationship or a shift in life circumstances that makes clearer the direction their life is taking. Thus, coming to terms with childlessness may not coincide with the actual cessation of menses. Clinically, it is apparent that the mourning process that has been thought to be an essential component of the menopause is quite variable and sometimes hardly noticeable. If one thinks of the menopause as occupying an expected place in a normal developmental sequence through life, then the time after childbearing is part of this normal sequence, a new phase when the monthly clock no longer dominates one's time and creates anxiety, as well as when anxiety about pregnancy can be put aside. With each new life phase, a woman's capacities change; there are cognitive as well as emotional shifts (Gutman, 1981), and new self-representations emerge and consolidate. Unfortunately, "normal" postmenopausal self-concepts have not been systematically described.

The following case histories illustrate the great variety of meanings and experiences of menopause.

CASE HISTORY: HB

HB is a 46-year-old woman with a long history of sexual difficulty with her husband, whom she described as an emotionally distant and unresponsive man. He is a successful businessman, and for many years she lived the part of a contented wife, socially active, with a pleasant lifestyle; she has adapted to many changes of cities. She has two children in their early 20s. About a year ago the family moved again because the husband was recruited for a new job that offered them both many advantages. After the move, she found that she was very restless, irritable, and depressed. She thought she might be menopausal. Many of her friends had been put on replacement estrogens, and the idea of approaching menopause was on her mind. She saw her gynecologist and told him she thought she was menopausal and that she was upset about a number of things. He did not find any clinical confirmation that she was menopausal but referred her to a therapist who counsels menopausal women.

For a long time HB had been dissatisfied with her marriage. Actually, while she and her husband were living the life of a contented couple, she was unhappy about their lack of intimacy and his remoteness from the children. She had worked but had not been free to follow a career until now. Recently, she said, she had fallen in love with a woman, and in this relationship she felt she found an intensity and fulfillment she had missed in her marriage. She was struggling with the implications of these feelings and was confused about what to do next.

HB had had a history of "crushes" on women during adolescence and early adulthood but had never considered any other possibilities but marriage. She had then protected her marriage until her children were adults. The move to a new city jarred her loose from familiar supports and relationships and left her free to form new ones.

When she was eight, she lost her mother after a long illness that had followed her parents' divorce. Her father remarried when she was 12. At 22 she married a fellow student with whom she had a romantic love affair; only later did she realize that he did not offer her enough warmth. Her father and stepmother died suddenly in an accident when she was already married. She was aware that she had not fully reacted to this shock and loss, but had instead developed some physical symptoms. She realized that in the relationship with her new lover she was seeking to replace her mother or to find a new mother. She realized that the new lover might be the mother figure she had wished for, and she accepted this possibility. In fact, it seemed to HB that she was being kind and loving to herself by accepting her need for a mother and finally having found such a person.

In a sense, her new relationship is a "midlife" development. That she fell in love at this time and not earlier was understandable as a consequence of the feeling that she was now at a time in her life when she needed to fulfill her own deep wishes and passions. She no longer wanted to put up with the emotional constraints of her marriage without some other source of gratification. HB's falling in love could be considered a midlife crisis in that she wanted to change the circumstances of her life, and it was a response to disappointment and to a reevaluation. However, the surge of feelings and their expression in the new relationship did not occur because she was menopausal. HB was upset and worried about breaking up her marriage and worried that if it did come to an end, she would feel abandoned by her husband, who had been a caring and thus "motherly" person. She had shifted from one kind of mother to another in her current love affair. She recognized the deep feelings evoked in this relationship but she, as well as the gynecologist, had been prepared to mislabel them.

CASE HISTORY: TM

TM is a 47-year-old lawyer. Several months before she came for a consultation, a longstanding relationship that she had hoped would lead to marriage began to deteriorate. She felt she had finally recognized that it was not going anywhere. She was disappointed and bitter, particularly since she recognized that it was now extremely unlikely that she would have children. She had a satisfying career and warm friendships, but also strong conscious and unconscious wishes to be a mother.

She began bleeding between her periods and was advised to have a D&C. Reluctantly, she agreed; she worried whether the bleeding was an irregularity in her periods heralding menopause. When she signed the informed-consent form for the D&Cshe felt she was giving away some power to protect herself by agreeing to any surgery at all. She was putting herself in the hands of the gynecologist. The gynecologist, who joked with her about the procedure, frightened her. That night TM dreamed she had given permission for a hysterectomy, that now her childbearing chances were gone. She awoke in a panic, not sure what she had actually signed when she signed the informed-consent form. She berated herself for not reading the fine print, felt she was slipping into senescence. A consultation helped her recognize the symbolic as well as the actual significance of the irregular bleeding and the diagnostic procedure. A period of depression and mourning followed, from which she emerged more able to terminate her disappointing relationship. She became very involved with children in the extended family, and her anxiety cleared without residual depression, although she consciously regretted that her chances for having her own children were gone. She was not actually menopausal, but the symptoms had mobilized her awareness that another relationship was unlikely, and having a child even less likely.

CASE HISTORY: PT

PT came into therapy when she was 48 years old. She felt that, although she was doing everything the way it should be done and things were going well in her life and with her family, she was not enjoying herself. She felt out of touch with her feelings and vague and distant from people, although her relationships with her husband and four children seemed on the surface to be smooth.

She was the only child of parents who each had had a previous marriage. Her father, a businessman, was often away. Her mother was busy and preoccupied; her grandparents, who brought her up, were warm and protective. A conspiracy of positive thinking seemed to envelop her childhood, and unpleasant events, even world events, were not mentioned. She knew little of the turbulence of World War II, even though her father was called into the Army. She had few childhood memories, except of being a family favorite. She was bright and explorative; she had been the first girl in her social circle to go away to college. Shortly after college she met her husband. They had a wonderfully exciting courtship and then married. She was aware that her explorative, assertive, and leadership qualities had become more subdued after marriage. Her four children were in school away from home.

Therapy during the first two years centered on recovering some awareness of her feelings. A crisis with one of her sons about a girlfriend stirred up in her anxiety about having caused the difficulties he was having. She readily felt guilty, was perfectionistic, anxious if she lost control. Feeling angry, particularly with her therapist, was much more difficult. Even though her feelings seemed positive and hard to reach, her dreams were elaborate, often filled with violent imagery—perilous encounters, hazardous roads, car accidents, even acrobatic mishaps. Associations to her dreams were sparse, if there were any at all. As therapy progressed, she recognized emerging discontent with her mother, discrepancies between her agreeable social self and her actual feelings, and moments of rage.

PT had many dreams of babies. Sometimes she rescued them; sometimes she was a nurse in a ward full of babies. Sometimes she was given a baby to care for. Her thoughts did not lead to depression or regret. Although she loved babies, she was consciously relieved that her childbearing days were over, and she was waiting to be a grandparent.

Her periods had always been irregular. Before her marriage, a gynecologist had wrongly predicted infertility. She did not react to the prediction with alarm, although she recognized the possibility. She remained unaware of her feelings, by and large, which protected her and permitted her to remain optimistic.

In the third year of therapy, she began to describe sensations resembling hot flashes. She consulted a gynecologist, who confirmed them and said she could not be treated with hormones because of uterine fibroids. She was given the choice of having a hysterectomy or waiting, and she chose to wait. She was told that menopause, with its diminished hormone levels, would shrink the fibroids. The next year was difficult, with hot flashes of unpredictable duration interrupting her sleep. Heavy, unpredictable bleeding interfered with her work and social commitments and with sexual relations.

Her dreams contained symbols of lost objects and blood, which she connected with the profuse menstrual flow. She and her gynecologist carefully considered the pros and cons of a hysterectomy for fibroids; such an operation would relieve her heavy bleeding. She feared surgery and preferred to tolerate the symptoms, including the hot flashes. Although uncomfortable, she did not feel depressed.

PT's relationships with her best friend and with her husband became more strained as she grew more aware of and expressive of her anger. She was concerned about one son whose relationship to his girlfriend was a stormy one. Gradually, PT listened to the family's descriptions of her behavior: that she was turning them off and would not listen to or hear conflict between family members, but instead tuned it out. A few years earlier, she had told the friend of one of her children that marriage improves with every year, an assessment she later retracted. She could see how she had always been inclined to smooth things over and had paid for the peace thus achieved with her sense of vitality and the vividness of her feelings.

She felt an acute need to go back to work; she had taken time off after leaving her last job. But it was difficult for her to make decisions about what moves to make next because she was in the process of reevaluating all her former ideas about her goals and sense of purpose.

After some time and further diagnostic surgical procedures, her hot flashes began to abate. Yet her severe and unpredictable menstrual period persisted, causing her to continue to feel awkward and embarrassed. At the same time, she clarified several areas of conflict.

PT had struggled with weight gain for many years. Although not obese, she was overweight and would engage in orgies of cookie baking and eating, first baking for her children, then for community causes, and then without excuse. The lack of control she felt over this behavior added to her feelings of lack of control of her periods and her hot flashes.

One day while shopping, she found herself at a candy counter, buying chocolate. She recalled in her therapy session that the event that had immediately preceded this action was a complicated decision about selecting a gift for a relative. PT had experienced conflict in regard to this rather distant and affluent woman. On one hand, PT wanted her gift to express her good taste and, on the other, she wanted not to overdo her desire to please by buying something too elaborate. She felt anxious. She resolved her conflict by buying a gift that she was sure was in good taste but, she thought, overly fancy and expensive. She felt dissatisfied with this solution. It was at this point that she found herself going to the candy counter. She saw the connection between the conflict and anxiety about the gift and buying chocolate. This insight was illuminating. She recognized that when she felt anxious she soothed herself by eating. At other times, her feelings remained distant from her. This connection seemed to provide some control over her eating and to allay to some degree her feelings of being out of control of her periods and of her body. She extended this control and began to exercise more regularly. She reported that she felt "more desirable, more alive and more in tune."

PT is in a perimenopausal stage, that is, the period of time surrounding the menopause. Her dreams, her approach to the next phase of her life, and relationships with her children and other family members indicate a shift from active mothering to a more distant relationship with her children. Despite the distancing, feelings of loss or depression are not prominent. She expects changes in her relationships with the children to come with their marriages and their independence, but she is looking forward to these shifts and to improved relationships. Her concern over her son's troubles with his girlfriend may represent a displacement from her earlier investment in childbearing and mothering, but it is appropriate to the reality of his life and hers.

CASE HISTORY: EV

EV, a woman almost 50 years old, was brought for a consultation by her 25-year-old daughter. She had become preoccupied with the idea that when she turned 50 she would become undesirable and superfluous to her husband and family. No amount of reassurance could shake this conviction. Her family planned an elaborate birthday party as a demonstration of their love and her ongoing important place in their lives. Although her four daughters planned a "grandmother tribute," and her husband bought her a new ring, she was not reassured. Her conviction, which had the firmness of a delusion, was, in fact, the beginning of a psychotic depression. EV's mother had had a difficult menopause, with headaches, hot flashes, and a depression for which she had to be hospitalized, and she never regained her premorbid liveliness. EV, who had read that the average age of onset of menopause is 50, remembered her mother's depression and became increasingly convinced she was heading inexorably along the same path. She herself had not yet become menopausal. Later, she was treated with antidepressant medication. When her psychotic depression improved, her preoccupation with her 50th birthday subsided.

This is a woman for whom the fantasy of the changes occurring in her body and her life fixed on the age of 50 as the turning point into an old woman, like her depressed mother. The mother's symptoms, which certainly the daughter and probably the mother attributed to menopause, made this change concrete in her mind. After "the change of life," she would not be the same. When her depression abated, the physical symptoms did not seem so inevitably to represent her damaged, "changed" status. The psychotic depression was symbolically, but not realistically, connected to the menopause.

CASE HISTORY: DJ

DJ was a 52-year-old woman who sought treatment because of depression. She thought her depression was due to her "empty nest" or to menopause. Her two children were both in college, and she had begun to feel old. When she caught unexpected glimpses of herself in the mirror or in store windows, she was dismayed. Her chin sagged, her hair looked unattractive. Sometimes, she thought, she looked like her mother. Sometimes she wondered "Who is that old woman?"

She examined herself for signs of aging and found varicose veins, a pot belly and the need for reading glasses. Her waning menstrual period confirmed her fears. She wondered what the mysterious estrogens really did and if it was menopause that was the matter with her. Her doctor prescribed estrogen maintenance therapy. DJ was ambivalent about taking pills all her life; to do so only confirmed her feelings of infirmity. But she did not want to develop osteoporosis. Would she lose sexual desire? Would she gain weight? Was her sense of disorientation at the shrunken household really a response to hormonal changes? She described a shopping trip in which she tried on many dresses and found that all of them looked "too young." She didn't know what was appropriate to wear. Should she be wearing those dark, limp dresses that middle-aged schoolteachers wore in her childhood? Was it befitting an "old" person to wear bright colors and short skirts?

Her husband wanted to retire. He was looking forward to going on long sailing trips when he retired. She panicked. She had begun to work when her youngest child had begun high school, and she had just been promoted to the position of office manager. She would have to stop working if he retired and they moved. She did not think she could start again, feeling as shaky as she did now.

She wanted to look good and appear competent but found her hot flashes to be embarrassing. She was ashamed to reveal to anyone what was going on in her body. It seemed to betray her sexual life, diminish her sexual status, emphasize her age and her weakness, and nullify the competence she wanted to convey.

DJ had a longstanding problem with blushing, which she found extremely embarrassing because it revealed feelings she wanted to conceal. Blushing made her feel out of control. She felt that her hot flashes revealed to others her embarrassing and unfortunate state of life. On the other hand, once when she ran for a bus on a cold day the exertion brought on a bout of hot flashes. She felt warmed by the flushes, appreciative of her body's coming to her aid.

Help was provided by a friend. DJ had moved from a large house to a condo development that included a tennis court. She had never thought of herself as an athlete and was convinced it was too late for her to try to learn. Her body, which had shown so many signs of aging, did not seem up to anything new. Her friend persuaded her to play tennis, and after much hesitation, she agreed to try. She found that she enjoyed the activity and also had a latent talent for tennis. It was an enormous pleasure to feel the sense of accomplishment and the feeling of competence with her physical self. The hot flashes seemed less disturbing and less revealing of a devalued body. Her rigid concept of a limited range of possibilities yielded in the face of a newly acquired skill.

In her therapy DJ found herself recalling family members and experiences. She was the younger of two sisters. Her father had died when she was 14, and her mother had remarried. Her stepfather brought his 12-year-old son into the family. He was much doted on, seeming able to get away with anything, and DJ resented him. It was clear that he would go to college, although her grades were better than his. He was given a bigger allowance and had more freedom than she and her sister had. He went to law school, had a mediocre career but still depended on his father. She never dared express her competitive rage. Her sister had also done brilliantly—went to a better college than she, made a fine marriage. Although DJ married a doctor, he was less accomplished than her brother-in-law was. Her two sons both had graduated college and were in business.

Gradually, she developed a sense that it was now "her turn." Tennis permitted her to "play to win," a desire, she realized, she had never been able to express without feeling guilty and selfish. She also felt some relief at not having to look youthfully attractive. If she was going to be treated like a nonsexual being because she was older and did not fit the youthful stereotypes, she could act the part. She allowed herself to gain some weight and worried less about her hair, allowing it to go gray. She did feel she had had a "change of life" and regretted lost opportunities, but she also felt comfortable, able to speak her mind, and take strong positions.

All these women were experiencing menopause. It was not an event to be ignored, but neither was it necessarily the central focus of their lives. As a marker for the passage from one phase to another, menopause can have powerful symbolic meanings. But it is also only one of many markers, a gradual transition to another set of concerns and interests.

Femininity, identity, and self-esteem are achieved as a result of a complex process of integration of many influences—identification with parents and others, internal representation of the body and its functions, patterns of relationships with many layers from both past and present, and elements of personality that remain constant. This integration is not undone by changes in reproductive function, although the factors that go into it do contribute in important ways to a woman's feelings about herself.

REFERENCES

Bibring, G., Dwyer, T., Huntington, D. & Valenstein, A. (1961), A study of the psychological processes in pregnancy and of the earliest mother-child relationship. *The Psychoanalytic Study of the Child,* 16:9–72, New York: International Universities Press.

Deutsch, H. (1945), *The Psychology of Women,* Vol. 2. New York: Grune & Stratton.

Erikson, E. (1963), *Childhood and Society,* 2nd ed. New York: Norton.

Gutman, D. (1981), Psychoanalysis and aging: A developmental view. In: *The Course of Life Vol III,* ed. S. Greenspan & G. Pollock. Mental Health Study Center, NIMH. Bethesda, MD: Dept. of Health and Human Services.

McKinlay, J. B., McKinlay, S. M. & Brambilla, D. J. (1987), Health status and utilization behavior associated with menopause. *Amer. J. Epidemiol.,* 125:110–121.

Neugarten, B. (1975), Adult personality. In: *The Human Life Cycle,* ed. W. Sze. New York: Aronson.

_____ Wood, V., Krainer, R. & Loomis, B. (1968), Women's attitudes toward the menopause. In: *Middle Age and Aging,* ed. B. Neugarten. Chicago: University of Chicago Press, pp. 193–200.

Notman, M. (1979), Midlife in women: Finiteness and expansion. *Amer. J. Psychiat.,* 136:1270–1274.

_____ Nadelson, C. (1982), Changing views of the relationship between femininity and reproduction. In: *The Woman Patient,* Vol. 2, ed. M. Notman & C. Nadelson. New York: Plenum Press, pp. 31–42.

Weisman, M. & Klerman, G. (1977), Sex difference and the etiology of depression. *Arch. Gen. Psychiat,* 34:98–111, 1977.

10

Portraits of Menopausal Women in Selected Works of English and American Literature

MARILYN MAXWELL

The search for menopausal women in early English and American fiction reveals two formidable barriers: first, the taboo that silenced all overt talk about sexuality, especially female sexuality; and, second, the culture's reduction of women to their reproductive function. The first condition clouds the middle-aged woman in obscure images, while the second all but eliminates her from the landscape of English and American literature. Together both reflect an abiding refusal to acknowledge women as complex human beings whose desires, dreams, talents, and overall behavior continually overflow the restrictive, artificial definitions that equate women with their sexuality.

The first barrier—the taboo that recoils from any overt discourse about topics connected with female sexuality, whether it be menstruation or menopause—leaves the literary critic with the problematic task of decoding cryptic messages about the few middle-aged women to appear on the literary landscape prior to the 20th century. As we shall see, Chaucer's Wife of Bath and the Prioress, and Shakespeare's Lady Macbeth and Gertrude, are all middle-aged women whose behavior is encoded by assumptions that seemingly connect middle age in women with heightened sexuality, madness, or both, a connection that finds explicit expression in Robert Burton's (1621) *The Anatomy of Melancholy*.

The second problem—the culture's reduction of women to their reproductive function in youth or their reproductive nonfunction in old age—leaves the critic confronting the veritable absence of middle-aged women in literature written prior to 1900. The aforementioned women are some of the few visible members of an otherwise invisible literary population. Perhaps the absence of middle-aged women in earlier fiction reflects, as one critic argues, the culture's confusing the end of fertility with the end of sexuality, thereby denying the process of aging in women (Kincaid-Ehlers, 1982). Or, perhaps, as I suspect, it points to a nervous denial and dismissal of women who are both sexual and nonreproductive. For during the medieval and Renaissance periods, women were perceived as insatiably lusty creatures and as dangerous to men; their rampant carnality, at times, even threatened to "devour patrimonies" (Burton, 1651). Consequently, sexually active women who served no reproductive function—who did not perpetuate patrilineal power—were conveniently made to disappear, if not from real life, at least from fiction. Not surprisingly, the few middle-aged women who do appear in earlier fiction are depicted as one-dimensional, idiosyncratic caricatures rather than vibrant, flesh-and-blood characters.

Once we turn our gaze to more modern literature we find that the cryptic messages inherent in earlier fiction give way to a more explicit treatment of menopause, but that many of the old assumptions and caricatures linger. Edith Wharton's (1986) *Ethan Frome*, R.P. Warren's (1946) "Blackberry Winter," and William Faulkner's (1932) *Light in August* portray women in middle age who suffer physical or emotional traumas *because they are menopausal.* Even the middle-aged woman whose dramatic monologue informs Robert Frost's (1914) poem "A Servant to Servants" displays a neurotic compulsion to talk and reveal her prior confinement to a mental institution. Although more complex than their fictional predecessors, the middle-age women who populate much of modern drama also reflect society's stereotypic image of the sad and emotionally distraught menopausal woman who has, for the most part, outlived her usefulness as both a nurturing mother and a sexual partner. This chapter's discussions of two plays, Arthur Miller's (1949) *Death of a Salesman* and Eugene O'Neill's (1956) *Long Day's Journey into Night* reveal two middle-aged women who have been socialized into abdicating power over their own lives and who now face the loneliness and isolation of middle age.

The images of middle-aged women in early English literature jump into clearer focus when viewed against the backdrop of the popular social, ethical, and medical ideas of the period. Robert Burton's (1965) *The Anatomy of Melancholy* provides one of the most effective guides by which a critic can decode the significance and implications of women's roles and images in early English literature. Combining ethics, physiology, psychology, and social comment, this treatise on disease and cure reveals the societal view of women as creatures of unnatural lust, who, at all ages, pose a threat to men. Burton argues that one can find contentment only when reason rules the passions through moderation and self-control. While he does criticize men who overindulge their carnal appetites, he unleashes his harshest censure against lusty women of all ages: "I will say nothing of the vices of their minds, their pride, envy, inconstancy, weakness, malaise, self-will and insatiable lust" (p. 445).

Later, when speaking of older women, Burton affirms the notion that "insatiable lust" is both characteristic of the female and yet unnatural: "Of women's unnatural, insatiable lust, what country what village doth not complain . . . What breach of oaths and vows, dotage and madness might I reckon up" (p. 445). And still again, when complaining about the impropriety of sexual activity in older people, Burton reveals his distinct double standard:

"Worse it is in women then in men, when she is an old widdow, a mother so long since, she doth very unseemly seek to marry" (p. 445).

Significant in these passages is an undercurrent of prejudice against women in which female sexuality is depicted as a vice—rampant, unnatural, and potentially dangerous to men. Agitated by uncontrollable sexual urges, the woman emerges, for Burton, as a creature of passion whose carnal appetites continually threaten to topple reason, to weaken her self-control, and to deny her peace of mind. Most repulsive in Burton's schema, of course, is the older woman, a creature of incongruity, whose sexual desires seemingly outlast her physical desirability. Warning men who are contemplating marriage about the disappointments that await them, Burton presents a dismal scenario of the aging process in women, invoking images that today are stereotypically linked with menopause:

After she has been married a small while and the ox hath trodden on her toe, she will be so much altered and grow out of favor thou wilt not know her. (She) grows too fat . . . and fulsome, stale, heavy dull, sour and all at last out of fashion. Those fair sparkling eyes will look dull, her soft coral lips will be pale, dry, cold, rough and blue, her skin rugged [p. 320].

The older woman, then, emerges as a sexually voracious and physically unattractive creature, open to scorn and derision. Furthermore, it is her rampant sexuality that defines her most clearly and that, given her age, alludes to an unnatural proclivity in the older woman. Given Burton's compilation of the prevailing knowledge of illness and his profile of the middle-aged woman, one that, in reality, caricatures and ridicules women, it is not surprising to find early fictional females being portrayed as the fun-loving, bawdy creatures of Chaucerian satire or the lascivious and unnatural moral monsters of Shakespearean tragedy.

Chaucer's (1387) portraits of the Wife of Bath and the Prioress are consistent with the prevailing attitude of medieval and Renaissance England, which viewed women primarily in terms of their sexuality. Although the satiric thrust of the author's pen here is mild, playful, and far less pointed than the vituperative condemnation leveled at some of the other pilgrims (e.g., the Summoner, the Pardoner), Chaucer depicts both the Prioress and the Wife of Bath as middle-aged women who are preoccupied with gratifying their carnal appetites.

Chaucer's subtle disclosure of the incongruity between the ideal nun's spiritual calling to serve God and to renounce the pleasures of the flesh and his Prioress' delight in all things physical clearly focuses on the sensuality associated with the prevailing female stereotype. Her coquettish disposition—"hir smylyng was ful symple and coy"—her poorly uttered French, spoken "ful faire and fetisly/After the schole of Stratford atte Bowe" (p. 18); and her affected table manners, all reveal a worldly woman interested more in social climbing than in soul-saving. In addition to her courtly pretentiousness, the nun's sensuality is revealed through a number of critical, though initially cryptic, descriptive images. For example, unlike most nuns, who, upon entering the convent, adopt the name of a revered saint, Chaucer's Prioress is "cleped madame Englentyne," having selected the name of a secular heroine from *Romance of the Rose*, a popular medieval love story. Highly conscious of the latest fashions, she rejects the simple, unadorned nun's habit and facial linen covering in favor of a stylish cloak and costume jewelry ("She wore a coral trinket on her arm/A set of beads, the gaudies tricked in green"); the linen veil, traditionally worn by nuns to cover the forehead, which in medieval times was viewed as an erotic part of a woman's body, is replaced by a fashionably pleated wimple that exposes a sensually broad and high forehead. Chaucer completes his description of the Prioress with a subtle satiric detail that highlights her lustful nature: bedecked in rosary beads, a relatively new idea of the time, the Prioress displays a "broach on which ther was first write a crowned A/And after AMOR VINCIT OMNIA" (p. 18).

Chaucer's Prioress is a middle-aged woman whose sensual nature is underscored by virtue of its being so at odds with her professed religious vows. Turning to the Wife of Bath, however, we encounter a woman who unabashedly impugns all religious authority and whose eroticism, therefore, requires a more blatant exposure by the author. Consequently, it is not surprising to find the Wife of Bath, an openly secular character, depicted as highly sexual, having gone through five husbands and only too ready to take on the sixth. Invoking the popular literary convention of the much-married, merry widow who is sexually active and fun loving, Chaucer endows his Wife with certain physical attributes that, to a medieval audience, would have signaled a highly sexed woman: her face is "reed of hewe" (is red of hue); "she is "gat-tothed" (gap-toothed), and she has "hipes large" (large hips) (p. 21). Much more complex than the Prioress, the Wife of Bath is a character seemingly rich with modern, feminist implications. She does, after all, reject patriarchal religious authority in favor of her own life experience when justifying women's sexuality; and, faced with limited options in a world where young women were either subjugated in marriage or in the convent, she does manage to gain sovereignty over her husbands, despite suffering physical and emotional abuse (her deafness in one ear is the direct result of her fifth husband's inflicting a blow to her head after reading her passages from misogynist literature). For the modern sensibility, her plight takes on the all-too-familiar tragic theme of the abused woman who must at times work within oppressive institutions. A lusty, clever survivor, the Wife of Bath has garnered the admiration of many modern readers and critics.

The fact remains, however, that Chaucer emphasizes her sexual appetites and lust for younger men, and, in effect, creates another farcical caricature of the erotic, middle-aged woman that was so popular in the literature of his day:

So help me God I was a lusty one [p. 78];

But in our bed he was so fresh and gay
So coaxing, so persuasive . . .
Whenever he wanted it-my bell chose . . .
he could still wheedle me to love [p. 80].

Furthermore, the reversal of sexual roles, whereby the Wife asserts her desire to control her husbands, would have connoted for a medieval audience an element of shrewishness about her character:

I never would abide
In bed with them if hands began to slide
Till they had promised ransom, paid a fee:
And then I let them do their nicety [p. 80].

The older wife, Burton warns, is at best a "commanding servant" who will reduce her husband to a beggar in his own household. Finally, the Wife's selective citing of biblical scripture to justify her sensuality (Solomon, she tells us, had many wives) is a carnal burlesquing of the traditional Biblical exegesis rather than a serious philosophical argument. All in all, Chaucer's Wife of Bath, despite her modern sympathizers, is consonant with the comic figure of the ineluctably sensual middle-aged widow who populates other medieval fiction.

The unchecked carnality of the middle-aged woman, so humorously portrayed in Chaucer's Wife of Bath, takes on tragic implications in two of Shakespeare's plays, *Hamlet* (1623) and *Macbeth* (1623). For both Gertrude and Lady Macbeth, middle age seems to represent a stage of life during which passion and excess usurp reason and moderation. As was noted in the discussion of Burton's *Anatomy*, such an overthrow of the rational faculty would indicate to a Renaissance audience a character's spiritual degradation and diseased state of mind, both of which threaten moral chaos. Gertrude's heightened sexuality is directly associated with her female nature, while Lady Macbeth's rampant lust for power openly violates prescribed gender roles, thus plunging her into unqualified madness.

In *Hamlet* Gertrude emerges as a middle-aged woman whose immersion in sexual pleasure so obscures her perception and understanding that she cannot see the horrifying truth that she is sleeping with her husband's murderer. As one critic notes:

> the Queen is one of the most poorly endowed human beings which Shakespeare ever drew. Very often he creates fools, but there is a richness in their folly, whereas Gertrude is simply a stately defective. The whole play depends on her not noticing and not understanding [West, 1963, p. 261].

She neither notice nor understands because her reasoning power has been so poisoned by her lust that her moral insight is rendered blind. As Hamlet implies in his first soliloquy, Gertrude has fallen to a level beneath that of the "beast that wants discourse of reason" (I,ii). Whereas Claudius too has succumbed to his baser passions, having murdered Hamlet's father to satisfy his lust for power and the Queen, it is *Gertrude's* sexual appetites that are most emphatically linked with the images of impropriety, weakness, and unnatural behavior. For it is her insatiable sexual drive that is apparently responsible for her rather hasty marriage to Claudius (occurring less than two months after her husband's death), a union fraught with incestuous implications: "O most wicked speed, to post/with such dexterity to incestuous sheets" (I,ii). Hamlet's angry observation here is well taken and would have been understood by a Renaissance audience, who viewed in-laws as family members. That she has quickly married her brother-in-law, Hamlet's uncle, imparts a tinge of moral stain to Gertrude's sexuality. Furthermore, it is her lustful nature that weakens her reasoning and moral faculties and triggers Hamlet's now famous pronouncement, "Frailty, thy name is woman" (I,ii), whereby he identifies all womanhood with potentially dangerous carnality. The sexuality of his middle-aged mother is called into moral question most notably when he suggests that her physical attraction to Claudius is unnatural for a woman *of her age:*

Have you eyes?
You cannot call it love, for at your age
the heyday in the blood is tame, it's humble [III,iv].

If Gertrude is acting unnaturally, she is also acting immorally, for the
Renaissance mind viewed moral behavior as a reflection of God's
natural order. If sexual activity in middle-aged women is, as Hamlet
implies, inappropriate in the natural scheme of things, then Gertrude
is morally defective and diseased. Claudius's sexual activity, too, is
base and immoral, not because he is a sexually active middle-aged
man, but rather because he is guilty of regicide and is sleeping with the
wife of the man he murdered. Despite his heinous crime, Claudius is
allowed to display a moral sensitivity to the laws of heaven that he has
transgressed; he attempts to pray for forgiveness. Gertrude, however,
remains a morally flat, one-dimensional sexual creature; a middle-aged
woman defined by an insatiable lust, she appears as almost an
aberration of nature, a "stately defective."

The morally defective sensuality of Gertrude takes on monstrous
proportions in the character of Lady Macbeth, whose lust for power is
couched frequently in sexual innuendos. A careful reading of the text
suggests a reversal of gender roles that is reminiscent of the Wife of
Bath but that is here presented with tragic implications. Arguing that
gender ambiguity is the keynote of the play, one critic notes that the
very opening scene depicting the three witches (who are middle-aged
women with beards!) foreshadows the gender confusion later apparent
in Lady Macbeth (French, 1981, p. 242).

Lady Macbeth first appears on stage in a state of intense expectation. Titillated by the prospect of her husband's becoming king, she
begins to characterize Macbeth in terms of female qualities and
feminine weakness. Lamenting the fact that he is "too full of the *milk*
of human kindness" (I,v, italics added) to expedite the witches' prediction and murder the king, Lady Macbeth invokes evil spirits to "Come
to my woman's breasts/And take my milk for gall" (I,v). That is to say,
she is imploring the spirits to transform her *milk* of human kindness,
a stereotypically female trait, into bitter gall, the fluid associated with
malignity. That she associates this bitterness with masculine behavior
becomes more evident when she asks the evil spirits to defeminize her,
thereby enabling her to enter the male domain of political intrigue

where codes of malevolent expediency often guide conduct and shape kingdoms:

> Come, you spirits
> That tend on mortal thoughts! unsex me here,
> And fill me from the crown to the toe top full
> Of direct cruelty; make thick my blood [I,v].

Pleading with the spirits to be "unsexed" and divested of her womanly qualities, Lady Macbeth is, in effect, asking to be endowed with the masculine capacity to kill. For, within the scope of the play, the warrior mentality, an exclusively male mind-set, is praised and rewarded. For example, Macbeth's ability to hack apart his enemies on the bloody battlefield elicits the unqualified appreciation of his king and wins him a promotion to Thane of Cawdor. Knowing, however, that her husband's capacity for slaughter will be diluted by his milky, feminine kindness when she suggests regicide, Lady Macbeth psychologically prepares herself to enter the male domain of political action, in which killing is sanctioned and, at times, rewarded.

In conjunction with her desire to be "unsexed," Lady Macbeth also asks to have her blood made thick, a request that would have had a special meaning for a Renaissance audience. Turning again to Burton's *Anatomy*, we discover that the Elizabethan viewed all of creation as a vast network of correspondences. For example, the four elements of nature (the macrocosm)—earth, air, water and fire—corresponded to the four humours in the human being (the microcosm)—black bile, phlegm, blood, and choler. Burton isolated black bile, the dark, thick, earthlike substance, as the physiological cause of melancholy in both men and women. An excess of black bile, that is, can manifest itself in various types of melancholic behavior, from depression and withdrawal to rowdiness, violence, and madness. Now, the Elizabethan considered normal blood to be thin; blood that is thickened by the black humour of melancholy is blood that is literally made earthy, that is, cold, dry, thick, and black (Irving, 1970 p. 78). Lady Macbeth's request to the spirits to thicken her blood, then, seems to entail a desire to engage in the more bizarre forms of melancholic behavior outlined by Burton.

Also significant in Burton's schematic is the fact that women are subject to a distinct form of melancholy because of the presence of menstrual blood; thick, dark and smoky, this abnormal blood in more "ancient maids, widows and barren women" has "offended the heart and mind with its vicious vapors" and often leads to a "brutish," untamed kind of behavior fraught with" terrible dreams and preposterous judgment" (Sect III, Mem II Subs IV). Implicitly associated with female sexuality, the thickening of the blood in women takes on the added connotation of that insatiable, unnatural carnality that for Burton is apparently inherent in female nature.

By summoning a melancholic lust for male power, Lady Macbeth begins to cross gender boundaries and prepares to assume the masculine role of the political provocateur. Although it is Macbeth who in fact kills Duncan, Lady Macbeth's prodding is indeed the "spur that pricks the sides of (his) intent" (I,vii). For it is her manly attack against his manhood, coupled with his ambition, that motivates Macbeth to commit murder and that sustains him afterward. For example, when, out of fear, Macbeth cannot bring himself to return to the murder scene to replace the bloody daggers, Lady Macbeth responds, "Give me the dagger . . . tis the eye of childhood that fears a painted devil" (II,ii). When he claims to have seen the ghost of the murdered Banquo, Lady Macbeth again attacks his manhood, accusing him of displaying a woman's weakness by telling a tale that "would well become a woman's story at a winter's fire" (III,iv).

Lady Macbeth is portrayed, then, as assuming the male role in order to satisfy her own lust for power. As French (1981) notes, by indirectly entering the world of political action, Lady Macbeth aligns herself with the male principle (p. 244). Again, as in *Hamlet*, male figures violate moral law whereas female figures transgress the natural order. Like Claudius, Macbeth is guilty of regicide and will be punished. However, in her lust for political power, Lady Macbeth crosses gender lines; like Gertrude, who unnaturally indulges her sexual lust, she, too, violates the natural order. Consequently, Lady Macbeth plunges into spiritual chaos, or madness, and eventually commits suicide. For the madness of this middle-aged woman is the mark of a "mind diseased" (V,iii); her sleep-walking a "great perturbation in nature" (V,i) and her inability to wash the imaginary blood from her hands a physical manifestation of a stained morality and perverse nature.

The popular images of middle-aged women in early literature reflect societal notions that linked female sexuality with unnatural lust, melancholic disorders, and illness. Though often more direct and explicit in their portrayals of menopausal women, many works of modern fiction still shroud the middle-aged woman in stereotypical images of disease, mental instability, lust, weakness, and deficiency. Again, such projections reflect the prevailing societal attitudes, attitudes that were, to a great extent, shaped by the powerful male medical establishment of 19th-century England and America, which viewed all females vulnerable to pathological functioning. (See Formanek, this volume.) Implicit in these attitudes is the notion that middle age is a particularly pathological period in a woman's life, characterized, at times, by unnatural lust and the loss of emotional and rational control. As Smith-Rosenberg (1985) observes, the medical establishment's view "succeeded in denying women the two cardinal Victorian virtues of control and rationality" (p. 196). Defined by her no longer functioning uterus, the middle-aged woman arrived on the societal scene as a pathetic, superfluous figure. She is the creature of "lack," of vacuity and barrenness, who "no longer" produces or nurtures the young. Having outlived her reproductive usefulness and tottering always on the edge of emotional and mental collapse, she requires the care of a more stable husband and doctors; unable to make clear, rational decisions, she must relinquish what little power she had over her own life to others. She emerges as the person whose sexuality is both suspect and vulnerable to the punitive wrath of more powerful men; defined as unstable, weak, and sick, the menopausal woman becomes a social isolate, a misfit. In short, the middle-aged woman is presented to us as the perpetual *invalid* whose individual and social worth has been *invalidated* by a culture that reduces women to their reproductive value.

Many of the stereotypic images just enumerated find their way into modern fiction. Although the word "menopause" never appears in *Ethan Frome* (1911), Edith Wharton's portrait of Zenobia, Ethan's older, "sickly" wife, is rich with stereotypic images of female middle age. Seen through the eyes of a male narrator, Zenobia (Zeena) is presented to the reader as a cold, stern, and reclusive woman who has retreated into the constricted world of her bedchamber. Plagued by the "sickliness" (p. 53), she leaves the house only for occasional excursions to her doctors.

Throughout the novel, Zeena is most intimately associated with the bleak, infertile, harsh New England winter landscape of Starkfield: "the bank of snow made her face look more than usually drawn and bloodless" (p. 48); she "drones" in a "flat whine" like the winter wind, and whatever room she inhabits takes on the "deadly chill of a vault" and "the dry cold of the night" (p. 40). In contrast to her young, passionate, and vibrant cousin Mattie, who is visiting the Fromes and with whom Ethan has fallen in love, Zeena looms over the household as a figure of death who has "faded into an insubstantial shade" (p. 29). "Flat-chested," withdrawn, and lifeless, Zeena, although only 36 years old, "was an old woman" (p. 48). According to Ethan, she has succumbed, as all women eventually do, to the "sickliness": "He recalled his mother's growing taciturnity and wondered if Zeena were also turning 'queer.' Women did, he knew. . . . At times, looking at Zeena's shut face, he felt the chill of such forebodings" (p. 54).

Ethan fears her falling prey to that "queerness" of middle age in which women passively withdraw into the silence of "sullen, self-absorption" (p. 87). However, her "alien" appearance threatens him also with a more active power against which he feels helpless and which intensifies his hatred for her: at times she was a "mysterious alien presence, an evil energy secreted from the long years of silent brooding. It was this sense of helplessness which sharpened his antipathy . . . he abhorred her" (p. 87). Zenobia's sporadic bursts of "powerful mastery" over Ethan awaken in him a profound fear and hatred of her as a woman, perhaps reflecting his implicit awareness of what Carroll Smith-Rosenberg (1985) calls the "sometimes ominous force of female sexuality" (p. 196), however displaced or disguised this force may be in Zenobia's case. For it is during one of these energized moments that Ethan perceives Zenobia as exacting a sadistic revenge upon him when she orders Mattie to be sent away. Her decision was "like a knifecut across the sinews and he felt suddenly weak and powerless" (p. 87). Viewed through the eyes of the male narrator, female middle age appears as a period of withdrawal, melancholy, and ominous expressions of sadistic power. Such stereotypic "symptoms" or "diseases" reflect societal attitudes that associate menopause with "queer" behavior and perceive the "crisis" of middle age as the harbinger of an early death.

The stereotypic images of infertility, strange behavior, and early death that characterize Zenobia also attend the figure of Dellie in

Robert Penn Warren's (1946) short story "Blackberry Winter." Recalling a critical summer during his childhood on a Tennessee farm, the 44-year-old narrator focuses on two characters whose strange behavior served to initiate him into the ways of evil and death in the world. One such character is Dellie, the black cook who lives with her common-law husband, Jebb, in their own cabin down the road from nine-year-old Seth. Viewed by the local whites as clean, neat, and stable—as "white folks' niggers"—Dellie, Jebb, and Little Jebb represent for Seth a surrogate family that provide him with more emotional warmth and freedom than he experiences in his own home.

Yet, during this critical summer, the familiar, loving figure of Dellie becomes strange and alien to Seth; he sees her "sick in bed" and barely recognizes her:

> It did not look like Dellie, or act like Dellie, who would grumble and bustle around our kitchen talking to herself, scolding me or Little Jebb, clanking pans . . . now Dellie just lay there up in bed, under the patchwork quilt, and turned the black face, which I scarcely recognized [p. 144].

When Dellie slaps Little Jebb for talking too loudly, Seth runs in fear from the house and seeks Jebb for an explanation for her unusual behavior. That Dellie is in menopause is made quite clear to the reader in the following exchange between Seth and Jebb:

> "Dellie says she's mighty sick," I said.
> "Yeah," he said.
> "What's she sick from?"
> "Woman-mizry," he said.
> "What's woman-mizry?"
> "Hit comes on em," he said . . .
> "What is it?"
> "Hit the change," he said, "Hit the change of life and time."
> "What changes?"
> "You too young to know."
> "Tell me."
> "Time come and you find out everything." [p. 146].

Jebb's vague and evasive responses do little to assuage Seth's concerns and only strengthen the idea that menopause is a mysterious illness that somehow transforms loving, familiar women into ominous strangers.

In addition to Jebb's overt reference to and description of "woman mizry," it is the pervasive imagery and implicit symbolic linking of nature's cycles to Dellie's condition that also subliminally reinforce stereotypic attitudes about female middle age. For example, even before Seth encounters the ailing, menopausal Dellie in her sick bed, he is struck by the unusually filthy appearance of her front yard. Due to a flood, "a lot of trash and filth" washed out from under Dellie's house: "Old pieces of rags, two or three rusted cans, pieces of rotten rope, some hunks of old dog dung, broken glass, old paper and all sorts of things like that washed out from under Dellie's house to foul her clean yard" (p. 143).

Here the house is explicitly referred to as "Dellie's house" and symbolically represents her body as the structure that houses the physiological turmoil often associated with female middle age, the gushes of menstrual blood that at times mark a woman's passage through menopause. Through such images as "rags," "rotten rope," and "dung," the female body, again, takes on the connotation of filth, of a "foulness" that is purged in middle age, when all of the stained fragments of a fading sexuality are washed away.

Furthermore, the very title of the story metaphorically connects a cold spell in nature with the idea of menopause as a cessation of fertility and a prelude to death. For the local population, "blackberry winter" denotes a brief cold spell in the middle of June, that is, only a temporary suspension of an otherwise fertile season. It is Jebb, however, who suggests to Seth that this particular cold spell is not in fact a "blackberry winter" at all, but rather a permanent freeze in nature heralding the end of the earth when "everything and everybody" will die. In Jebb's mind, mother earth, like Dellie, is finally too tired to create anymore: "this here old yearth is tahrd. Hit is tahrd and ain't gonna perduce" (p. 147). For Jebb, the earth, like Dellie, needs to rest, but it is, for him, the sleep of death. Reflecting the patriarchal attitudes of his society, Jebb views menopause as the termination of a woman's essential function and precedes death. Jebb's subtle connection between menopause and early death would later resonate more clearly for young Seth, whose mother would die "right in middle-age" (p. 150).

Ethan Frome and "Blackberry Winter" not only reflect the stereo-types that link female middle age with disease, peculiar behavior, and early death, but also illuminate male responses to women in meno-pause. In both texts, the significant male figures absent themselves from the "ailing" woman, Ethan retreating into an emotional entan-glement with Mattie and Jebb withdrawing into his own morbid, reflective solitude. Each response belies the male's confusion about and fear of "the ominous force of female sexuality" and represents, to a certain extent, his covertly hostile rejection of the indecipherable woman of middle age. Consistent with society's perception of the problematic middle-aged woman is the depiction in both texts of the woman in menopause as alone, as having been either emotionally or physically abandoned by men; both texts tend to reinforce the image of the menopausal woman-as-isolate. Such acts of abandonment in literature are emblematic of the culture's perception of the menopausal woman as functionally obsolete, a perception that serves to under-mine her worth and relegate her to the periphery of social relevance.

The latent hostility inherent in the societal rejection of the middle-aged woman is fictionally realized in an act of horrifying violence in William Faulkner's (1932) *Light in August*. *Light in August* is the story of Joe Christmas, whose alleged mixed racial ancestry leaves him futilely struggling to establish an identity in the American South. Left at an orphanage when a child, Joe meanders through a variety of unfulfil-ling experiences, living at times as a white and at other times a black man. When he arrives in Jefferson at the age of 33, he becomes involved with a middle-aged white woman, a recluse named Joanna Burden. When Joanna eventually tries to impose her newly acquired religious conviction upon him, Joe brutally murders her, slashing her throat and then burning down her house.

Clearly the focal character of the novel is Joe Christmas, whose inability to find his place in a racist culture explains much of the hostility and bitterness that inform his personality and precipitate his violent behavior. Yet it is also Joe's deep-seated misogyny that allows him to unleash his aggression against a middle-aged woman whose menopausal condition intensifies his rage and contributes to her death. For, throughout the novel, Joe manifests an abhorrence of female sexuality; he recoils particularly from any idea or situation associated with menstrual blood. As a youth, he views menstruation as "periodic filth" and violently strikes a young woman who declines his sexual overtures because "it was that day of the month" (p. 209). Her more detailed explanation leaves him "vomiting in the woods" as he associates menstrual blood with the "deathcolored, foul liquid" oozing from the tree trunks (p. 210). For Joe Christmas female sexuality is an ominous, nauseating force that underscores a "woman's affinity for casting a faint taint of evil about the most trivial and innocent of actions" (p. 185). For a man who likes "to smell horses because they are not women" (p. 119), the bloody mutilation of Joanna Burden, a menopausal woman, is a fitting culmination of Joe's violent responses to female sexuality.

The portrayal of Joanna Burden reflects the culture's stereotype of the woman in menopause. Physically, she is a woman who is "cold-faced, almost manlike" (p. 283) and who is beginning "to get fat" (p. 286), having "gained thirty pounds" (p. 289) since her relationship with Joe began. Emotionally, she initially appears as a sexually voracious woman whose insatiable appetite would leave her in the "wild throes of nymphomania" that threatened to "suck [Joe] down into a bottomless morass" (p. 285). When that sexual passion begins to give way to religious fervor, Joe begins to view her as approaching the "autumn" of her life when "summer died" and something "threatful and terrible occurred" (p. 288–289). He comes to see her as old and obsolete. When he discovers that her missed periods are a sign of menopause and not of pregnancy, he responds violently:

'You haven't got any baby,' he said. You never had one. There is not anything the matter with you except being old. You just got old and it happened to you and now you are not any good anymore. That's all that's wrong with you.' He released her and struck her again. . . . She lay on the bed looking up at him across her bleeding mouth [p. 304].

Perceiving her as functionally obsolete, as "sexless" and "not any good any more," Joe lashes out against female middle-age: "Perhaps that is where outrage lies. Perhaps I believe that I have been tricked, fooled. That she lied to me about her age, about what happens to women at a certain age" (p. 119). While it is Joanna's religious impulse that ignites his final murderous rage, it is her menopausal condition that leaves her vulnerable to Joe Christmas's fatal repudiation of female sexuality.

Male responses to women in menopause are characterized by varying degrees of rejection, humiliation, and abandonment. Portrayed as "ill" or "queer," the fictional middle-aged woman emerges as an ultimately powerless creature whose fading sexuality and loss of reproductive value leave her vulnerable to physical and emotional disorders and subsequently to the alienation by more powerful men. While the extreme nature of Joe Christmas's violent reaction may be atypical of male responses to women in menopause, his hostile behavior reflects a patriarchal oppression of women that does typify many other fictional portraits in both poetry and drama.

In Robert Frost's dramatic monologue "A Servant to Servants," a lonely, middle-aged woman desperately tries to detain a group of people who have camped out on her family's property by riveting them with her incessant talk. Conveyed in the unrhymed iambic pentameter of blank verse, the woman's anxiety tumbles out in a torrent of run-on ideas and fragmented thoughts:

> I didn't make you know how glad I was
> To have you come and camp here on our land.
> I promised myself to get down some day
> And see the way you lived but I don't know!
> With a houseful of hungry men to feed
> I guess you'd find . . . It seems to me
> I can't express my feelings, any more
> Than I can raise my voice or want to lift
> My hand. (Oh I can lift it when I have to)
> Did you ever feel so? I hope never.

In the 177 lines that constitute the poem, the speaker reveals herself as an emotionally-distraught woman who knows, however, that she is suffering from the tedium and meaninglessness of her stereotypic role as a "servant" to the men in her life:

> It's rest I want—there—I have said it out—
> From cooking meals for hungry hired men

And washing dishes after them — from doing
Things over and over that just won't stay done.

The poignancy of her subjection is intensified by the clarity of her
perception, for she understands only too well that middle-aged women
are often rendered "invisible":

We have four here to board, great good for-nothings,
Sprawling about the kitchen with their talk
While I fry bacon. Much they care!
No more put out in what they do and say
Than if I weren't in the room at all.

She also senses that it is more than a change of scenery that she needs.
Having moved out of her parents' house, where she and her husband
had been living, the speaker is still haunted by her childhood memory
of the cage in their attic in which her "mad" uncle was confined like an
animal. She is keenly aware of the "punishment" awaiting those who
do not conform to expected modes of behavior. Despite the fact that
she and her husband are now living in their own home, the speaker
remains unhappy, yet is reluctant to express her discontentment to
her husband. Having been sent away once by her husband to the
State Asylum, she knows that she must keep silent.

The seemingly incessant chatter that informs "A Servant to Servants" is, in effect, a profound psychological portrait of an oppressed
woman. Attracted to the campers, whose less conventional life style
contrasts with her own stifled existence, the speaker considers but
quickly dismisses the possibility of following their example:

I almost think that if I could do like you,
Drop everything and live out on the ground—
. . . I haven't courage for a risk like that.

Despite the lucid insights into her own malaise, this woman remains
powerless to ameliorate her situation, to free herself from the restrictive role of the "servant" that has been imposed on her by more
powerful men.

It is this image of powerlessness in the face of male domination that also characterizes two middle-aged women in modern drama. Both Linda Loman in *Death of A Salesman* and Mary Tyrone in *Long Day's Journey into Night* emerge as the paradigmatic female whose middle-aged status leaves her impotent within the confines of the traditional family. In each play, the middle-aged woman is trapped within a family crisis from which she cannot escape and over which she exercises very little power of resolution. Hemmed in on all sides by three powerful and at times abusive male family members, both Linda Loman and Mary Tyrone retreat inward into the claustrophobic space of their own fabricated worlds of denial.

In *Death of a Salesman*, Arthur Miller portrays Linda Loman as a sensitive and compassionate middle-aged woman who has devoted her entire adult life to her husband, Willy, and their two sons, Biff and Happy. While it becomes apparent, through the play's many flashbacks, that Linda has never occupied a position of respect and authority in the Loman household, her peripheral existence as a middle-aged woman underscores her vulnerability and impotence within the family structure. Powerless now in the face of a family crisis, Linda Loman becomes the target of the men's sporadic outbursts of abuse and scorn. Her psychological dependency on the traditional family structure leaves her completely bereft of a sustaining sense of self when, at the tragic end of the play, Willy dies and the Loman family unit falls apart.

Earlier, when the sons return home for a family visit, it becomes immediately apparent that each of the Loman men is profoundly "lost" in his life. A worn-out salesman, Willy faces the disillusionment of having failed to realize his "massive dreams" and will suffer the humiliating dismissal from a company for which he has worked for 40 years; Biff, the former high school football star, is "lost" also and at the age of 35 is still wandering aimlessly out West from one low-paying job to another, a painful reminder to Willy of the family's propensity for failed promise. Finally, the life of Happy Loman comprises shady business transactions, visits to prostitutes, and parties. Very much like his father, Happy finds himself caught up in the meaninglessness of a life built upon smooth talk, phony smiles, and little substantive talent or hard work. It is within this potentially explosive setting that Linda Loman attempts to function as the traditional wife and mother. Her efforts to retain the integrity of the deteriorating family unit prove to be futile, however, as Willy succumbs to his depression and commits suicide.

Clearly the focal point of the play is Willy Loman and his two sons. Often excluded from the male triad, Linda hovers on the periphery of their traditional masculine talk and action. The following exchange at the kitchen table reveals Willy's cruel exclusion of his wife from the men's discussion of a possible business venture:

> Biff: I'll see Oliver tomorrow. Hap, if we could work that out . . .
>
> Linda: Maybe things are beginning to—
>
> Willy: (wildly enthused, to Linda)—Stop interrupting (to Biff) But don't wear sports jacket and slacks when you see Oliver.
>
> Biff: He did like me. Always liked me.
>
> Linda: He loved you.
>
> Willy: (to Linda) Will you stop . . .
>
> Linda: Oliver always thought the highest of him.
>
> Willy: Will you let me talk!
>
> Biff: Don't yell at her Pop, will ya! [pp. 141–142].

As a woman, she has no business venturing into the masculine world of commercial transactions. Furthermore, she remains the only character in the play who is never viewed in any other setting than that of the home, and when the three Loman men decide to meet for dinner to celebrate their anticipated business deal, she is not invited. Linda's inability to penetrate male conversation or the outside world is emblematic not only of her subordinate position in the family structure but also of the disparaging stereotypes of women that pervade the play.

Throughout *Death of a Salesman* women are presented as either the saintly, loyal nurturer (Linda) or the sullied "chippie." The two prostitutes who meet Biff and Happy at the restaurant represent for them nothing more than a night's entertainment; the secretary with whom Willy has an affair earns a pair of nylon stockings while he uses her to get in to see the buyers. Happy sleeps with the fiancées of business rivals out of an "overdeveloped sense of competition" and enjoys "ruining" them (p. 107.) This exploitive reduction of women to male objects of pleasure and advancement obviously reflects a derogatory view of all women and underscores the men's rather cruel treatment of Linda Loman at times.

In addition to being periodically silenced by Willy throughout the play, Linda Loman also suffers disparaging remarks from both of her sons. While Biff is probably the person most sensitive to his mother's concerns about Willy, he is also, at times, the most hurtful to her. Aware of his father's extramarital affair, Biff angrily responds to Linda's protective concern for her husband: "Stop making excuses for him! He always, always wiped the floor with you. Never had an ounce of respect for you" (p. 134). Happy's treatment of Linda belies his general disdain for women. In a very revealing scene, Happy insultingly offers his mother some flowers to assuage her angry response to their abandoning their father in a restaurant:

> Linda: Get out of here, both of you, and don't come back! I
> don't want you tormenting him anymore. . . . (She
> starts to pick up the flowers and stops herself) Pick up
> this stuff, I'm not your maid any more. Pick it up,
> you bum, you!
>
> (Happy turns his back to her in refusal . . .) [p. 194].

Either through abrasive remarks or insensitive behavior, each of the Loman men, in effect, turns his back to Linda Loman at some point in the play.

Furthermore, since it is clear throughout the entire play that Linda Loman's sense of self-worth and fundamental identity reside in her role as the traditional wife and mother, the rejection by her family is all the more tragic. Willy's suicide, the ultimate act of rejection, leaves her understandably devastated and confused about returning to a house where "nobody is home." Aware that Willy had been contemplating suicide, Linda Loman remains powerless to prevent it; her own process of denial allows her to rationalize away his despair and blame his depression on exhaustion and unfair treatment in the business world. Yet, like Mary Tyrone in *Long Day's Journey into Night*, Linda Loman's power to effect positive change in the home environment is also undermined by the disdain with which male family members view women in general and by the fading significance of the middle-aged woman in the traditional family.

O'Neill's (1956) *Long Day's Journey into Night* depicts the middle-aged woman as a lonely, depressed, and emotionally unstable character who is faced with the problem of drug addiction. Having just returned from a sanitarium, Mary Tyrone reenters an Irish Catholic family that has remained basically unchanged in its traditional assumptions. Fraught with the same sexist dynamics that prompted Mary's initial escape into morphine oblivion, the Tyrone family structure clearly subjugates Mary to the will and desires of her husband, Tyrone, and their two adult sons, Edmund and Jamie.

Despite their solicitous remarks concerning her health and comfort throughout the play, the three Tyrone men gradually replace their initial support and understanding of her condition with moral condemnation and rejection. When it becomes clear to her family that Mary has slipped back into morphine dependency, each of the Tyrone men unleashes harsh criticism aimed at her failure to conform to their image of her as the traditional wife and mother. Her younger son, Jamie, associates drug use with prostitution and moral decadence: "I thought only whores were drug addicts" (p. 163). Edmund, echoing Dr. Hardy's sentiments at the sanitarium, preaches sermons on will power to his mother (pp. 74, 92), while her husband complains that Mary could have conquered the addiction if only she had prayed and not forgotten her faith (p. 78). As one critic notes, "Mary is perceived by the men not as a victimized, complex being in distress, but as a shattered ideal or a fallen Madonna" (Maxwell, 1987).

While it is undoubtedly true that the Tyrone men condemn Mary primarily because of her drug addiction, the fact remains that her middle-aged status in the traditional family hierarchy leaves her vulnerable to their critical remarks and alienating gazes. At age 54, Mary is quick to perceive the men's awareness of her aging process, of her changing physical attributes, which in this society signal a loss of feminine appeal:

> Tyrone: You're a fine armful now, Mary, with those 20 pounds you've gained.
> Mary: I've gotten too fat, you mean, dear. I really ought to reduce [p. 14].

Under the constant scrutiny of the three men, who are, in effect, waiting for her to succumb again to the morphine, Mary has internalized the culture's negative view of the aging process in women:

> Mary: Is my hair coming down? It's hard for me to do it up properly now. My eyes are getting so bad and I never can find my glasses [p. 20].

And later, when reminiscing about her hair:

> Mary: It was a rare shade of reddish brown and so long it came down below my knees. . . . It wasn't until after Edmund was born that I had a single grey hair. Then it began to turn white [p. 28].

Weight gain, failing eyesight, and greying hair are accompanied by continual references to her rheumatoid hands, images that stereotypically complete the portrait of the middle-aged woman.

If her changing physical appearance heralds the onset of middle age for Mary Tyrone, it is her growing insignificance in the affairs of the family that clearly solidifies her position as a superfluous figure in society. Throughout the play, each male character leaves the house to engage in some activity in the outside world, whether it is gardening, transacting business, or just drinking with the boys. Mary, alone, remains indoors for the entire play, the implication being, again, that women in general had no business outside the home. However, for Mary Tyrone, a woman whose children are grown and whose husband is more of a watchdog than a partner, the home becomes an empty psychological prison to which she has been abandoned in middle age. It is not surprising to hear her comment on her growing sense of loneliness and alienation: "It is so lonely here. Why do I feel so lonely" (p. 95)? For this middle-aged woman, as for many, there is no longer any business to tend to in the inside world of the home.

Divested of her significance as wife and mother and condemned as a moral reprobate by her former support system, Mary Tyrone is left emotionally impoverished and mourning her loss of self: "None of us can help the things that life has done to us. They're done before you know it . . . until at last . . . you've lost your true self forever" (p. 61).

Having devoted her life to the traditional role of wife and mother, Mary Tyrone walks through middle age facing not only alienation from the outside world of male activity, but also the loneliness of an empty home and the devastating loss of self-identity.

CONCLUSION

In a diary entry dated March 1, 1937, Virginia Woolf writes:

> I wish I could write out my sensations at this moment. They are so peculiar and so unpleasant. Partly T[ime] of L[ife] I wonder? A physical feeling as if I were drumming slightly in the veins: very cold, impotent and terrified. As if I were exposed on a high ledge in full light. Very lonely . . . very useless. No atmosphere around me. No words. Very apprehensive. . . . And I know that I must go on doing this dance on hot bricks till I die [in Bell, 1972, pp. 198–199].

Despite the use of the euphemistic label "T of L," Woolf's comments about menopause are significant, for here a *woman* speaks directly about a *woman's* feelings during a biological stage in a *woman's* life. In doing so, Woolf anticipates one of the most positive literary effects of the Women's Movement, namely, the appearance of novels that illuminate the complexity of female middle age and that replace caricatures with flesh-and-blood characters. Doris Lessing's *The Summer Before the Dark*, May Sarton's *Crucial Conversations* and Grace Paley's short stories are just a few of the many works of fiction to portray the critical emotional and intellectual issues facing women in middle age. It is probably safe to say that many of the female characters in feminist fiction succeed, after much pain and struggle, in emerging from that "dance on hot bricks" to a celebration of middle age and an acknowledgment of self-worth.

However, for the prefeminist fictional woman discussed in the present study, middle age remains veiled in stereotypic images of disease, unnatural sexuality and irrational behavior. From Chaucer's satiric caricatures of the bawdy Wife of Bath to O'Neill's poignant portrayal of the dependent, "fallen" Mary Tyrone, females in middle age fall prey, at times, to male ridicule, suspicion, and outright abuse and violence. While Virginia Woolf's diary entry looks forward to feminist fiction, it also speaks to the women considered in this study, who, like Woolf, internalize the oppressive stereotypes of "the menopausal woman" and come to view themselves as "useless" and "impotent."

REFERENCES

Bell, Q. (1972), *Virginia Woolf: A Biography*. New York: Harcourt Brace Jovanovich.

Burton, R. (1621), *The Anatomy of Melancholy*, ed. L. Babb. Michigan: Michigan State University Press, 1965.

Chaucer, G. (1387), The Canterbury tales. In: *The Works of Geoffrey Chaucer*, ed. F.N. Robinson. New York: Houghton Mifflin, 1957.

Faulkner, W. (1932), *Light in August*. New York: Random House, 1987.

French, M. (1981), *Shakespeare's Division of Experience*. New York: Summit.

Frost, R. (1914), A servant to servants. In: *The Poetry of Robert Frost*, ed. E.C. Latham. New York: Henry Holt, 1969.

Irving, E. (1970), *Shakespeare, Medicine and Psychiatry*. New York: Philosophical Library.

Kincaid-Ehlers, E. (1982), Bad maps for an unknown region: Menopause from a literary perspective. In: *Changing Perspectives on Menopause*, ed. A.M. Voda. Austin: University of Texas Press, pp. 24–38.

Maxwell, M. (1987), Socialization of women: A view from literature. In: *Women and Depression*, ed. R. Formanek & A. Gurian. New York: Springer, pp. 222–237.

Miller, A. (1949), Death of a salesman. In: *Arthur Miller: Eight Plays*. New York: Nelson Doubleday, 1981.

O'Neill, E. (1956), *Long Day's Journey into Night*. New Haven, CT: Yale University Press.

Shakespeare, W. (1623), *Hamlet* (ed. C. Hoy). New York: Norton, 1963.

_____ (1623), *Macbeth* (ed. B. Groom). Oxford: Oxford University Press, 1939.

Smith-Rosenberg, C. (1985), *Disorderly Conduct*. New York: Oxford University Press.

Warren, R.P. (1946), Blackberry winter. In: *A Robert Penn Warren Reader*, ed. A. Erskine. New York: Random House, 1988.

West, R. (1963), The nature of will. In: *Hamlet*, ed. C. Hoy. New York: Norton.

Wharton, E. (1911), *Ethan Frome*. New York: New American Library, 1986.

11

Reflections of Self and Other

Men's Views of Menopausal Women

SUZANNE B. PHILLIPS

The tangible evidence of loss of youth and approaching old age, as biological givens, represent facts of life which shake the unconscious ego's cherished illusion of being ageless and timeless [Bergler, 1954, p. xi].

For women, menopause bears such evidence. It is a physiological reality that implies change and aging—the menses cease, a woman's reproductive capacity ends. As a diagnosis, menopause refers precisely to the cessation of the menses and is made retrospectively after a year has elapsed, with the average age for women in the U.S. being 49 years. As a normal phase of life, menopause actually spans a number of years during which signs and symptoms of change gradually occur in conjunction with other developmental, psychological, and socio-cultural events of midlife (Perlmutter, 1978). The term menopausal women used here refers to women who are physically and emotionally addressing this phase of life.

Although there is no specific marker like menopause to connote a man's midlife, there is nonetheless a gradual accumulation of life events, role transitions, and physiological changes that lead a man to experience himself as having become middle aged. He reckons with the conscious and unconscious experience of parenting his parents,

281

disengaging from his children, and realigning with his spouse. He compares where he is in his career with where he expected to be. Physiologically he is aware of the undeniable signs—the limitations, the differences between now and earlier times, the death of peers.

Theories of adult development (Erikson, 1959; Levinson, 1986), suggest that the process and resolution of midlife tasks involve a redefinition of one's place in the outside world and in the context of one's relationship with significant others. Erikson (1982) proposes that the positive resolution of earlier stages allows the adult to achieve a sense of personal integrity and competence, coupled with empathy for and care of others. Levinson (1986) holds that the rebuilding of a new life structure in midlife facilitates a step in individuation. It permits one to be more compassionate, reflective, and judicious, more loving of self and others.

If one considers that men are often the significant others in women's lives, then men's perceptions of women during the meno-pausal years figure as an important aspect of women's redefinitions of self. The question of how men view menopausal women, however, is seldom asked by women and is almost never answered by men.

Whereas the literature on menopause is relatively sparse and incon-clusive (McKinlay and McKinlay, 1973; Parlee, 1978; Kaufert et al., 1986), formal consideration of men's views, their perceptions of and reactions to menopausal women, is almost nonexistent. Only brief references to menopause as a possible factor influencing marital relationships and dysfunction exist (Bergler, 1954; Farrell and Rosen-berg, 1981; Willi, 1982; Scarf, 1987).

This absence of theoretical formulation and empirical study may reflect a long-standing cultural bias portraying the menopause as the end of the female's usefulness (Deutsch, 1945; Posner, 1979). It may also derive from a tradition of male medicalization of menopause, which invites trivialization or even dismissal of this stage as an area of study (Cowdan, Warren, and Young, 1985; Formanek, 1987); lack of interest by men in an event for which there is no male counterpart; denial of and dissociation by men from an event that clearly connotes change and aging (Farrell and Rosenberg, 1981); and collusive permis-sion by women to dismiss this aspect of self, which they may fear as unacceptable or unattractive.

This chapter asks the question, How do men view menopausal

women? It also pursues an answer. It considers menopause to be for women a physical and emotional event that becomes relevant to men only in the context of their physical, social, and emotional exchange with women.

In the pursuit of men's views of menopausal women, I drew upon three sources: theoretical views of men in midlife, clinical observations of men in individual and marital treatment, and results from a questionnaire examining male and female attitudes in midlife. This questionnaire was mailed to 100 men and women over 40 years old and returned by 25 men and 26 women (Phillips, 1988).

I propose that men's views of menopausal women are a function of four dimensions:

1. The parallel posture of men and women as they face midlife issues.
2. Gender differences, which complicate men's and women's understanding and response to each other in midlife.
3. Preexisting personality traits that underscore response to changes in self and other.
4. Interaction patterns that characterize the context of men's and women's relationships.

PARALLEL POSTURE

At the time of young love it seemed appropriate and rather an advantage for the boy and the girl to be nearly identical ages. A quarter of a century later woman's biological fate and man's psychological conflict coincide [Bergler, 1954, p. 3].

Although Bergler conceptualizes men and women in archaic extremes as the vulnerable menopausal woman and the confused masochistic man, he speaks to the reality that in our society the marriage of contemporaries leads to synchrony at midlife.

Consciously and unconsciously a man's response to his partner's menopause is influenced by his own midlife changes. Although in our society only 39% of menopausal women seek medical intervention for physiological symptoms or problems (Cowdan et al., 1985), there is a cultural expectation that menopause implies change, aging, reduced

attractiveness, and lessened sexual interest. Accordingly, men anticipate their partners' menopause with concern, empathy, anxiety, and
sometimes anger. Whether a man is in a loving or a strained relationship, his partner's menopause becomes an added emotional component of his already saturated midlife picture.

In their comprehensive study of men in midlife, Farrell and Rosenberg (1981) propose that, although a midlife crisis may or may not
occur, the problems of confronting middle age for men are inevitable
and ubiquitous. Relevant to the parallel posture of men and women at
midlife, men often experience a shrinkage of career possibilities at a
time when women are expanding theirs; a shift in power as children
become less dependent and women's earning potential increases; a
sense of isolation, even neglect, as bodily changes occur but are less
defined and attended to than menopausal symptoms (Farrell and
Rosenberg, 1981).

In many cases the man's derisive comments, or dismissal of his
partner's menopausal concerns, mask feelings of hurt or anger for real
or anticipated neglect. As reflected by a majority of questionnaire
respondents (96% of men and 80% of the women), both middle-aged
men and women feel that they are not understood by the other sex.
Whereas women (68%) feel understood by other women, only 35% of
the men feel understood by other men (Phillips, 1988).

Such attitudes are consistent with the recent findings of more
formal gender comparison studies (Smith et al., 1988), which reveal
that men differ from women in their hesitancy to share feelings or
personal difficulties—even with one another. This reluctance leaves
them emotionally isolated, possibly more stressed, and less likely to
understand or be understood by others. As McGill (1985) suggests in
his book on male intimacy, one of the contributing factors to male
midlife crisis is the absence of intimate others with whom to share
midlife concerns. Men often feel that they are the ones struggling with
the midlife issues without the "institutionalized moratorium," the
luxury of time, space, and freedom from obligations they believe
women have (Farrell and Rosenberg, 1981, p. 30).

In reality neither men nor women feel they have the time, space, or
support they want or may have had at earlier junctures of identity
formation. The occasional impatience or overt anxiety with each
other's midlife issues bespeaks the unconscious wish for time out and

someone who will remain constant and available. As a matter of fact, middle-aged male and female respondents both list time as their most pressing need (50% of responses). Men (62%) as well as women (84%) identify mother more often as the parent they think of most during midlife (Phillips, 1988).

Men's responses to women's menopause are influenced not only by their own parallel midlife issues but by the manner in which they respond to those issues. Farrell and Rosenberg (1981) found that by midlife men have been conditioned to deny, or socialized to ignore, the stress they feel. Proposing that midlife crisis implies facing the anxieties aroused by death, Klemme (1970) suggests that men often have a depressive reaction that generates coping methods like denial, projection, regression, or use of alcohol. Lowenthal, Thurnher, and Chiriboga (1975), in an extensive study of men and women throughout the four stages of life, found that men tend to repress or avoid negative feelings. A man will report as acceptable the same marriage that his wife sees as deadening. Further evidence of men's use of denial is suggested by the sharp increase of psychosomatic ailments – peptic ulcer, hypertension, and heart disease – reported to peak among males during their 40s and 50s (Farrell and Rosenberg, 1981, p. 20). Accordingly, for some men, denial or lack of response to their partner's menopause is less a reflection of their feelings about menopause and more a function of their own coping style.

Recognizing the parallels of their midlife tasks, men and women in the best of circumstances empathize and invite each other forward. In the worst, they minimize the other's unresolved conflicts, project blame, find fault, abandon or feel abandoned themselves. The influence of these parallels in men's views of menopausal women is reflected in the case of Trent and Mary:

For Trent, involvement in work had always served to stabilize identity and to defend against fears of criticism and inadequacy. At 48, Trent's involvement in work reached a driven and compulsive pitch. He had expected to be more successful and was impatient with himself and envious of others who were financially and professionally ahead of him. Despite his social contacts, his secret sense of shame precluded discussion of his feelings with anyone but his spouse. There was thus little oppor tunity to dilute his expectations or to foster other avenues for validation. Implied in his relationship with his spouse was the wish for her to be there, but to wait. Reflected even in the content of the eventual marital therapy were his compulsive ruminations about work while defensively putting wife and personal life on hold. His conflict was implied in angry outbursts and feelings of deprivation about missing out in life. He could not understand his wife's desire for his attention or her anger at his lack of emotional support and involvement.

Paralleling Trent's midlife race against time was Mary's own midlife. Facing menopausal changes as well as identity issues, Mary at 47 rushed toward other sources of emotional support and validation. Her focus dramatically turned from traditional home and family roles to independent pursuits in the outside world. As her needs were no longer congruous with Trent's, he complained that he could no longer depend on her. He was both anxious and frustrated that she was emotionally unwilling to maintain the status quo while he dealt with midlife. He felt that he had lost the predictable partner who aided him in handling emotional upheavel. He assumed that Mary's menopause was the cause for her change, his loss, and their stress.

In Trent's response to Mary lies the wish to keep the partner constant so as to reduce the anxiety associated with his own and her changes. Much of this anxiety is underscored by the midlife reactivation of unresolved issues of rage, loss, and oedipal conflict. Trent's experience with successful, demanding, but uninvolved parent figures was reflected in his difficulty in trusting that his partner could be more independent and yet remain nurturing and committed. The heightening of defensive patterns at such vulnerable times contributes to the male's tension and overreaction to the menopause.

GENDER DIFFERENCES

The case of Trent and Mary also demonstrates gender differences in reconciling a basic human dilemma—the seemingly contradictory demands between affiliation and self-actualization (Singer, 1988).

According to Singer, affiliation refers to the need for closeness, belonging, "attachment to parents, to friends, to lovers, eventually to community, religious group, or nation" (p. 103). Self-actualization refers to the constructive striving for autonomy, self-realization, self-concern, competence, uniqueness, and power. Singer suggests that historically, from the Freudian perspective, the affiliation need was equated with sexual desire. The gratification of this sexual need became associated with threat of death, loss of reason and loss of individuality. Aggression emerged as the second major drive. Ultimately the conflict between the drives was genderized by Freud as the "femaleness" of sexuality and the "maleness" of aggression (Bergler, 1981, p. 125). Recognizing the importance of object relations considerations and acknowledging the influence of cognition and affect on motivation, Singer (1988), broadening the definition of such drives and the nature of the conflict, maintains that most people seek a balance in life between the need to actualize, on one hand, and the need to affiliate, on the other.

I propose that men and women differ with respect to this balance. By midlife, although chronologically in parallel positions, men and women are developmentally, emotionally, and interpersonally in different places with respect to the balance of self-actualization and affiliation needs. Women have traditionally been expected to be more emotional, to disclose feelings, and to be attuned to the feelings of others. Women often achieve a capacity for intimacy and a grasp of the complexity of relationships at an earlier age than men do. Having spent most of their life affiliated with others, women often have a definition of self in terms of others' needs. Their sense of self, even their sense of competence, is as someone's daughter, wife, or mother. They have often feared or given up the opportunity to develop a separate, self-determined identity. In midlife the need to find and express this separate self becomes clearer and more pressing (Notman, 1979; Farrel and Rosenberg, 1981; Sheehy, 1981).

Men, on the other hand, have been conditioned to actualize, to put aside their feelings—expressions of stress, pain, or loneliness—in order to succeed. They reach midlife inflated with success, obsessed with the challenge, or wearied from the pursuit. Often they have achieved a sense of identity vis-à-vis their work-related roles, but without resolution of intimacy issues (Farrell and Rosenberg, 1981). Taking stock of their lives in middle age, men often feel emotionally distant. In an effort to pursue their affiliation needs, they now value, idealize, scrutinize, sometimes demand attachments.

In this light, the clash of male and female needs in midlife is often inevitable and confusing. Both men and women are perplexed by the other's expectations. Consistent with gender differences in dealing with stress and confusion, men often seek an external cause for the couple's discord (Smith et al., 1988). If in the earlier years of the relationship interpersonal stress was accounted for by the female's being "premenstrual," then it is likely that the woman's midlife strivings and changes will be attributed to her being "menopausal."

Women, on the other hand, often respond to the clash of needs and emotional stress by self-blaming or reading stress as an index of trouble in their relationships (Smith et al., 1988). Consistent with their sociocultural heritage, they expect that self-actualization will jeopardize their attachments. In the present questionnaire, 46% of the women identified their spouse as a source of daily worry, compared with only 8% of the men (Phillips, 1988).

Notwithstanding such differences, most men and women are able to accept and support themselves and their partners in dealing with broader midlife needs and redefinitions. Most are able to address the anxieties of midlife and accept the life cycle as inevitable, thus permitting movement with hope rather than despair. Eighty-eight percent of men and women respondents reported feeling loved and appreciated by their partners (Phillips, 1988).

PERSONALITY TRAITS

Certain traits in a man's personality seem to be of particular significance in his perception of, and response to, the menopausal partner. For both men and women, response to midlife issues seems to be a function of personality and prior life patterns (Benedek, 1950; Bart, 1971; Perlmutter, 1978; Farrell and Rosenberg, 1981; Lax, 1982; Notman, 1984).

For the man, the menopause of his partner—wife, lover, love object—is an event that has an impact on his own sense of self. Depending on his development and unconscious dynamics, this "changing" female partner may be experienced as a separate but emotionally related person or as an emotional extension – a merged, idealized, or devalued selfobject (Kohut, 1971). Their relationship may be characterized by cohesion or collusion, sexual relating, or sexual addiction (Willi; 1982, McDougall, 1985). There may be tolerance for change in self and in the female partner, or panic and a narcissistic need to maintain the other as a type-cast self-extension – a regulator of the man's sense of self.

The negative effect that delayed or pathological development has on a man's view of self in middle age and consequently on his response to his partner has been formulated as psychic masochism (Bergler, 1954), identity diffusion (Erikson, 1959), or pathological narcissism (Kernberg, 1980). For those with a poorly integrated self-concept and impaired sense of relating, relationships serve unconscious identity needs. A predictable partner is needed to maintain cohesiveness, stability, and positive affective coloring of the self (Stolorow and Lachmann, 1980). Menopause is perceived as changing this partner and can be consciously and intrapsychically threatening. As one man asked, "What happens to me now?"

Such reactions to the physical event of the woman's menopause often reflect an inability to relate in depth to all dimensions of this partner. In the case of Todd, his wife's menopause, as evidenced in her occasional report of hot flashes and irregular menses, was experienced as total change. She began to be perceived by him as a different person, unavailable and unempathic. The projection of his own misunderstanding and fear regarding her change was evident.

At 45, Jay's wife, who had been obese most of her life, resolved to find a new self. She began a supervised diet and exercise program and over the course of a year lost thirty pounds. This was a crisis for Jay, who could not tolerate her change, much less empathize with or applaud it. Her positive self-regard was emotionally stressful to him because it was experienced as cause for doubt, and loss. He began to accuse her of not loving him when she was not by his side. Unable to grasp that his demands provoked her need for distance, he felt validated in his fear of her ultimate abandonment of him.

Sometimes a man's assumption that his menopausal partner will no longer be as accepting or as available becomes an inevitable reality. A woman's midlife striving toward separation and conflict resolution often permits a differentiation and integration of self that was formerly impossible. Following such changes, she may actually be less suitable and less willing to be emotionally available as a selfobject (Kohut, 1971).

For a man who cannot come to terms with his own fears of inadequacy, aging, separation, and death, connection to the meno-pausal partner may be emotionally untenable. Her menopause con-founds his continuous need for mirroring by an idealized object to solidify his own sense of self (Kohut, 1971). In response, a man may have an affair with a younger, conventionally attractive female. As Kernberg (1980) describes in his consideration of pathological narcis-sism in middle age, ". . . eternally youthful bodies are needed compul-sively, regardless of the face, the person, the attitudes with which such bodies even relate . . ." (p. 144).

McDougall (1985) suggests that for such men sexual relating tends to be an addictive, unrelated, ritualized use of the partner to maintain "libidinal homeostasis" as well as "narcissistic homeostasis" (p. 251). Fearing that menopause will rob the partner of sexual interest and desirability, such men seem to panic because of the feared loss of control in the couple's sexual relating. Their demands often become excessive and are met with lack of interest and distance, leaving them anxious and in greater need of narcissistic recovery.

In those situations where a midlife affair is more a function of unresolved conflict than of conscious adult choice, there is often the unrealistic expectation that the original partner will remain constant and available despite overt devaluation and sexual replacement. In such cases, the man engages in a desperate struggle to have both the affair, which permits idealized gratification, and the midlife partner, whose presence permits projection of the split-off image of aging and imperfection. Unconsciously, the menopausal partner may represent the asexual maternal object, whose existence figures as an unconscious determinant in the acting out. At times, the man may feel an inappropriate need to provide his partner with the details of the affair and may express the wish that she understand, be pleased, even proud. The inevitable disappointment of this regressive need is met with despair and rage toward self and the partner who rejects this projection of the accepting maternal object.

INTERACTIVE PATTERNS

Men's views of menopausal women interact with women's views of themselves. When a woman's own personality precludes integration of a new image and role for self as a result of menopause, she may impart this difficulty to her partner. For example, a man's view of the menopausal woman's sexual function is both a conscious and unconscious response to the woman's view of her own sexuality. According to Eisenbud (1987), for women, being wanted is the sexual turn-on. During the menopausal years, a woman may anticipate being wanted less. Her anticipation of not being sexually desirable because of her loss of certain physical characteristics, inability to bear children, or fear of sexual dysfunction, can preclude her sexual responsiveness or willingness to take sexual risks. She may, for example, stop initiating sex. Her psychological inhibition is then experienced by her partner as a loss of sexual drive or lack of interest in him. A vicious cycle of rejection results, and her menopausal status is viewed as the cause of sexual difficulties and marital stress.

Women who equate the loss of their reproductive capacity with the loss of their primary identity tend to experience the menopausal years with great dread (Bart, 1971). If a man is overidentified with his partner's need to parent children, such that parenting is his primary role and source of status, her menopause may be cause for anxiety and despair both in terms of partner and self.

Any major change in a couple's life bears evidence of their patterns of relating as they struggle consciously and unconsciously to assimilate the change, to respond to the crisis. A common example of this is the use of "collusion" (Willi, 1982). This interactive pattern is defined as the unconscious interplay of two partners, concealed from both and based on similar, unresolved central conflicts. Essentially the common unresolved conflict is acted out through different roles, which gives the appearance of each partner's being the exact opposite of the other. Often one partner's behavior is progressive or overcompensating while the other's is regressive. In reality, their behaviors are polar variants of the same theme. In the long run, the collusive solution fails—each partner's repressed elements return, often as symptoms. The following case demonstrates this:

Rose was the "sensitive one." Historically, in her family and in her marriage, she was the one who worried for everyone and was easily upset. It was almost impossible for her to express anger or frustration without tears. Over the course of six months prior to individual treatment, Rose found herself overly anxious, unable to relax, experiencing early morning wakefulness and insomnia. She described herself as hopeless, without purpose. When physiological symptoms of menopause appeared, she decided, in collusion with her spouse, that the cause of her difficulties was menopausal. She sought psychological help. In the early psychological consultation, Rose was almost too eager to take on the role of the helpless, sensitive, troubled one. What perplexed her was that consciously many of the goals and aspects of her own personal identity and life were in progress. It was in her associations to her spouse that she became most emotional, reporting guilt for causing him such worry.

Soon after treatment began, it became evident that Rose's anxiety and depression of the prior months were associated with her spouse's decision to change jobs once again in search of higher pay and more responsibility. While Rose was promoted and was offered more and more status in her professional career, her spouse was actually experiencing more difficulty. The treatment revealed a collusion to deny his difficulties at the cost of producing her symptoms.

For a year Rose's spouse had informed her of the problems at work without further discussing them. When she pursued discussion of those problems, she was reminded by him of how easily she was upset and how the problems were best left undiscussed. She colluded in not wanting to hear more, and together they avoided the recognition and fear that he was not as successful as they had both hoped he would be. As long as she remained the sensitive, helpless one to whom he could direct his pain or anxiety without responsibility, they could both maintain the illusion of his being the stronger of the two. Her increasing feelings of helplessness and rage at his failure to take responsibility, and her willingness to contain such feelings began to be expressed in anxiety and depression. When at the same time she began to experience menopausal symptoms, she gladly offered them as a rationale for her conflicts. He willingly colluded since her menopause served their common unconscious defense. Menopause provided a problem of hers, not his, for the fear, disappointment, and anger they both felt. Here the man's view of the menopausal woman—as one in turmoil and physiological stress—served his needs as well as hers.

Collusive patterns sustain midlife issues, but other interactive patterns may facilitate their resolution. When a woman embraces the adult dimensions of self, integrating the existing, the different, and the lesser known potentials of self, she invites a man to know *her*. When she is able to feel individuated, she can remain connected while, at the same time, she is "less tyrannized by inner conflicts and external demands" (Levinson et al., 1978, p. 5). When she turns to herself for redefinition, she comes to know who she was, who she wished to be, and who she can still be. A man—even the significant man in her life—cannot know this for her. It will be her own self-resolution that will inform him. His perspective may then become mutually validating, reaffirming a view of self that she can readily accept. And his perspective may lend credibility and promise to his own view of self.

SUMMARY

Menopause implies change. As a physical event, it is evidence of aging. As a phase of life, it spans the years of midlife, demanding a dismantling of the old and a building of the new, a resolution of internal conflicts and integration of all. It is an event that calls for re-definition of self. For the menopausal woman, some part of this self-definition includes the sense of self she gleans in the eyes of the significant others in her life. For many women the significant other is a man. How does this man view her?

In seeking an answer to this question, this chapter has considered men's views of menopausal women in the light of men's parallel positions to women in midlife, gender differences, preexisting personality traits, and the conscious and unconscious interactive patterns between men and women in close relationships.

From a review of theoretical formulations, clinical material, and questionnaire data has emerged evidence of confusion, crisis, collusion, as well as concern, empathy, and complement. How men view menopausal women is a complex question. It calls forth a recognition of the interplay of object relations issues, conflict resolutions, developmental changes, and sociocultural aspects of life's major tasks. It reflects men's and women's capacity to believe in self while at the same time trusting the other:

> . . . the most powerful and profound awareness of ourselves occurs with our simultaneous opening up with another human. This is the most deeply and directly we humans are capable of experiencing our real selves in the world. It is the most meaningful and courageous of human experiences [Malone and Malone, 1987, pp 19–20].

REFERENCES

Bart, P.B. (1971), Depression in middle-aged women. In: *Women in Sexist Society*, ed. V. Gornick & B.K. Moran. New York: Basic Books, pp. 99–117.

Benedek, T. (1950), The functions of the sexual apparatus and their disturbances. In: *Psychosomatic Medicine*, ed. F. Alexander. New York: Norton, pp. 239–240.

Bergler, E. (1954), *The Revolt of the Middle-Aged Man*, New York: International Universities Press, 1985.

Cowdan, G., Warren, L. & Young, J. (1985), Medical perceptions of menopausal symptoms. *Psychol. Women Quart.*, 9:3–14.

Deutsch, H. (1945), *The Psychology of Women*. New York: Grune & Stratton.

Eisenbud, R.J. (1987), Gender in the service of ego. Presented at annual meeting of the American Psychological Association, New York City.

Erikson, E.H. (1959), Identity and the life cycle. *Psychological Issues*, Monogr. 1. New York: International Universities Press.

———— (1982), *The Life Cycle Completed*. New York: Norton.

Farrell, M. & Rosenberg, S. (1981), *Men at Midlife*. Dover, MA: Auburn House.

Formanek, R. (1987), *Women and Depression*. New York: Springer.

Kaufert, P., Lock, M., McKinlay, S. & Beyene, Y. (1986), Menopause research: The Korpilampi workshop. *Soc. Sci. & Med.* 22:1285–1289.

Kernberg. O. (1980), *Internal World and External Reality*. New York: Aronson.

Klemme, H.L. (1970), Midlife crisis. *Menn. Perspect.*, 1:2–6.

Kohut, H. (1971), *The Analysis of The Self*. New York: International Universities Press.

Lax, R. (1982), The expectable depressive climacteric reaction. *Bull. Menn. Clin.*, 46:151–167.

Levinson, D. (1986), A conception of adult development. *Amer. Psychol.*, 41:3–13.

_____ Darrow, C., Klein, E., Levinson, M. & McKee, B. (1978), *The Seasons of a Man's Life.* New York: Knopf.

Lowenthal, M.F., Thurnher, M. & Chiriboga, D., (1975), *Four Stages of Life.* San Francisco, CA: Jossey-Bass.

Malone, T. & Malone, P. (1987), *The Art of Intimacy.* New York: Prentice Hall.

McDougall, J. (1985), *Theaters of the Mind.* New York: Basic Books.

McGill, M. (1985), *The McGill Report on Male Intimacy.* New York: Holt, Rinehart, Winston.

McKinlay, S. & McKinlay, J. (1973), Selected studies of the menopause: an annotated bibliography. *J. Biosoc. Sci.,* 5:533–555.

Notman, M.T. (1979), Midlife concerns of women: Implications of menopause. *Amer. J. Psychiat.,* 136:1270–1274.

_____ (1984), Psychiatric disorders of menopause. *Psychiat. Annals.* 14:448–453.

Parlee, M.B. (1978), Psychological aspects of the climacteric in women. *Psychiat. Opin.,* 15:36–40.

Perlmutter, J.F. (1978), A gynecological approach to menopause. In: *The Woman Patient,* ed. M. Notman & C. Nadelson. New York: Plenum Press, pp. 323–335.

Phillips, S.B. (1988), The midlife questionnaire. Unpublished survey.

Posner, J. (1979), It's all in your head: Feminist and medical models of menopause (strange bedfellows). *Sex Roles,* 5:179–190.

Scarf, M. (1987), *Intimate Partners.* New York: Random House.

Sheehy, G. (1981), *Pathfinders.* New York: Morrow.

Singer, J. (1988), Psychoanalytic theory in the context of contemporary psychology: The Helen Block Lewis memorial address. *Psychoanal. Psychol.,* 5:95–125.

Smith, D., O'Leary, V., Shields, S., Morokoff, P. & Isenberg, N. (1988), Two different worlds: Men, women and emotion. Presented at annual meeting of the American Psychological Association, Atlanta, GA.

Stolorow, R.D. & Lachmann, F.M. (1980), *Psychoanalysis and Developmental Arrests.* New York: Aronson.

Willi, J. (1982), *Couples in Collusion.* New York: Aronson.

Author Index

Subject Index

A

ACTH, *See Adrenocorticotrophic hormone*
Adaptation, subjective, 84, 85f
Adipose tissue, 184
  reduction of, 220
Adolescent females, attitude toward
    menopause, 162
Adrenal cortex, 184
Adrenocorticotrophic hormone
    (ACTH), 141, 184
Adult development, theories of, 282
Affiliation
  contradiction with self-actualization,
    286–288
  needs, 287
Age
  attitude toward menopause and, 91,
    92, 93
  at menopausal onset, 134, 137–139
Aggression, 287
Aging
  menopause and, 39
  menopause versus, 186–187
Aging women, "proper" role of, 58–59

Amenorrhea, 4, 6
  19th century physicians' approach to,
    9
American Medical Dictionary, 46
American women, menopausal symp-
    toms in, 83
Anatomy of Melancholy, The (Burton),
    257
Androgen(s)
  peripheral conversion of, 183
  production of, 182, 183
Androstenedione, 182
  peripheral conversion of, 184
  synthesis of, 183
Anthropological methods, 146
"Anticipated climacteric," 98
Anxiety, in menopause, 80t
Anxiety neurosis, 67–68
Appendicular bone mass, 203
Arab women, menopausal attitudes of,
    124
Atrophic vaginitis, *See* Vaginitis,
    atrophic
Attitude(s)
  toward menopause, 97t

311